# Epilepsy

NEUROLOGY IN PRACTICE

SERIES EDITORS:

ROBERT A. GROSS, DEPARTMENT OF NEUROLOGY, UNIVERSITY OF ROCHESTER MEDICAL CENTER, ROCHESTER, NY, USA

JONATHAN W. MINK, DEPARTMENT OF NEUROLOGY, UNIVERSITY OF ROCHESTER MEDICAL CENTER, ROCHESTER, NY, USA

# Epilepsy

EDITED BY

## John W. Miller, MD, PhD

*Director, UW Regional Epilepsy Center*
*Professor of Neurology and Neurological Surgery*
*University of Washington*
*Seattle, WA, USA*

## Howard P. Goodkin, MD, PhD

*The Shure Professor of Neurology and Pediatrics*
*Director, Division of Pediatric Neurology*
*Department of Neurology*
*University of Virginia*
*Charlottesville, VA, USA*

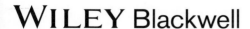

This edition first published 2014
© 2014 by John Wiley & Sons, Ltd

*Registered Office*
John Wiley & Sons, Ltd, The Atrium, Southern Gate, Chichester, West Sussex, PO19 8SQ, UK

*Editorial Offices*
9600 Garsington Road, Oxford, OX4 2DQ, UK
The Atrium, Southern Gate, Chichester, West Sussex, PO19 8SQ, UK
111 River Street, Hoboken, NJ 07030–5774, USA

For details of our global editorial offices, for customer services and for information about how to apply for permission to reuse the copyright material in this book please see our website at www.wiley.com/wiley-blackwell

*Library of Congress Cataloging-in-Publication Data*

Epilepsy (Miller)
   Epilepsy / edited by John W. Miller, Howard P. Goodkin.
     1 online resource.
   Includes bibliographical references and index.
   Description based on print version record and CIP data provided by publisher; resource not viewed.
   ISBN 978-1-118-45695-8 (Adobe PDF) – ISBN 978-1-118-45697-2 (ePub) – ISBN 978-1-118-45694-1 (cloth)
I.  Miller, John W. (John William), 1951– editor of compilation.   II.  Goodkin, Howard P., editor of compilation.   III.  Title.
   [DNLM:   1.  Epilepsy. WL 385]
   RC372
   616.85′3–dc23
                             2013044450

A catalogue record for this book is available from the British Library.

Wiley also publishes its books in a variety of electronic formats. Some content that appears in print may not be available in electronic books.

Cover images: background – © iStockphoto.com/Eraxion; inset – courtesy of Mark Quigg
Cover design by Sarah Dickinson

Set in 8.75/11.75pt Utopia by SPi Publisher Services, Pondicherry, India
Printed and bound in Singapore by Markono Print Media Pte Ltd

1   2014

# Contents

Color plate section between pages 80 and 81

# Contributor List

**Bassel W. Abou-Khalil, MD**
Professor of Neurology
Director of the Epilepsy Center
Vanderbilt University School of Medicine
Nashville, TN, USA

**Gail D. Anderson, PhD**
Professor of Pharmacy, Pharmaceutics (adj) and
Neurological Surgery (adj)
Department of Pharmacy
UW Regional Epilepsy Center
University of Washington
Seattle, WA, USA

**Jacquelyn L. Bainbridge, PharmD, FCCP**
Professor of Clinical Pharmacy and Neurology
University of Colorado Skaggs School of Pharmacy
and Pharmaceutical Sciences and School of
Medicine
Anschutz Medical Campus
Aurora, CO, USA

**Jane G. Boggs, MD**
Associate Professor of Neurology
Wake Forest University School of Medicine
Comprehensive Epilepsy Center
Winston Salem, NC, USA

**Jeffrey Bolton, MD**
Staff Physician
Department of Neurology
Boston Children's Hospital Division of Epilepsy
Instructor of Neurology
Harvard Medical School
Boston, MA, USA

**Jessica L. Carpenter, MD**
Assistant Professor
Department of Neurophysiology
Children's National Medical Center
George Washington University
Washington, DC, USA

**Mary B. Connolly, MB BCh**
Division of Pediatric Neurology
Department of Pediatrics
British Columbia's Children's Hospital
Vancouver, British Columbia, Canada

**Elizabeth J. Donner, MD, FRCPC**
Associate Professor of Paediatrics
Division of Neurology
Department of Paediatrics
University of Toronto
The Hospital for Sick Children
Toronto, Ontario, Canada

**Daniel L. Drane, PhD**
Assistant Professor of Neurology and Pediatrics
Departments of Neurology and Pediatrics
Emory University School of Medicine
Atlanta, GA, USA
Department of Neurology
University of Washington School of Medicine
Seattle, WA, USA

**Dana Ekstein, MD**
Senior Neurologist
Department of Neurology
Epilepsy Center
Hadassah-Hebrew University Medical Center
Jerusalem, Israel

**Edward Faught, MD**
Professor of Neurology
Emory University
Atlanta, GA, USA

**Paul A. Garcia, MD**
Professor of Clinical Neurology
Director of Clinical Epilepsy Services
Department of Neurology
University of California San Francisco
San Francisco, CA, USA

**Nicolas Gaspard, MD, PhD**
Postdoctoral Research Associate
Division of Epilepsy and EEG
Neurology Department
Yale University School of Medicine
New Haven, CT, USA

**Howard P. Goodkin, MD, PhD**
The Shure Professor of Neurology and Pediatrics
Director, Division of Pediatric Neurology
Department of Neurology
University of Virginia
Charlottesville, VA, USA

**Renzo Guerrini, MD**
Professor and Director
Neuroscience Department
Children's Hospital A. Meyer
University of Florence
Florence, Italy

**Shahin Hakimian, MD**
Assistant Professsor of Neurology
Department of Neurology
UW Regional Epilepsy Center
University of Washington
Seattle, WA, USA

**Adam L. Hartman, MD**
Assistant Professor of Neurology, Pediatrics,
and Molecular Microbiology and Immunology
Divisions of Epilepsy and Pediatric Neurology
Co-Director, Neurosciences Intensive Care
Nursery
Johns Hopkins Medicine
Baltimore, MD, USA

**Sheryl R. Haut, MD**
Professor of Clinical Neurology
Director, Adult Epilepsy
Epilepsy Management Center, Einstein-Montefiore
Bronx, NY, USA
Department of Neurology, Montefiore Medical
Center
Albert Einstein College of Medicine
Bronx, NY, USA

**Sandra L. Helmers, MD, MPH**
Professor of Neurology
Department of Neurology
Emory University School of Medicine
Atlanta, GA, USA

**Lawrence J. Hirsch, MD**
Professor of Neurology
Chief, Division of Epilepsy and EEG
Yale Comprehensive Epilepsy Center
Yale University School of Medicine
New Haven, CT, USA

**John D. Hixson, MD**
Department of Neurology
University of California San Francisco
San Francisco, CA, USA

**Gregory L. Holmes, MD**
Department of Neurological Sciences
University of Vermont
Burlington, VT, USA

**J. Stephen Huff, MD**
Professor of Emergency Medicine and
Neurology
Departments of Emergency Medicine and
Neurology
University of Virginia
Charlottesville, VA, USA

**Autumn Klein, MD, PhD (Deceased)**
Department of Neurology
UPMC Presbyterian/Magee Women's Hospital
of UPMC
Pittsburgh, PA, USA

**Pearce J. Korb, MD**
Instructor Department of Neurology
Emory University School of
Medicine
Atlanta, GA, USA

**Allan Krumholz, MD**
Professor of Neurology
Department of Neurology
Director, Maryland Epilepsy Center
University of Maryland Medical Center
University of Maryland School of Medicine
Baltimore, MD, USA

**Jennifer Langer, MD**
Assistant Professor of Neurology
Department of Neurology
University of Virginia
Charlottesville, VA, USA

**Rūta Mameniškienė, MD, PhD**
Clinic of Neurology and Neurosurgery
Faculty of Medicine
Vilnius University
Vilnius, Lithuania
Epilepsy Centre
Department of Neurology
Vilnius University Hospital Santariškių
Klinikos
Vilnius, Lithuania

**John W. Miller, MD, PhD**
Professor of Neurology and Neurological
Surgery
Departments of Neurology and Neurological
Surgery
University of Washington
Seattle, WA, USA
Director, UW Regional Epilepsy Center
Harborview Medical Center
Seattle, WA, USA

**Valeria M. Muro, MD**
Division of Pediatric Neurology
Department of Pediatrics
British Columbia's Children's Hospital
Vancouver, British Columbia, Canada

**Aidan Neligan, MD**
Clinical Research Fellow
Department of Clinical & Experimental
Epilepsy
UCL Institute of Neurology
London, UK
Epilepsy Society
Chalfont St Peter, Buckinghamshire, UK

**Katherine C. Nickels, MD**
Assistant Professor of Child Neurology
and Epilepsy
Mayo Clinic
Rochester, MN, USA

**Frances J. Northington, MD**
Professor of Pediatrics
Division of Neonatology
Director, Neurosciences Intensive Care Nursery
Neonatal Research Laboratory
Johns Hopkins Medicine
Baltimore, MD, USA

**Edward J. Novotny, Jr., MD**
Professor of Neurology, Pediatrics, Radiology and
Neurosurgery
Director of Pediatric Epilepsy Program | Child
Neurology
Alvord, Gerlich and Rhodes Family Endowed Chair
in Pediatric Epilepsy
University of Washington
Seattle Children's Hospital
Seattle, WA, USA

**Caleb Y. Oh, PharmD**
Clinical Research Fellow in Neurology
Department of Clinical Pharmacy
University of Colorado Skaggs School of Pharmacy
and Pharmaceutical Sciences
Anschutz Medical Campus
Aurora, CO, USA

**Heather E. Olson, MD**
Fellow in Epilepsy Genetics
Division of Epilepsy
Department of Neurology
Boston Children's Hospital
Boston, MA, USA
Department of Neurology
Harvard Medical School
Boston, MA, USA

**Kimberly L. Pargeon, MD**
Epilepsy Management Center
Einstein-Montefiore
Bronx, NY, USA
Department of Neurology, Montefiore
Medical Center
Albert Einstein College of Medicine
Bronx, NY, USA

**Philip N. Patsalos, FRCPath, PhD**
Professor of Clinical Pharmacology
Department of Clinical and Experimental
Epilepsy
UCL-Institute of Neurology
London, UK
Epilepsy Society
Chalfont Centre for Epilepsy
Chalfont St Peter, Buckinghamshire, UK

**Phillip L. Pearl, MD**
Professor of Pediatrics, Neurology, and Music
The George Washington University School of
Medicine and Columbian College of Arts
and Sciences
Division Chief, Department of Child Neurology,
Children's National Medical Center
Washington, DC, USA

**Vaishali S. Phatak, PhD**
Assistant Professor of Neurology
UW Regional Epilepsy Center
University of Washington
Seattle, WA, USA

**Annapurna Poduri, MD**
Division of Epilepsy
Department of Neurology
Boston Children's Hospital
Boston, MA, USA
Department of Neurology
Harvard Medical School
Boston, MA, USA

**Nicholas P. Poolos, MD, PhD**
Associate Professor of Neurology
Associate Director
Department of Neurology and UW Regional
Epilepsy Center
University of Washington
Seattle, WA, USA

**Mark Quigg, MD, MSc, FANA**
Department of Neurology
University of Virginia
Charlottesville, VA, USA

**Anna Rosati, MD, PhD**
Pediatric Neurology Unit and Laboratories
Neuroscience Department
Children's Hospital A. Meyer
University of Florence
Florence, Italy

**Jay Salpekar, MD**
Associate Professor of Psychiatry and Pediatrics
George Washington University School of
Medicine
Director, Neurobehavior Program
Center for Neuroscience and Behavioral
Medicine
Children's National Medical Center
Washington, DC, USA

**Ana M. Sanchez, MD**
Assistant Professor of Neurology
Department of Neurology, Maryland Epilepsy
Center
University of Maryland Medical Center
University of Maryland School of Medicine
Baltimore, MD, USA

**Josemir W. Sander**
Department of Clinical & Experimental Epilepsy
UCL Institute of Neurology
London, UK
Epilepsy Society
Chalfont St Peter, Buckinghamshire, UK
SEIN-Epilepsy Institute in The Netherlands
Foundation
Heemstede, The Netherlands

**Steven C. Schachter, MD**
Chief Academic Officer, Department of Neurology
Center for Integration of Medicine and Innovative
Technology
Beth Israel Deaconess Medical Center
Massachusetts General Hospital and Harvard
Medical School
Boston, MA, USA

**Joseph I. Sirven, MD**
Professor and Chairman, Department of Neurology
Mayo Clinic
Phoenix, AZ, USA

**Carl E. Stafstrom, MD, PhD**
Professor of Neurology and Pediatrics
Chief, Pediatric Neurology Section
University of Wisconsin
Madison, WI, USA

**Elaine C. Wirrell, MD**
Professor of Child Neurology and Epilepsy
Mayo Clinic
Rochester, MN, USA

**Peter Wolf, MD**
Danish Epilepsy Centre
Dianalund, Denmark

**Yuezhou Joe Yu, MD**
Department of Neurology
Children's National Medical Center
Washington, DC, USA
Departments of Neurology and Pediatrics
School of Medicine and Columbian College of Arts
and Sciences
The George Washington University
Washington, DC, USA

# Series Foreword

The genesis for this book series started with the proposition that, increasingly, physicians want direct, useful information to help them in clinical care. Textbooks, while comprehensive, are useful primarily as detailed reference works but pose challenges for uses at the point of care. By contrast, more outline-type references often leave out the *hows and whys* – pathophysiology, pharmacology – that form the basis of management decisions. Our goal for this series is to present books, covering most areas of neurology, that provide enough background information to allow the reader to feel comfortable, but not so much as to be overwhelming, and to associate that with practical advice from experts about care, combining the growing evidence base with best practices.

Our series will encompass various aspects of neurology, with topics and the specific content chosen to be accessible and useful.

Chapters cover critical information that will inform the reader of the disease processes and mechanisms as a prelude to treatment planning. Algorithms and guidelines are presented, when appropriate. "Tips and Tricks" boxes provide expert suggestions, while other boxes present cautions and warnings to avoid pitfalls. Finally, we provide "Science Revisited" sections that review the most important and relevant science background material and "Bibliography" sections that guide the reader to additional material.

We welcome feedback. As additional volumes are added to the series, we hope to refine the content and format so that our readers will be best served.

Our thanks, appreciation, and respect go out to our editors and their contributors, who conceived and refined the content for each volume, assuring a high-quality, practical approach to neurological conditions and their treatment.

Our thanks also go to our mentors and students (past, present, and future), who have challenged and delighted us; to our book editors and their contributors, who were willing to take on additional work for an educational goal; and to our publisher, Martin Sugden, for his ideas and support, for wonderful discussions and commiseration over baseball and soccer teams that might not quite have lived up to expectations. We would like to dedicate the series to Marsha, Jake, and Dan; and to Janet, Laura, and David. And also to Steven R. Schwid, MD, our friend and colleague, whose ideas helped to shape this project and whose humor brightened our lives, but he could not complete this goal with us.

Robert A. Gross
Jonathan W. Mink
*Rochester, NY, USA*

# Preface

Epilepsy is a common but heterogeneous neurological condition of children and adults, with variable manifestations, numerous etiologies, and diverse treatments. Every clinician frequently encounters this disorder in the emergency room, the hospital, and the outpatient clinic and needs to have a systematic approach for its evaluation and management.

In keeping with the goals of this series, this book summarizes the knowledge and practices of expert epilepsy specialists in a concise, practical pocketbook for everyday use by treating physicians. The main emphasis is on bedside clinical evaluation and treatment. The target audience is neurology residents and fellows, general neurologists, and primary care, ICU, and emergency room providers that frequently encounter seizures and epilepsy in their practices. This book is intended to make all of the major issues of the clinical evaluation and treatment of seizures and epilepsy accessible to the practitioner, and we believe the authors have covered these topics in a way that is useful for everyday clinical decisions.

The book opens with a discussion of the basics of epilepsy, including the definitions of seizures and epilepsy, their classification, and their causes. These concepts are the foundation of a rational approach to diagnosis and workup at the bedside. This is followed by a guide to treatment with antiepileptic drugs, addressing when and how to initiate medical therapy. Choice of antiepileptic medications in clinical practice is determined not only by possible efficacy, but also by issues of adverse effects, safety, drug interactions, and effects on comorbid conditions. Dose adjustments and transitions to alternate antiepileptic medications are also discussed, as are strategies for optimizing medication regimens and considering nonmedical treatments in patients who have drug-resistant epilepsy.

Specific common syndromes and conditions in children and adults are reviewed, with special emphasis on new information on treatable genetic and metabolic disorders. Another topic of great relevance to the practicing clinician is the treatment of acute seizures and status epilepticus in the home, emergency room, and ICU. A *hot topic* of special interest is the emergence of continuous video-EEG monitoring as a tool for the diagnosis and management of acute seizures in the ICU.

The book closes by reviewing the consequences of chronic epilepsy. Uncontrolled epilepsy has profound effects on the daily life of individuals and is associated with increased risk of injury and mortality. It affects the management of comorbid medical conditions and may have significant effects on mood and cognitions.

The complexities of this malady demand a nuanced and customized approach to diagnosis and management. One size does not fit all. We believe this book distils the most salient information on this protean disorder, which will allow the practitioner to devise a plan to appropriately evaluate and manage each individual patient. Although this book is dense with information, the authors have striven to organize the facts to place them at the fingertips of the busy practitioner, so that the most important points are presented in boxes and tables that jump out of the page. We hope that the readers will agree and that this book will find a favored place on the shelf of staff rooms and physician offices and in the pockets of their white coats.

During the editing of this book, we were saddened to learn of the passing of Autumn Klein, MD, PhD, who was renowned for her expertise and research in epilepsy in pregnant and postpartum women. She will be missed.

John W. Miller
Howard P. Goodkin

# Part I

# Epilepsy Basics

# Recognizing Seizures and Epilepsy: Insights from Pathophysiology

**Carl E. Stafstrom**

Pediatric Neurology Section, University of Wisconsin, Madison, WI, USA

## Introduction

This chapter provides a brief overview of seizures and epilepsy, with emphasis on pathophysiological mechanisms that determine seizure generation and how these differ from the mechanisms underlying paroxysmal neurologic events that are not epileptic in nature. Detailed discussion about the pathophysiology of epilepsy can be found in numerous reviews, so the question arises: why consider this topic in a book that focuses on the practical approach to seizure management? There are two major reasons. First, the choice of antiepileptic drug (AED) is often crucially dependent on the seizure type or epilepsy syndrome, and hence an understanding of the underlying pathophysiology can direct medication choice. Second, burgeoning knowledge of epilepsy genetics is revealing more and more syndromes with specific mutations that determine the seizure phenotype, sometimes suggesting drugs that should or should not be selected. In this chapter, important terms are defined, and some basics of seizure pathophysiology are discussed as an aid for the practicing physician. It is important to recognize that epilepsy is not a singular disease, but is heterogeneous in terms of clinical expression, underlying etiologies, and pathophysiology.

## Definitions

A *seizure* is a temporary disruption of brain function due to the hypersynchronous, abnormal firing of cortical neurons. Sometimes, the term *epileptic seizure* is used to distinguish it from a *nonepileptic seizure* such as a psychogenic ("pseudo") seizure (Chapter 6), which involves abnormal clinical behavior that might resemble an epileptic seizure but is not caused by hypersynchronous neuronal firing. The clinical manifestations of a seizure depend upon the specific region and extent of brain involved and may include an alteration in motor function, sensation, alertness, perception, autonomic function, or some combination of these. Anyone might experience a seizure in the appropriate clinical setting (e.g., meningitis, hypoglycemia, toxin ingestion), attesting to the innate capacity of a "normal" brain to support epileptic activity in certain circumstances. More than 5% of people will experience a seizure at some point during their lifetimes.

*Epilepsy* is the condition of *recurrent, unprovoked* seizures (i.e., two or more seizures). Epilepsy occurs when a person is predisposed to seizures because of a chronic pathological state (e.g., brain tumor, cerebral dysgenesis, or post-traumatic scar) or a genetic susceptibility. Approximately 1% of the population suffers from epilepsy, making it the second

*Epilepsy*, First Edition. Edited by John W. Miller and Howard P. Goodkin.
© 2014 John Wiley & Sons, Ltd. Published 2014 by John Wiley & Sons, Ltd.

most common neurologic disorder (after stroke), affecting more than two million persons in the United States.

An *epilepsy syndrome* refers to a group of clinical characteristics that occur together consistently, with seizures as a primary manifestation. Syndrome features might include similar seizure type, age of onset, electroencephalogram (EEG) findings, precipitating factors, etiology, inheritance pattern, natural history, prognosis, and response to AEDs. Examples of epilepsy syndromes are infantile spasms, Lennox–Gastaut syndrome, febrile seizures, childhood absence epilepsy, rolandic epilepsy, and juvenile myoclonic epilepsy. Many of these syndromes are discussed in Chapter 21.

Finally, *epileptogenesis* refers to the events by which the normal brain becomes capable of producing epileptic seizures, that is, the *process* by which neural circuits are converted from normal excitability to hyperexcitability. This process may take months or years, and its mechanisms are

poorly understood. None of the currently available AEDs have robust antiepileptogenic effects. Clearly, the development of antiepileptogenic therapies is a research priority.

## Classification of seizures and epilepsies

Epileptic seizures are broadly divided into two groups, depending on their site of origin and pattern of spread. Focal (or partial) seizures arise from a localized region of the brain, and the associated clinical manifestations relate to the function ordinarily mediated by that area. A focal seizure is called "simple" if the patient's awareness or responsiveness is retained, and "complex" if those functions are impaired during the seizure. Focal discharges can spread locally through synaptic and nonsynaptic mechanisms or distally to subcortical structures, as well as through commissural pathways to involve the whole brain, in a process known as *secondary generalization* (Figure 1.1). For example, a seizure arising from

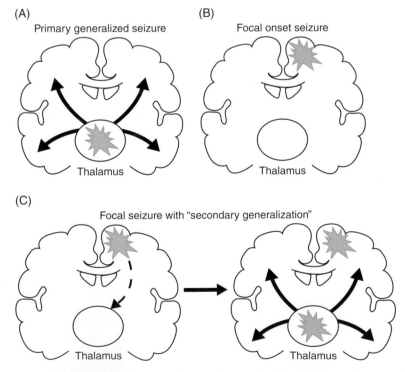

**Figure 1.1.** Coronal sections of the brain indicating patterns of seizure origination and spread. (A) Primary generalized seizure begins deep in brain (thalamus) with spread to superficial cortical regions (arrows). (B) Focal onset seizure begins in one area of the brain (star) and may spread to nearby or distant brain regions. (C) A focal onset seizure "secondarily generalizes" by spreading first to thalamus (left panel) then to widespread cortical regions (right panel).

the left motor cortex may cause rhythmic jerking movements of the right upper extremity; if the epileptiform discharges subsequently spread to adjacent areas and eventually encompass the entire brain, a secondarily generalized tonic–clonic convulsion may ensue.

In contrast, in a generalized seizure, abnormal electrical discharges begin in both hemispheres simultaneously and involve reciprocal thalamo-cortical connections (Figure 1.1). The EEG signature of a primary generalized seizure is bilateral synchronous spike-wave discharges seen across all scalp electrodes. The manifestations of such widespread epileptiform activity can range from brief impairment of responsiveness (as in an absence seizure) to a full-blown convulsion with rhythmic jerking movements of all extremities accompanied by loss of posture and consciousness.

Epilepsy syndromes have been divided historically by etiology (symptomatic vs. idiopathic; the majority of idiopathic epilepsies have a genetic basis) and site of seizure onset (generalized vs. focal or "localization-related"). This classification is being revised based on rapidly accumulating knowledge about the molecular genetic basis of epilepsies and new information gleaned from modern neuroimaging, as well as the realization that many epilepsy syndromes include both focal and generalized seizures. The newer classification scheme (Chapter 2) uses etiologic categories: genetic, structural/metabolic, and unknown. Undoubtedly, this scheme will be refined as further knowledge is gained. From the pathophysiological perspective, some mechanisms are likely to operate across epilepsy categories, and other mechanisms may be specific to certain epilepsy syndromes.

## Pathophysiology

At the cellular level, the two hallmark features of epileptiform activity are neuronal hyperexcitability and neuronal hypersynchrony. *Hyperexcitability* refers to the heightened response of a neuron to stimulation, so that a cell might fire multiple action potentials rather than single ones in response to a synaptic input. *Hypersynchrony* reflects increased neuron firing within a small or large region of cortex, with cells firing in close temporal and spatial proximity.

While there are differences in the mechanisms that underlie focal versus generalized seizures,

at a simplistic level it is still useful to view any seizure activity as a perturbation in the normal balance between inhibition and excitation in a localized region, in multiple discrete areas (seizure "foci"), or throughout the whole brain (Figure 1.2). This imbalance likely involves a combination of increased excitation and decreased inhibition (Table 1.1).

In addition to the traditional concept of excitation/inhibition imbalance, novel pathophysiological mechanisms for the epilepsies are also being discovered. For example, in febrile seizures, release of inflammatory mediators such as cytokines could contribute to neuronal hyperexcitability, an observation that might open new avenues of treatment.

## Seizure mimics

Many conditions resemble seizures clinically yet have a distinct etiology and therefore warrant treatment other than AEDs. Such seizure mimics are typically paroxysmal and recurrent, like seizures. Representative examples, listed in Table 1.2, illustrate the wide diversity of mechanisms and hence treatment modalities.

---

### ✭ TIPS AND TRICKS

Distinguishing epileptic from nonepileptic episodes relies on a detailed clinical history including precipitating triggers; careful description of the patient's behavior before, during, and after the episode; whether ictal movements can be suppressed manually; and the ability of the patient to recall the spell.

---

Response of a suspected seizure event to an AED does not necessarily mean that the episode was epileptic, as the ability of AEDs to reduce neuronal excitability are well recognized. Recording such an event on EEG or, preferably, video–EEG is often helpful in differentiating a seizure from a nonepileptic event. However, some epileptic seizures have a subtle or minimal electrographic correlate, especially if the focus is deep in the brain, such as in the temporal lobe. Therefore, a detailed clinical description should be combined with appropriately selected laboratory investigations in the evaluation of a seizure-like event.

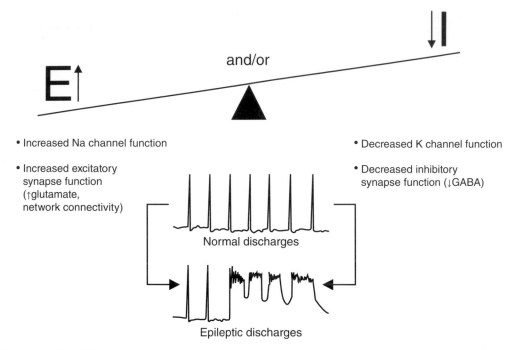

**Figure 1.2.** Simplified scheme indicating that seizure generation results from increased excitation (E), decreased inhibition (I), or both. Examples of intracellular recordings from normal and epileptic neurons are drawn next.

**Table 1.1.** Examples of pathophysiological processes leading to epilepsy.

| Level of dysfunction | Disorder | Pathophysiological mechanism |
|---|---|---|
| Ion channels | Benign familial neonatal convulsions<br>Dravet syndrome | Potassium channel mutations: impaired repolarization<br>Sodium channel mutations: enhanced excitability |
| Synapse development | Neonatal seizures | Depolarizing action of GABA early in development |
| Neurotransmitter receptors<br>  Excitatory | Nonketotic hyperglycinemia | Excess glycine leads to over-activation of NMDA receptors |
|   Inhibitory | Angelman syndrome | Abnormal GABA receptor subunits |
| Neurotransmitter synthesis | Pyridoxine (vitamin B6) dependency | Decreased GABA synthesis; B6 is a cofactor of GAD |
| Neuron structure | Down syndrome and other disorders with intellectual impairment and seizures | Abnormal structure of dendrites and dendritic spines: altered current flow in neuron |
| Neuronal network | Cerebral dysgenesis; post-traumatic scar; mesial temporal sclerosis (in TLE) | Altered neuronal circuits: formation of aberrant excitatory connections (sprouting) |

GABA, gamma-aminobutyric acid; GAD, glutamic acid decarboxylase; NMDA, N-methyl-d-aspartate; TLE, temporal lobe epilepsy.

**Table 1.2.** Some common seizure mimics.

| Seizure mimic | Underlying pathophysiology | Representative treatment |
|---|---|---|
| Benign paroxysmal positional vertigo | Labyrinth dysfunction | Head repositioning procedures |
| Breath-holding spells | Vasovagal | Reduce precipitant, reassurance |
| Migraine | Spreading cortical depression, neurogenic inflammation | Serotonin receptor agonists |
| Paroxysmal movement disorders | Multiple types and genetic basis; most are channelopathies | AEDs (e.g., carbamazepine) |
| Psychogenic seizure | Unknown; unresolved psychological conflicts | Counseling, behavior therapy |
| Sleep disorders | Multiple defects in regulation of arousal | Depends on type: e.g., reassurance for night terrors, arousal-promoting drugs for narcolepsy |
| Syncope | Vasovagal | Avoidance of triggers |
| Tics | Basal ganglia dysfunction | Dopamine receptor blockade |

AED, antiepileptic drug.

---

### ☝ CAUTION!

Epileptic seizures and seizure mimics can occur in the same patient, making their differentiation particularly challenging.

### ☆ TIPS AND TRICKS

The best practice is to use a single agent (monotherapy) to avoid side effects due to multiple AEDs. If it is necessary to treat a patient with more than one AED, drugs with *differing* mechanisms of action should be chosen to minimize adverse effects and drug–drug interactions.

## Overview of medication mechanisms of action

Knowledge of pathophysiological mechanisms of seizures and epilepsy is helpful in choosing the best AED for a given seizure type or epilepsy syndrome. Many AEDs work at specific cellular or molecular targets (Table 1.3). For instance, agents that enhance γ-aminobutyric acid (GABA) function include benzodiazepines and phenobarbital. Other drugs, such as phenytoin, carbamazepine, and lacosamide, decrease repetitive neuronal firing by altering sodium channel function. Still others (e.g., valproate, topiramate) act at multiple sites, endowing the AED with a broad spectrum of action. In clinical practice, it is optimal to choose an AED that has a specific action in the given epilepsy syndrome, if possible (Chapter 11). For example, ethosuximide is preferable for absence seizures due to its blockade of a calcium channel subtype that underlies the rhythmic, reciprocal epileptic firing between neocortical neurons and thalamic neurons.

Two examples illustrate how knowledge of pathophysiological principles informs clinical practice. In neonates, there is a reversed chloride ion gradient across the neuronal membrane, such that binding of the neurotransmitter GABA to its receptor may paradoxically cause excitation rather than inhibition, as occurs in the mature brain. Thus, the clinical consequence of treating neonatal seizures with GABAergic agents (phenobarbital, benzodiazepines) might be to exacerbate seizures, due to increased excitation rather than inhibition. Alternative treatments for neonatal seizures are not yet validated, though bumetanide, a diuretic that speeds up the maturation of GABAergic inhibition, is undergoing clinical trials.

The second example is Dravet syndrome (DS), previously called severe myoclonic epilepsy of infancy. In DS, mutation of sodium channels results

**Table 1.3.** Mechanisms of commonly prescribed antiepileptic drugs (see also Chapter 19).

| AED | Mechanism |
| --- | --- |
| Phenobarbital | Activates GABA$_A$ receptors |
| Phenytoin | Blocks Na channels |
| Carbamazepine | Blocks Na channels |
| Valproate | Multiple – enhances GABA action, blocks Na and Ca channels |
| Ethosuximide | Blocks T-type Ca channels |
| Benzodiazepines | Activate GABA$_A$ receptors |
| Levetiracetam | Modulates synaptic vesicle protein SV2A |
| Topiramate | Multiple – blocks AMPA-type glutamate receptors and Na channels, enhances GABA action |
| Vigabatrin | Inhibits GABA transaminase |
| Zonisamide | Multiple – blocks Na and Ca channels, alters neurotransmitter transport |
| Oxcarbazepine | Blocks Na channels |

AMPA, 2-amino-3-(3-hydroxy-5-methyl-isoxazol-4-yl) propanoic acid; Ca, calcium; GABA, gamma-aminobutyric acid; Na, sodium; SV, synaptic vesicle.

in impaired closure of sodium channel gates and increased neuronal firing. In this disorder, agents that further block sodium channels are best avoided, and in fact, lamotrigine can worsen seizures in children with DS. Many other examples are likely to emerge whereby understanding the underlying epilepsy pathophysiology and pharmacological mechanisms of action will directly impact patient care. In addition, as more epilepsies yield to molecular genetic elucidation, the application of patient-specific pharmacogenetic profiles may guide therapy.

## Conclusion

This book provides a practical approach to the diagnosis and management of seizures and epilepsy. The principles outlined in this introductory chapter stress the importance of understanding the pathophysiology of seizure generation for optimal management. Details can be found in the references, and many of the concepts introduced here are expanded on in subsequent chapters.

## Bibliography

Berg AT, Scheffer IE. New concepts in classification of the epilepsies: Entering the 21st century. *Epilepsia* 2011; **52**:1058–1062.

Ceulemans B. Overall management of patients with Dravet syndrome. *Dev Med Child Neurol* 2011; **53**(Suppl. 2):19–23.

Chang BS, Lowenstein DH. Epilepsy. *N Engl J Med* 2003; **349**:1257–1266.

D'Ambrosio R, Miller JW. What is an epileptic seizure? Unifying definitions in clinical practice and animal research to develop novel treatments. *Epilepsy Curr* 2010; **10**:61–66.

Dubé CM, Brewster AL, Baram TZ. Febrile seizures: Mechanisms and relationship to epilepsy. *Brain Dev* 2009; **31**:366–371.

Helbig I, Scheffer IE, Mulley JC, Berkovic SF. Navigating the channels and beyond: Unraveling the genetics of the epilepsies. *Lancet Neurol* 2008; **7**:231–245.

Johnson MR, Tan NC, Kwan P, Brodie MJ. Newly diagnosed epilepsy and pharmacogenomics research: A step in the right direction? *Epilepsy Behav* 2011; **22**:3–8.

Noebels JL, Avoli M, Rogawski MA, Olsen RW, Delgado-Escueta AV (eds.). *Jasper's Basic Mechanisms of the Epilepsies*. New York: Oxford University Press, 2012.

Obeid M, Mikati MA. Expanding spectrum of paroxysmal events in children: Potential mimickers of epilepsy. *Pediatr Neurol* 2007; **37**:309–316.

Pitkanen A, Lukasiuk K. Molecular and cellular basis of epileptogenesis in symptomatic epilepsy. *Epilepsy Behav* 2009; **14**:16–25.

Rakhade SN, Jensen FE. Epileptogenesis in the immature brain: Emerging mechanisms. *Nat Rev Neurol* 2009; **5**:380–391.

Stafstrom CE. The pathophysiology of epileptic seizures: A primer for pediatricians. *Pediatr Rev* 1998; **19**:335–344.

Stafstrom CE. Epilepsy: A review of selected clinical syndromes and advances in basic science. *J Cereb Blood Flow Metab* 2006; **26**:983–1004.

Stafstrom CE, Rho JM. Neurophysiology of seizures and epilepsy. In: Swaiman KF, Ashwal S, Ferreiro DM, Schor NF, eds. *Pediatric Neurology: Principles and Practice*, 5th ed. Edinburgh: Elsevier Saunders, 2012, 711–726.

# Classifying Epileptic Seizures and the Epilepsies

**Valeria M. Muro and Mary B. Connolly**

Division of Pediatric Neurology, Department of Pediatrics, British Columbia's Children's Hospital, Vancouver, British Columbia, Canada

## Introduction

The first classification of epileptic seizures was proposed by Henri Gastaut in 1964, with modifications by the Commission on Classification and Terminology of The International League Against Epilepsy (ILAE) in 1981 and 1989. The original purpose of classifying seizures and epilepsy, as stated by Engel, was to "provide a universal vocabulary that not only facilitated communication among clinicians, but also established a taxonomic foundation for performing quantitative clinical and basic research on epilepsy." The classification was based on expert opinion of the electroclinical features of seizures. Gastaut and colleagues recognized the imperfection of their system due to limited knowledge of the underlying pathophysiology of epilepsy. With advances in neuroimaging, neurophysiology, genetics, and neuroimmunology, classification needed to evolve further.

The International League Against Epilepsy (ILAE) organization of the epilepsies in 2010 was a major update of terminology to incorporate scientific advances. The term *organization*, rather than *classification*, was proposed, as the new term enables epilepsies to be organized by different parameters such as seizure type, age at onset, electroencephalogram (EEG), or neuroimaging. This new system, with its limitations, is "a work in progress" that will continue to develop as knowledge of the underlying pathophysiology and etiologies of epilepsies evolves.

## Generalized and focal seizures

In all classification schemes, the distinction between focal and generalized seizures is critical, since this distinction determines possible etiologies (Chapter 3) and choice of medical and surgical treatments (Chapters 11 and 27). In the updated nomenclature (2010), *generalized seizures* (Chapter 24) originate

> at some point within and rapidly engage bilaterally distributed networks. Such networks can include cortical and subcortical structures but do not necessarily involve the entire cortex. Although individual seizure onsets can appear localized, the location and lateralization are not consistent from one seizure to another. Generalized seizures can be asymmetric.

The subtypes are summarized in Table 2.1, with the main changes from the 1981 classification being the addition of subtypes of absence and myoclonic seizures.

*Focal seizures* originate "at some point within networks limited to one hemisphere. Focal seizures may originate within subcortical structures." Focal seizures may be classified as focal without

*Epilepsy*, First Edition. Edited by John W. Miller and Howard P. Goodkin.
© 2014 John Wiley & Sons, Ltd. Published 2014 by John Wiley & Sons, Ltd.

**Table 2.1.** Classification (organization) of epileptic seizures.

| |
| --- |
| Generalized seizures |
|   Tonic–clonic (in any combination) |
|   Absence |
|     Typical |
|     Atypical |
|     Absence with special features |
|     Myoclonic absence |
|     Eyelid myoclonia |
|   Myoclonic |
|     Myoclonic |
|     Myoclonic-atonic |
|     Myoclonic-tonic |
|   Clonic |
|   Tonic |
|   Atonic |
| Focal seizures |
| Epileptic spasms |

impairment of consciousness (clonic, autonomic, and hemiconvulsive), focal with subjective sensory or psychic phenomena (aura specific), focal dyscognitive with impairment of consciousness, and focal evolving to a bilateral convulsive seizure.

The terms *simple partial*, *complex partial*, and *partial seizures with secondary generalization* have been embedded in the epilepsy lexicon for decades. There is considerable resistance to letting go of these terms. However, *simple* (without alteration of awareness) and *complex* (with altered awareness) are often used incorrectly. *Complex partial* has been replaced by the term *focal dyscognitive*, describing seizures with disturbed cognition as the prominent feature. The term *secondarily generalized seizure* is replaced by *focal seizure evolving to a bilateral convulsive seizure*.

Neonatal seizures (Chapter 20) are no longer regarded as a separate entity. Seizures in neonates can be classified within the new scheme.

Epileptic spasms (Chapter 21) were not acknowledged in the 1981 classification. *Epileptic spasms* is preferred to *infantile spasms* because they may continue or begin after the first year of life. Because there is insufficient knowledge to classify these seizures as focal, generalized, or both, they have been placed in

their own group, unknown. In some patients, there is evidence that epileptic spasms can arise from surgically treatable focal brain lesions.

## Generalized and focal epilepsies

Many patients can be classified as having focal or generalized epilepsy based on clinical features (Chapter 5), EEG (Chapter 7), and MRI (Chapter 8). Generalized epilepsies are associated with generalized spike wave discharges on EEG while focal epilepsies are associated with focal slowing or epileptiform discharges and sometimes focal structural abnormalities (Chapters 7 and 24).

However, some patients do not fit exactly into the generalized or focal epilepsy categories and instead have features of both. Children with Dravet syndrome are an example.

> ⭐ **TIPS AND TRICKS:**
>
> Changes in terminology and concepts
>
> | New terminology | Old terminology |
> | --- | --- |
> | Focal seizures | Simple and complex partial seizures |
> | Evolving to bilateral convulsive seizure | Secondarily generalized seizure |
> | Self-limited | Benign |
> | Epileptic encephalopathy | Catastrophic |
> | Structural/ metabolic/immune | Symptomatic |
> | Genetic | Idiopathic |
> | Unknown | Cryptogenic |

## Electroclinical syndromes or epilepsy syndromes

The classification of epilepsy syndromes has great usefulness in clinical practice, as it guides the choice of antiepileptic drugs (Chapter 11) and other treatments. There are no major differences in the classification of epilepsy syndromes between the 2010 nomenclature and the earlier system of 1989 except that several new epilepsy syndromes have been added. These include the very common febrile seizures plus, autosomal dominant frontal lobe epilepsy, and autosomal dominant temporal lobe epilepsy with auditory features due to mutations in the leucine-rich, glioma-inactivated 1 (*LGI1*) gene.

**Table 2.2.** Electroclinical syndromes arranged by age at onset and related conditions.

**Neonatal period and infancy**

  Benign familial neonatal epilepsy (BFNE)

  Early myoclonic encephalopathy (EME)

  Ohtahara syndrome

**Infancy**

  Epilepsy of infancy with migrating focal seizures

  West syndrome

  Myoclonic epilepsy in infancy (MEI)

  Benign infantile epilepsy

  Benign familial infantile epilepsy

  Dravet syndrome

  Myoclonic encephalopathy in nonprogressive disorders

**Childhood**

  Febrile seizures plus (FS+)

  Panayiotopoulos syndrome

  Epilepsy with myoclonic-atonic (previously astatic) seizures

  Benign epilepsy of childhood with centrotemporal spikes (BECTS)

  Autosomal dominant nocturnal frontal lobe epilepsy (ADNFLE)

  Late-onset childhood occipital epilepsy (Gastaut type)

  Epilepsy with myoclonic absences

  Lennox–Gastaut syndrome

  Epileptic encephalopathy with continuous spikes and waves during slow sleep (CSWS)

  Landau-Kleffner syndrome (LKS)

  Childhood absence epilepsy (CAE)

**Adolescence and adulthood**

  Juvenile absence epilepsy (JAE)

  Juvenile myoclonic epilepsy (JME)

  Epilepsy with generalized tonic–clonic seizures alone

  Progressive myoclonic epilepsies (PME)

  Autosomal dominant epilepsy with auditory features (ADEAF)

  Other familial temporal lobe epilepsies

**Less specific age relationship**

  Familial focal epilepsy with variable foci (childhood to adult)

  Reflex epilepsies

Table 2.2 presents a partial list of epilepsy syndromes categorized by age at onset. A particular epilepsy syndrome may have a number of possible causes, as exemplified by West syndrome (epileptic spasms and hypsarrythmia), which may be due to brain malformations, brain injury due to hypoxic-ischemic encephalopathy, infection, hypoglycemia, neurocutaneous disorders, or gene defects (Chapter 3).

Electroclinical syndromes include a range of epileptic encephalopathies (Chapter 21), which begin early in life and are characterized by generalized and/or focal seizures or epileptic spasms, persistent severe EEG abnormalities, and cognitive dysfunction or decline (Table 2.3). The term *epileptic encephalopathy* refers to the concept that the epileptic activity itself contributes to severe cognitive and behavioral impairments above and beyond what might be expected from the underlying pathology alone. It is important to identify patients with epileptic encephalopathy because early effective intervention may improve seizure control and developmental outcome in some cases.

Idiopathic focal epilepsies comprise a group of syndromes characterized by focal onset seizures, no detectable brain lesion, and a characteristic EEG signature. These syndromes (Chapter 21) include

**Table 2.3.** Age-related epileptic encephalopathies.

**Neonatal period**

  Early myoclonic encephalopathy

  Ohtahara syndrome

**Infancy**

  Epilepsy of infancy with migrating focal seizures

  West syndrome

  Dravet syndrome

  Myoclonic encephalopathy

**Childhood**

  Epileptic encephalopathy with continuous spikes and waves during slow sleep (CSWS)

  Lennox–Gastaut syndrome

  Myoclonic-atonic epilepsy

**Other severe epileptic encephalopathies**

  Rasmussen's syndrome

  Fever-induced refractory epileptic encephalopathy

  Hemiconvulsion-hemiplegia epilepsy syndrome

benign epilepsy with central temporal spikes, benign occipital lobe epilepsy (early and late subtypes), and idiopathic occipital lobe epilepsy with photosensitivity. The term *benign* implies that these conditions have an excellent prognosis, with no cognitive or behavioral disturbances and easily controlled seizures. However, in reality these syndromes have a wide spectrum of clinical presentations and comorbidity, so *self-limiting* is a better term than *benign*. Similarly, early-onset idiopathic occipital lobe epilepsy (Panayiotopoulos syndrome) may overlap with the later onset Gastaut syndrome, so this entity may be regarded as a subtype of a larger group, "autonomic" age-related epilepsy. Idiopathic occipital lobe epilepsy with photosensitivity also has features of both focal and generalized epilepsy.

## Etiology of epilepsy

The 1989 ILAE classification divided epilepsy etiology into idiopathic, cryptogenic, and symptomatic groups. Idiopathic epilepsies were presumed genetic; cryptogenic epilepsies were likely to have a cause, but it could not be identified; and symptomatic epilepsies had an identifiable cause. The new organization expands etiology into five categories: genetic, structural, metabolic, immune, and unknown. Chapter 3 provides extensive detail on the etiologies of the epilepsies. Because some structural lesions (e.g., tuberous sclerosis complex, tumors) and neurometabolic disorders (Chapter 23) are due to gene mutations, these categories are not mutually exclusive. Furthermore, it is likely that environmental and epigenetic factors influence the expression of seizures in an individual with genetic epilepsy.

### Genetic

Epilepsy is deemed genetic when it is the direct result of a known or presumed genetic disorder and seizures are the core symptom (Chapter 22). Less than 1% of epilepsies are monogenic; many such disorders arise from *de novo* gene mutations. Dravet syndrome is an example of an epileptic encephalopathy of single genetic origin, with 75% having an *SCN1A* gene abnormality. Mutations of several other genes such as *CDKL5*, *PCDH19*, *SLC2A1*, and *STXBP1* can result in epileptic encephalopathies. To date, there are over 300 genes associated with the development of epilepsy, although not all are causative.

The genetic generalized epilepsies, previously called idiopathic generalized epilepsies, have a complex inheritance pattern. Some susceptibility variants may be inherited but alone are insufficient to cause epilepsy. Furthermore, a genetic etiology does not exclude the fact that environmental factors such as head injuries may play a role in the development of epilepsy.

### Structural

A structural cause implies the presence of MRI abnormalities that are the likely cause of the individual's epilepsy (Chapter 8). Examples are malformations of brain development, tumors, scars, and vascular malformations. Some structural lesions may be genetic, such as those caused by tuberous sclerosis complex. Some types of MRI findings, such as arachnoid cysts, nonspecific white matter signal changes, or nonspecific atrophy, may be found, but these are not typically the cause of epilepsy.

### Metabolic

Many metabolic disorders are associated with epilepsy; most have a genetic basis. As discussed in detail in Chapter 23, appropriate treatment of some neurometabolic disorders that cause treatment-resistant epilepsy can prevent neurological deterioration. Glucose transporter deficiency syndrome may present with focal seizures in young children; the ketogenic diet may prevent neurological regression in these patients. Other important rare treatable neurometabolic causes of epilepsy are pyridoxine-dependent epilepsy, folinic acid-responsive seizures, creatine disorders, serine disorders, and molybdenum cofactor deficiency.

### Immune

In recent years, the importance of immune mechanisms—that is, autoimmune-mediated inflammation in the central nervous system that causes epilepsy—has been recognized. Epilepsies caused by immune mechanisms may respond to treatment with immunomodulatory agents. These disorders include anti-NMDA receptor encephalitis that presents with neuropsychiatric features and limbic encephalitis with antibodies to voltage-gated potassium channels such as LGI1 and CASPR2.

### Unknown

In about one third of individuals with epilepsy, the cause is unknown, even though clinical and EEG features may allow localization of the epileptic focus. Advances in neuroimaging should continue to improve the detection of subtle brain abnormalities such as cortical dysplasia and atrophic lesions in many of these patients. It is also possible that new genetic methods, such as epilepsy gene panels or whole exome or genome sequencing, as well as identification of new neurometabolic and neuroimmunological conditions, may reduce the number of patients with epilepsy of unknown cause.

## Conclusions

The new system of nomenclature for epileptic seizures and the epilepsies expands and clarifies the terminology we use in clinical practice. This system remains imperfect and will continue to require refinement as new knowledge emerges. Correct classification is essential for understanding this complex and diverse condition, and for making correct decisions regarding its evaluation and management.

## Bibliography

Berg AT, Berkovic SF, Brodie MJ, et al. Revised terminology and concepts for organization of seizures and epilepsies: Report of the ILAE Commission on Classification and Terminology, 2005–2009. *Epilepsia* 2010; **51**(4):676–685.

Blume WT, Luders HO, Mizrahi E, Tassinari C, van Emde Boas W, Engel J, Jr. Glossary of descriptive terminology for ictal semiology: Report of the ILAE task force on classification and terminology. *Epilepsia* 2001; **42**:1212–1218.

Commission of Classification and Terminology of the International League Against Epilepsy: Proposal for revised clinical and electroencephalographic classification of epileptic seizures. *Epilepsia* 1981; **22**:489–501.

Commission on Classification and Terminology of the International League Against Epilepsy: Proposal for revised classification of epilepsies and epileptic syndromes. *Epilepsia* 1989; **30**: 389–399.

Engel J, Jr. ILAE classification of epilepsy syndromes. *Epilepsy Res* 2006; **70**(Suppl. 1):S5–S10.

Fisher RS, van Emde Boas W, Blume W, et al. Epileptic seizures and epilepsy: Definitions proposed by the International League Against Epilepsy (ILAE) and the International Bureau for Epilepsy (IBE). *Epilepsia* 2005; **46**:470–472.

Gaillard WD, Cross JH, Duncan JS, Stefan H, Theodore WH, Task Force on Practice Parameter Imaging Guidelines for International League Against Epilepsy, Commission for Diagnostics. Epilepsy imaging study guideline criteria: Commentary on diagnostic testing study guidelines and practice parameters. *Epilepsia* 2011; **52**(9):1750–1756.

Gastaut H, Caveness WF, Landolt W, et al. A proposed international classification of epileptic seizures. *Epilepsia* 1964; **5**:297–306.

Gloor P. Consciousness as a neurological concept in epileptology: A critical review. *Epilepsia* 1986; **27**(Suppl. 2):S14–S26.

Scheffer IE. Epilepsy: A classification for all seasons? *Epilepsia* 2012; **53**(Suppl. 2):6–9.

# What Causes Epilepsy?

**Anna Rosati and Renzo Guerrini**

Pediatric Neurology Unit and Laboratories, Neuroscience Department, Children's Hospital A. Meyer, University of Florence, Florence, Italy

## Introduction

There are many possible causes for epilepsy, including genetic, acquired, and provoking factors. Epilepsy can be classified into four categories based on presumed etiology:

1. *Idiopathic epilepsy* does not have a detectable neuroanatomical or neuropathological abnormality. These epilepsies are caused by a complex genetic predisposition or, infrequently, single-gene inheritance. Idiopathic epilepsy is not just the absence of obvious causative factors; it also features specific clinical and electroencephalogram (EEG) characteristics.
2. *Symptomatic epilepsy* has an acquired or genetic cause associated with neuroanatomical or neuropathological abnormalities indicative of an underlying disease or condition. When the cause is genetic (e.g., a genetic brain malformation), the epilepsy is the result of the interposed brain abnormality rather than the direct consequence of the genetic abnormality.
3. *Provoked epilepsy* has a specific systemic or environmental factor as the apparent etiology of seizures with no obvious causative neuroanatomical or neuropathological abnormalities.
4. *Cryptogenic epilepsy* is of presumed symptomatic nature but the cause has not been identified. The use of this term is no longer advised because of the possibility of confusion with the term *idiopathic.*

The causes of epilepsy differ by age. In children and adolescents, epilepsy is more often genetically determined, whereas adult epilepsy is more often due to acquired structural causes. At every age, the cause of epilepsy is unknown for about half of individuals. Identification of the etiology of epilepsy has practical implication for both prognosis and treatment.

## Idiopathic epilepsies

Idiopathic epilepsies are common, constituting about 40% of the epilepsies worldwide. They are characterized by generalized or partial seizures in otherwise normal infants, children, adolescents, and young adults with normal brain MRI and no previous relevant medical history. Response to antiepileptic drugs is usually satisfactory, but it is unproven that treatment changes ultimate outcome.

In most cases, idiopathic epilepsies exhibit a complex pattern of inheritance in which various genes act in a different way in each patient to produce

**Table 3.1.** Idiopathic generalized and focal epilepsies.

| | Specific syndromes | Age at onset | Age at remission | Prognosis |
|---|---|---|---|---|
| Idiopathic generalized epilepsies | Idiopathic myoclonic epilepsy in infancy | 3 months to 3 years | 3–5 years | Variable |
| | Epilepsy with myoclonic-atonic seizures | 3–5 years | Variable | Variable |
| | Childhood absence epilepsy | 5–6 years | 10–12 years | Relatively good |
| | Epilepsy with myoclonic absences | 1–12 years | Variable | Guarded |
| | Juvenile absence epilepsy | 10–12 years | Usually lifelong | Relatively good |
| | Juvenile myoclonic epilepsy | 12–18 years | Usually lifelong | Relatively good |
| | Epilepsy with generalized tonic-clonic seizures only | 12–18 years | Usually lifelong | Relatively good |
| Idiopathic focal epilepsies of infancy and childhood | Benign infantile seizures (nonfamilial) | Infancy | Infancy | Good |
| | Benign epilepsy of childhood with centrotemporal spikes | 3–13 years | 16 years | Good |
| | Early-and late-onset idiopathic occipital epilepsy | 2–8 years; 6–17 years | 12 years; 18 years | Good |

the specific phenotype or syndrome. The various syndromes of idiopathic epilepsies differ in age of onset. Idiopathic epilepsies with complex (presumed polygenic) inheritance are divided into the idiopathic generalized epilepsies (IGEs) and the idiopathic partial epilepsies of childhood (Table 3.1).

A few idiopathic epilepsy syndromes have a familial distribution with simple inheritance, usually autosomal dominant with reduced penetrance, and are usually caused by mutations in single genes that encode for ion channels or their accessory subunits. This has led to the concept that idiopathic epilepsies are channelopathies, even though the link between molecular deficit and clinical phenotype is still insufficiently characterized and non-ion channel genes are now emerging as causes of sporadic or familial early-onset focal, seemingly idiopathic seizure disorders. It is notable that mutations in the same gene can cause different epilepsy syndromes (phenotypic heterogeneity) and the same syndrome can be caused by mutations in different genes (genotypic heterogeneity). Phenotypic variability has been putatively attributed to modifier genes or polymorphisms determining the phenotypical expression or, alternatively, to environmental factors. Recent genetic insights have been gained through the discovery that monogenic idiopathic epilepsies may be comorbid with disorders such as paroxysmal movement disorders, hemiplegic migraine, broad-spectrum encephalopathies, learning difficulties, and psychiatric conditions. "Monogenic idiopathic epilepsies" are summarized in Table 3.2.

## Symptomatic epilepsies

Symptomatic epilepsies are associated with structural brain abnormalities indicating an underlying disease or condition. This category includes (1) developmental and congenital disorders associated with genetic or acquired cerebral pathological changes, and also (2) acquired conditions. In symptomatic epilepsies, the underlying genetic conditions are responsible for either clear neuropathological abnormalities (e.g., epilepsy due to neurocutaneous diseases) or more subtle changes at the subcellular or molecular pathology level (e.g., the epilepsies due to Angelman syndrome, Rett syndrome, *CDKL5* gene mutations).

### Symptomatic epilepsies due to genetic or congenital disorders

*Single-gene disorders*

In most of the single-gene disorders that cause epilepsy and manifest primarily in childhood, seizures are only one symptom of a much broader clinical picture characterized by learning disabilities and other neurological features (Chapter 22). The seizures have variable characteristics and

**Table 3.2.** Monogenic idiopathic epilepsies.

| Syndrome | Gene | Locus | Age at onset | Phenotype | Prognosis |
|---|---|---|---|---|---|
| BFNS | KCNQ2 KCNQ3 | 20q13 8q24 | First days of life | Focal, tonic–clonic convulsions | Excellent |
| BFNIS | SCN2A | 2q24 | Neonatal period until 3–6 months | Focal and generalized convulsions | Excellent |
| BFIS | SCN2A PRRT2* | 2q24 16p11.2 | 3–12 months | Focal seizures with or without generalized tonic-clonic seizures | Good |
| GEFS+ | SCN1A SCN1B SCN2A GABRD GABRG2 | 2q24 19q13 2q24 1p36 5q31 | Early infancy or childhood | Febrile seizures, generalized tonic-clonic seizures, absences, atonic seizures, focal seizures, myoclonic seizures | Good |
| JME | EFHC1 GABRA1 | 6p12 5q34 21 | Adolescence | Myoclonic seizures on awakening; generalized tonic-clonic seizures | Good |
| ADNFLE | CHRNA2 CHRNA4 CHRNB2 KCNT1 | 8p21 20q13 1q21 9q34.3 | Markedly variable (2 months to 56 years); peak at 11 years; 90% <20 years | Sleep-related focal seizures with frontal semiology | Variable; lifelong with spontaneous remission and relapses |
| ADPEAF | LGI1 | 10q24 | 4–50 years | Focal seizures with auditory or visual hallucinations | Variable |

ADFNLE, autosomal dominant nocturnal frontal lobe epilepsy; ADPEAF/ADLTE, autosomal dominant partial epilepsy with auditory features/autosomal dominant lateral temporal epilepsy; BFIS, benign familial infantile seizures; BFNIS, benign familial neonatal–infantile seizures; BFNS, benign familial neonatal seizures; HM, hemiplegic migraine; JME, juvenile myoclonic epilepsy; PKD, paroxysmal kinesigenic dyskinesia; PS, partial seizures.

*Episodic ataxia, HM, migraine, PKD.

severity. These single-gene disorders are usually associated with variable and complex phenotypes. The epilepsy is distinctive, or is a predominant and consistent feature, in only a few of these conditions (Table 3.3).

*Chromosomal disorders*

Epilepsy is frequently observed in chromosomal disorders (Chapter 22). These syndromes are associated with behavioral and intellectual disabilities, and characteristic dysmorphic features. In some, the clinical presentation and EEG abnormalities are characteristic (e.g., Angelman syndrome, ring chromosome 20 syndrome, and 4p-syndrome); in

others, the manifestations appear nonspecific and are not diagnostic of the particular chromosomal abnormality. Often, seizure onset is during the neonatal period or in infancy (Table 3.4).

*Inherited metabolic and mitochondrial disorders*

Seizures are often part of the clinical picture of inherited metabolic and mitochondrial disorders, particularly when these conditions begin early in life (Chapter 23). Unfortunately, the clinical presentation of seizures is seldom distinctive enough to allow immediate diagnosis. Nevertheless, clinical phenotypes, epilepsy syndrome, and especially the characteristic times of presentation narrow

**Table 3.3.** Complex single-gene disorders with epilepsy.

| Disease | Gene | Age at onset | Phenotype |
|---|---|---|---|
| ARX disorders | *ARX* | Neonatal and infancy | Epileptic encephalopathy, infantile spasms |
| Familial epilepsy and MR limited to females | *PCDH19* | Infancy | Generalized or focal seizures highly sensitive to fever, brief seizures occurring in clusters, mental retardation |
| Angelman syndrome | *UBE3A* | Infancy | Learning difficulties, ataxia, seizures, myoclonus, subtle dysmorphic facial features, sociable disposition |
| Rett syndrome | *MECP2* | Infancy | Severe cognitive impairment, distinctive hand stereotypies, early-onset epilepsy (60% of cases) |
| CDKL5 gene-related epilepsy | *CDKL5* | Infancy | Severe cognitive impairment, early-onset epilepsy, infantile spasms, epileptic encephalopathy (100% of cases) |
| FOXG1 gene-related epilepsy | *FOXG1* | Infancy | Severe cognitive impairment, dyskinesia, early-onset epilepsy (100% of cases) |
| Tuberous sclerosis | *TSC1, TSC2* | Variable | Focal or generalized epilepsy (80%), infantile spasms |
| Neurofibromatosis type 1 | *NF1* | Variable | Focal seizures (5–10%) |
| Unverricht–Lundborg disease | *CTSB* | Adulthood | Progressive myoclonic epilepsy (PME) |
| Lafora body disease | *EPM2A, NHLRC1* | Adolescence | PME |
| Neuronal ceroid lipofuscinoses | *TPP1* *CLN3* *CLN5* | Variable | PME |
| Sialidosis | *NEU1* | Adulthood | PME |
| MERRF | *MT-TK, TL1, TH, TS1* | Variable | PME |

CLN3, CLN5, ceroid lipofuscinosis gene; EPM2A, gene encoding laforin phosphatase; FOXG1, forkhead box G1; MERRF, myoclonic epilepsy with ragged red fibers; MR, mental retardation; MT-TK, mitochondrially encoded tRNA lysine; MT-TL1, mitochondrially encoded tRNA leucine 1; MT-TS1, mitochondrially encoded tRNA serine 1; NEU1, N-acetyl-alpha-neuraminidase; NF1, neurofibromin 1 gene; NHLRC1, NHL repeat-containing protein 1; PCDH19, protocadherin; TPP1, tripeptidyl peptidase 1; TSC, tuberous sclerosis complex; UBE3A, ubiquitin-protein ligase.

diagnostic possibilities. EEG findings may also facilitate recognition of the more common diagnoses. All infants and young children seen with unexplained epilepsy and neurological disability (e.g., intellectual disability) should be evaluated for inherited metabolic disorder. A positive family history may provide an important clue, and careful studies of blood, urine, and cerebrospinal fluid (CSF) may reveal characteristic abnormalities. More common metabolic and mitochondrial diseases and associated epilepsy syndromes are reported in Table 3.5 and in Chapter 23.

**Table 3.4.** Chromosomal disorders.

| Syndrome | Frequency of epilepsy | Age at onset | Type of seizures | Prognosis |
|---|---|---|---|---|
| Ring chromosome 20 syndrome | 95–100% | Infancy to 14 years | NCSE, FS | Poor |
| 4p-syndrome | 80–90% | 5–23 months | AS, SE, GCS | Good |
| 1p36 deletion syndrome | 50–58% | Infancy or childhood | IS, GCS, FS, MyS, AS | Variable, rarely intractable |
| Fragile X syndrome | 13–44% | Childhood | Focal epilepsy | Good |
| Distal deletion of the long arm of chromosome 6 | 25% | 4 months to 10 years | IS, FS | Good |
| Klinefelter syndrome | 5–17% | 3 months to 3 years | FC, FS, GCS, AS | Good |
| Down syndrome | 8% | Variable | IS, FS, GCS | Variable |
| Trisomy 13 (Patau syndrome) | Rare | Neonatal | FC, FS, Multifocal or photosensitive MyS | Poor |
| Trisomy 12p | Rare | Childhood | Myoclonic absences | Good |
| Ring chromosome 14 syndrome | Rare | Infancy | GCS, MyS, FS | Variable |

AS, absence seizure; FC, febrile convulsion; FS, focal seizure; GCS, generalized convulsive seizure; IS, infantile spasm; MyS, myoclonic seizures; NCSE, nonconvulsive status epilepticus; SE, status epilepticus.

## Malformations of cortical development

Malformations of cortical development include a wide range of disorders that commonly cause neurodevelopmental delay and epilepsy, especially in children. They account for at least 40% of drug-resistant childhood epilepsies. Abnormalities of neuronal and glial proliferation or programmed cell death, neuronal migration, synaptogenesis, and cortical organization result in distinct or partially overlapping entities. Some malformations are associated with mutations of specific genes, but others result from environmental influences such as intrauterine infection or perfusion failure. Although in many cases, the cause remains unclear, exome sequencing studies are revealing that *de novo* mutations of genes that encode for proteins regulating centrosome activity, vesicle trafficking, and cell adhesion are responsible for the majority of sporadic malformations. There is also emerging evidence that some regional malformations, such as hemimegalencephaly, are caused by somatic mosaic mutations that are present only in the malformed tissue.

The most common malformation of cortical development is *focal cortical dysplasia* (FCD). This term designates a spectrum of abnormalities of the laminar structure of the cortex, variably associated with cytopathological features including giant (or cytomegalic) neurons, dysmorphic neurons, and balloon cells. A developmental lineage model has been proposed in which balloon cells and dysplastic neurons are derived from radial progenitor cells in the telencephalic ventricular zone. The abnormal area is not usually sharply defined from the adjacent tissue. The close cytoarchitectural similarities between FCD and the cortical tubers of tuberous sclerosis has prompted the hypothesis of a common pathogenetic basis. Histopathologic similarities between FCD, hemimegalencephaly, and the dysembryoplastic neuroepithelial tumors, two highly epileptogenic developmental lesions, further support the hypothesis of a developmental origin.

A classification system with distinct clinicopathologic FCD variants has been proposed based on clinical presentation, imaging findings, and histopathologic features. FCD Type I refers to isolated lesions with either radial (FCD Type Ia) or tangential (FCD Type Ib) dyslamination of the

**Table 3.5.** Metabolic and mitochondrial disorders.

| |
|---|
| *Metabolic disorders in the newborn* |
| Nonketotic hyperglycinemia |
| Pyridoxine dependency |
| Molybdenum cofactor deficiency |
| Sulfiteoxidase deficiency |
| Peroxisomal disorders (Zellweger syndrome, neonatal adrenoleukodystrophy, acyl-CoA oxidase deficiency) |
| Urea cycle disorders |
| Maple syrup urine disease |
| Organic acidurias |
| Fatty acid oxidation defects |
| Defects of mitochondrial energy metabolism (pyruvate dehydrogenase deficiency, pyruvate carboxylase deficiency, Leigh syndrome) |
| Disorders of carbohydrate metabolism (fructose-1,6-bisphosphatase deficiency, early-onset multiple carboxylase deficiency) |
| *Metabolic disorders of early infancy* |
| Lysosomal disorders (GM2 gangliosidoses, GM1 gangliosidosis type I and type II, Krabbe disease) |
| Disorders of vitamin metabolism (biotinidase deficiency, methylenetetrahydrofolate reductase deficiency, congenital folate malabsorption) |
| GLUT1 deficiency syndrome |
| Organic acidurias |
| Aminoacidurias (phenylketonuria, hyperphenylalaninemias, tyrosinemia type III) |
| Urea cycle disorders (arginase deficiency) |
| Disorders of GABA metabolism |
| Menkes disease |
| *Metabolic disorders of late infancy* |
| Metachromatic leukodystrophy |
| Deficiency of α-N-acetylgalactosaminidase |
| Mucopolysaccharidoses |
| Neuronal ceroid lipofuscinoses |
| Defects of mitochondrial energy metabolism (POLG disease) |
| Carbohydrate-deficient glycoprotein syndrome |
| *Metabolic disorders of childhood and adolescence* |
| Homocystinuria |
| Diabetes mellitus |
| Adrenoleukodystrophy |
| Lysosomal disorders (sialidosis type I and type II, Gaucher disease type III) |
| Neuronal ceroid lipofuscinosis |
| Lafora disease |
| Defects of mitochondrial energy metabolism (POLG mutations; MERRF; MELAS) |
| Dentatorubral-pallidoluysian atrophy |
| Unverricht–Lundborg progressive familial myoclonic epilepsy |

MELAS, mitochondrial myopathy, encephalopathy, lactic acidosis, and stroke; MERRF, myoclonic epilepsy with ragged red fibers; POLG, polymerase g.

neocortex, microscopically identified in one or multiple lobes. FCD Type II is an isolated lesion characterized by cortical dyslamination and dysmorphic neurons without (Type IIa) or with balloon cells (Type IIb). FCD Type III occurs in combination with hippocampal sclerosis (FCD Type IIIa) or with epilepsy-associated tumors (FCD Type IIIb). FCD Type IIIc is found adjacent to vascular malformations, whereas FCD Type IIId is associated with epileptogenic lesions acquired in early life (i.e., traumatic injury, ischemic injury, or encephalitis).

The most frequent clinical presentation of FCD is a child or adolescent developing intractable partial epilepsy. However, infantile spasms may be the first manifestation. FCD is a frequent cause of focal status epilepticus. It is the most common pathological substrate in epilepsy surgery series, reaching up to 40%. FCD is rarely a restricted process. Surface and intracranial EEG recordings reveal focal positive spike discharges or high-frequency discharges, and ablation of tissue exhibiting these electrographic patterns correlates with outcome. Although patients can be operated on without invasive intracranial recordings, the best results are obtained when resections are guided by intracranial EEG investigations (Table 3.6).

### Neurocutaneous disorders

The neurocutaneous disorders are a group of distinct conditions characterized by congenital dysplastic abnormalities involving the skin and nervous system. Tuberous sclerosis complex (TSC) is a dominant disorder manifested primarily by abnormalities of the CNS, the skin, and the kidney. About 80% of TSC patients develop epilepsy with about two-thirds presenting with seizures before the age of 2 years, often with infantile spasms. Sturge–Weber syndrome (SWS) is a nonfamilial phakomatosis in which a venous angioma of the leptomeninges is accompanied by an ipsilateral nevus flammeus of the skin supplied by the trigeminal nerve. Seventy percent of patients with SWS develop seizures within the first year of life, and almost all have epilepsy before 4 years of age. Unilateral convulsive status epilepticus occurs in about 50%, leaving half with permanent hemiplegia. Another neurocutaneous disorder, neurofibromatosis, has only a 5–10% occurrence of epilepsy. Other, less frequent, neurocutaneous conditions include hypomelanosis of Ito, epidermal

**Table 3.6.** Malformations of cortical development.

| *Abnormalities of gyration* |
|---|
| Agyria–pachygyria subcortical band heterotopia spectrum (*LIS1, TUBA1A, RELN, ARX, DCX* genes) |
| Diffuse polymicrogyria (*TUBB2B* gene) |
| Multilobar polymicrogyria |
| Schizencephaly (*EMX2* gene) |
| Minor gyral abnormalities |
| *Heterotopia* |
| Periventricular nodular heterotopia (*FLNA* gene) |
| Subcortical nodular heterotopia |
| Subcortical band heterotopia (*DCX* and *LIS1* genes) |
| *Other gross malformations* |
| Megalencephaly and hemimegalencephaly |
| Agenesis of the corpus callosum |
| Anencephaly and holoprosencephaly |
| Microcephaly |
| *Cortical dysgenesis associated with neoplasia* |
| DNET |
| Ganglioglioma |
| Gangliocytoma |
| *Other cortical dysplasias* |
| Focal cortical dysplasia |
| Tuberous sclerosis (*TSC1* and *TSC2* genes) |

DNET, dysembryoplastic neuroepithelial tumor.

nevus syndrome, midline linear nevus syndrome, incontinentia pigmenti, and Klippel–Trenaunay–Weber syndrome.

### Symptomatic epilepsies due to acquired conditions

This category includes cerebral pathological processes as well as epilepsies due to external or environmental causes. Seizures can result from anything that injures the brain, with the types of injury depending on age. Seizures in children often are caused by birth traumas, infections such as meningitis, and congenital abnormalities. Nonaccidental brain injury, often under recognized acutely, is a relatively rare cause of symptomatic epilepsy in children. In the middle years, seizures are commonly caused by head injuries, infections, alcohol, stimulant drugs, and medication side effects. In the elderly, a higher proportion of seizures are caused by brain tumors and strokes.

## Cerebral palsy

Cerebral palsy is associated with epilepsy in about 50% of quadriplegic and hemiplegic forms, and in about 26% of spastic diplegic and in dyskinetic forms. Infantile spasms are observed in more than 15% of patients. Epilepsy is usually early-onset, may be focal or generalized, and has a variable course. Only 13% achieve a remission of 2 years or more. Children with cerebral palsy and epilepsy function at lower levels in terms of cognitive skills and memory than children with the same form of cerebral palsy without epilepsy. Those with smaller lesions and severe epilepsy do less well than those with larger lesions without epilepsy.

## Hippocampal sclerosis

The terms hippocampal sclerosis (HS), Ammon's horn sclerosis, and mesial temporal sclerosis designate subtly different entities featuring gliosis and neuronal loss in temporal structures. There are several pathologic subtypes of HS that are associated with additional pathologic changes, in some cases outside the hippocampus (dual pathology). The typical MRI features of HS are reduced volume, increased signal intensity on T2-weighted images, and abnormal morphology of hippocampus. There is no sex or side preference; 48–56% of cases are bilateral in postmortem studies. In children with temporal lobe epilepsy, MRI detected HS in 21% of those with new-onset seizures and in 57% of those with refractory seizures. HS is the most common pathological finding in mesial temporal lobe epilepsy (MTLE), accounting for approximately 70% of patients undergoing surgery for drug-resistant focal seizures. The clinical features of MTLE include an early initial injury (typically complicated febrile convulsions, but also central nervous system infections or head injury) followed by a variable *latent interval* of around 7–10 years before onset of spontaneous seizures in late childhood or adolescence. Seizures are characterized by a typical rising epigastric aura, followed by behavioral arrest, and a slowly progressing unresponsiveness, with a motionless stare or oroalimentary automatisms.

## Cerebrovascular diseases/stroke

Seizures are a frequent complication of a stroke and can even be the presenting symptom. Early seizures occur within 7 days of stroke symptoms onset; late seizures occur thereafter. The early, acutely symptomatic seizures can predict the later development of epilepsy. Pathophysiological mechanisms of early seizures differ between ischemic and hemorrhagic stroke and include sudden development of a space-occupying lesion with mass effect, focal ischemia, and blood breakdown products. Late seizures correlate with gliosis and development of meningocerebral scars.

*Intracranial hemorrhage* (ICH) is frequently the result of penetrating head trauma (see following text). Nontraumatic ICHs are more prominent in children and young adults and more common among men than women. Causes of nontraumatic ICH are aneurysms, vascular malformations (arteriovenous malformations, venous angiomas, cavernous angiomas, and telangiectasias), acute or chronic hypertension, amyloid angiopathy, venous thrombosis, primary and metastatic brain tumor, vasculitis, and bleeding disorders (hemophilia, sickle cell disease, thrombocytopenia, and leukemia). Vascular malformations may cause epilepsy even in the absence of overt bleeding; cavernous angiomas and arteriovenous malformations are the most epileptogenic forms. About 50–70% of seizures occur within the first 24 h of ICH, and 90% in the first 3 days, with the overall 30 day risk of seizures being about 8%. Factors predisposing to seizures include hemorrhagic size, cerebral cortex involvement, hydrocephalus, intracranial midline shift, low Glasgow Coma Scale, and severe neurological deficit. Continuous video–EEG monitoring is advised to recognize early electrographic seizures and nonconvulsive episodes, which represent an underestimated and frequent complication of ICH. Overall incidence after ICH is 4.2–20% for clinical seizures and around 30% for subclinical seizures. Frequency of status epilepticus ranges from 0.3% to 21.4%.

Epilepsy almost always develops within 2 years of the hemorrhage, and the risk of epilepsy is about 1%. In patients with an *ischemic stroke*, epilepsy occurs in about 6% of patients within 12 months and 11% within 5 years. Factors associated with a great risk of epilepsy are severity, greater size of infarct, hemorrhagic transformation, a cortical site of stroke, and embolism.

★ TIPS AND TRICKS

Between 5% and 10% of patients presenting with stroke have a history of recent prior epileptic seizures. In the adult, a screen for vascular risk factors with the aim of stroke prevention should be considered with new-onset seizures if other causes are not present.

*Cancer*

Primary brain tumors

Brain tumors account for 3.6% of all epilepsy and 12% of acquired epilepsy. Epilepsy from brain tumor occurs at all ages but in a higher proportion in the 25–64-years-old age group. Seizures are the most common presenting symptom of primary brain tumors. Some patients have one seizure leading to the tumor diagnosis and will never have another seizure after the tumor is resected. In others types of brain tumors such as dysembryoplastic neuroepithelial tumors, the natural course of the tumor is very benign, but the severity of epilepsy dictates the necessity for surgical intervention. Seizure incidence is lower (30–50%) in some of the most malignant brain tumors, such as glioblastoma and primary CNS lymphoma, and higher (50–80%) in some less malignant infiltrative lesions, such as WHO grade II diffuse gliomas. Location in the temporal lobe and cortical rather than white matter involvement are usually associated with a higher risk of seizures. In this regard, oligodendroglial tumors are often located at the cortical–white matter interface and cause seizures frequently, whereas primary CNS lymphomas more commonly grow in the white matter and are not usually diagnosed because of a seizure. In patients with primary brain tumors, seizures may also result from surgery, exposure to chemotherapy, or radiotherapy to the brain.

Systemic cancer

Seizures are also a frequent complication in patients with disseminated cancer, mostly because of parenchymal brain metastasis or leptomeningeal disease, but they can also be caused by cytotoxic chemotherapy and toxic–metabolic encephalopathy.

Solid brain metastases seem to cause seizures less frequently than do primary brain tumors, which may be explained by their less infiltrative growth. Lung cancer (both non-small cell and small cell) is the most common cancer associated with metastasis presenting with seizures, although seizures can also be seen with breast, skin, renal, pancreatic, thyroid, and colon cancers. The time between diagnosis of the primary tumor and occurrence of seizures due to metastasis depends on the propensity of the primary tumor to metastasize to the brain. Central nervous system (CNS) metastases occur early, often on presentation, in lung cancers and malignant melanoma, but may be delayed by as much as 2–3 years in breast cancers. New-onset seizures in patients with known brain metastases may indicate hemorrhage into a metastatic lesion, notably in patients with metastatic melanoma or tumor progression with associated edema.

When seizures occur for the first time in patients under treatment for cancer, the possibility of drug-induced seizures should be considered.

★ TIPS AND TRICKS

The initial evaluation of a first seizure in any patient with known systemic cancer must include neuroimaging, preferably MRI, to look for parenchymal or leptomeningeal involvement by cancer, and other neurological conditions such as cerebrovascular and infectious disorders. Concomitantly, a comprehensive metabolic investigation including serum or sometimes CSF drug assays, if available, should be undertaken.

*Head trauma*

Brain injury accounts for about 6% of all epilepsy and occurs at all ages. Post-traumatic seizures are traditionally subdivided into immediate, early, and late seizures. Similar to seizures observed with stroke, immediate seizures occur within 1–24 h after injury and represent the initial effect of the acute injury on the brain. Early seizures occur within the first week and late seizures occur after 1 week. About 50% of seizures occur within the first 24 h, 25% within the first hour. The overall risk of early seizures varies from 2% to 15%. Early seizures increase the risk for post-traumatic epilepsy. Several processes contribute to the development of early seizures – hypoxia, increased intracranial pressure, hypotension, brain edema, ischemia, electrolyte imbalance, and secondary infection. Late seizures reflect permanent neuropathological changes in the brain and tend to recur, and therefore signal the onset of post-traumatic epilepsy. The overall risk of post-traumatic epilepsy is approximately 5–7%. The greater the severity of the injury, the higher the risk of both early and late seizures. Early seizures occur in less than 5% of mild and moderate head injuries but are seen in more than 30% of those with an intracranial hematoma. Children younger than 5 years are more likely than adults to have seizures within the first hour after mild head injury. Adults older than 65 years are highly vulnerable to brain damage and late post-traumatic epilepsy from any type of head injury. Post-traumatic seizures may begin focally or secondarily generalize. The site of injury largely determines the type of focal manifestations. Approximately 10–20% of early seizures develop into status epilepticus, usually in children and most often in severe trauma. Focal motor status is most common with subdural hematoma or depressed skull fractures, and can be refractory to treatment.

## Cerebral infections

Acute symptomatic seizures, defined by the International League Against Epilepsy as occurring within 7 days of an acute CNS infection, are seen in 2–67% of patients with encephalitis. The incidence of acute symptomatic seizures and subsequent epilepsy varies with the cause of encephalitis, the patient's age, delays in starting treatment, and degree of cortical inflammation. The risk of developing chronic epilepsy is highest within the first 5 years following the encephalitis, but it can occur up to 20 years later.

The most common serious viral encephalitis is due to herpes simplex virus type-1 (HSV-1), and this infection frequently results in severe and intractable epilepsy; it is particularly important to make an early diagnosis of HSV in neonates, in whom encephalitis may be part of a disseminated infection. Other important causes of viral encephalitis include varicella zoster virus and enteroviruses. Immunocompromised people have an increased risk of infection from a wider range of pathogens, including viruses such as cytomegalovirus and small intracellular bacteria and parasites such as *Toxoplasma gondii*.

Pyogenic brain abscess is another uncommon but serious infection that causes epilepsy. Commonly isolated organisms are streptococci, including aerobic and anaerobic types. *Streptococcus pneumoniae* is a rare cause of brain abscess, often the sequella of occult CSF rhinorrhoea or pneumococcal pneumonia in elderly patients. Staphylococci account for 10–15% of abcesses and are usually caused by penetrating head injury or bacteremia secondary to endocarditis. Clostridial infections are most often post-traumatic. Neurocysticercosis is the most common parasitic disease of the CNS and a major cause of epilepsy in endemic areas such as Mexico, India, and China. In Africa, malaria is a particularly common cause of seizures and, typically, status epilepticus in the acute phase of cerebral malaria. There is a 9–11-fold increase in risk of chronic epilepsy in children with a history of malaria. Epilepsy is also frequently the presenting symptom of a cerebral tuberculoma.

## Immunological and inflammatory diseases

Epilepsy may occur in autoimmune disorders. Clinical presentations may vary among patients and include seizures, psychiatric features, movement disorders, amnesia, confusion, or loss of consciousness. These diseases can be associated with tumors, but they are more often nonparaneoplastic, and immunotherapy is often effective. In some epilepsy types, clinical and biologic data strongly support the pathogenic role of autoantibodies (e.g., limbic encephalitis, anti-NMDA receptor encephalitis), while in other types, immune-mediated inflammation occurs but the full pathogenic chain is unclear (e.g., Rasmussen's syndrome) or only hypothesized (idiopathic hemiconvulsion-hemiplegia syndrome and febrile infection-related epilepsy syndrome) (Table 3.7). Assessment of clinical phenotype and analysis of serum and sometimes CSF are crucial for identification of autoantibodies.

The frequency of epilepsy in patients with multiple sclerosis is about three times that of the general population. In one study, the cumulative risk of epilepsy in patients with multiple sclerosis was found to be 1.1% by 5 years, 1.8% by 10 years, and 3.1% by 15 years.

Epilepsy can occur in all other forms of large-, medium-, or small-vessel vasculitides, sometimes due to infarction. Seizures occur in about 25% of cases of systemic lupus erythematosus. Seizures can be the presenting symptom and are particularly common in severe or chronic cases and in lupus-induced encephalopathy. Epilepsy occurs less often in other vasculitides such as Behçet's disease and in other "connective tissue disorders" such as Sjögren's

**Table 3.7.** Autoimmune or presumed autoimmune and inflammatory epilepsies.

| Syndrome | Age at onset | Phenotype | Cancer | Prognosis |
|---|---|---|---|---|
| FIRES | Early childhood | Focal status epilepticus; cognitive impairment | None | Poor |
| Ramussen's syndrome | Childhood–adolescence; rare in adulthood | Focal status epilepticus; progressive hemiparesis and hemispheric atrophy | None | Poor |
| NMDAR encephalitis | Variable | Encephalitis; status epilepticus; movement disorders; F >> M | Ovarian teratoma (rare in children, present in 58% older than 18 years) | Variable; 20% relapse, higher in idiopathic cases |
| LGI1 encephalitis | Adulthood | Limbic encephalitis; faciobrachial seizures; hyponatraemia, M >> F | None | Variable |
| GABABR | Adulthood | Limbic encephalitis | SCLC (70%) | Variable |
| AMPAR | Adulthood | Limbic encephalitis | SCLC, breast, thymus (60%) | Variable |

AMPAR, α-amino-3-hydroxy-5-methyl-4-isoxazolepropionic acid receptor; FIRES, febrile infection-related epilepsy syndrome; GABABR, γ-aminobutyric acid-B receptor; LGI1, leucine-rich glioma inactivated 1; NMDAR, $N$-methyl-D-aspartate receptor; SCLC, small-cell lung cancer.

syndrome, mixed connective tissue disease, and Henoch–Schönlein purpura. Seizures are the most common neurological complication of inflammatory bowel diseases (ulcerative colitis and Crohn's disease), in one series occurring in 6% of cases. In celiac disease, the clinical spectrum of epilepsy ranges from benign syndromes to intractable epilepsy. Epilepsy is also a prominent feature of Hashimoto's thyroiditis, a relapsing encephalopathy associated with high thyroid antibody titers.

> ★ **TIPS AND TRICKS**
>
> Consider an immune-mediated condition in patients with unexplained subacute onset of seizures, particularly in the presence of MRI or CSF evidence of inflammation.

*Degenerative diseases*

Degenerative dementias, such as Alzheimer's disease, are associated with an increased incidence of seizures. The prevalence of seizures in patients with dementia ranges from 10% to 20%. Patients with seizures are usually younger and significantly more cognitively impaired than those with dementia only. Seizures also occur in prion disorders and some frontotemporal lobar degeneration syndromes, whereas Parkinson's disease and other parkinsonian conditions seem relatively seizure-free. The pathogenesis of seizures in these conditions is uncertain but may be related to neocortical and hippocampal hyperexcitability and synchronized activity.

## Provoked epilepsies

### Reflex epilepsy

Reflex epilepsy is a condition in which seizures can be provoked habitually by an external stimulus or, less commonly, internal mental processes. Some individuals with reflex epilepsy may have seizures only with specific stimuli, while others may have both reflex and spontaneously occurring seizures. Simple reflex seizures are precipitated by elementary sensory stimuli, (e.g., flashes of light, startle), while complex reflex seizures are precipitated by patient-specific, more elaborate stimuli (e.g., specific pieces of music). Photosensitive epilepsy is the most common type of reflex epilepsy. Clinical photoconvulsive seizures or subclinical photoparoxysmal responses occur when an individual is exposed to

**Table 3.8.** Metabolic and toxic conditions.

*Metabolic disturbances and systemic illness*

Hypoxia

Hypoglycemia

Nonketotic hyperglycemia

Hypocalcemia (with or without hypoparathyroidism)

Hyponatremia (inappropriate antidiuretic hormone syndrome and water intoxication)

Hypomagnesemia

Hypophosphatemia

Uremia

Hepatic failure

Thyroid disorders

Sickle-cell anemia

Thrombotic thrombocytopenic purpura

Whipple's disease

*Drugs and toxins*

Analgesics (fentanyl, mefenamic acid, meperidine, pentazocine, propoxyphene, tramadol)

Antibiotics (ampicillin, cephalosporins, imipenem, isoniazid, metronidazole, nalidixic acid, oxacillin, penicillin)

Antidepressants (amitriptyline, doxepin, bupropion)

Antineoplastics (carmustine, busulfan, methotrexate, vincristine, cytosine arabinoside, chlorambucil)

Antipsychotics (chlorpromazine, haloperidol, perphenazine, prochlorperazine)

Bronchial agents (aminophylline, theophylline)

General anesthetics (enflurane, methohexital)

Local anesthetics (procaine, lidocaine)

Sympathomimetics (ephedrine, phenylpropanolamine terbutaline)

Alcohol

Amphetamines

Anticholinergics

Antihistamine

Atenolol

Baclofen

Cyclosporin A

Domperidone

Flumazenil

Folic acid

Insulin

Lithium

Aqueous iodinated contrast agent

Methylphenidate

Oxytocin

Heavy metals

Carbon monoxide

visual stimuli, usually flashes of light of a particular frequency. Photosensitivity (strictly defined) is present in a population with a frequency of about 1.1 per 100,000 persons, 5.7 per 100,000 in the 7–19 years age range, and is strongly associated with epilepsy. About 3% of persons with epilepsy are photosensitive and have seizures induced by photic stimuli. Most patients with photosensitivity have an IGE, although photosensitivity also occurs in patients with focal epilepsy arising in the occipital region and occasionally in other conditions.

### Toxic-metabolic conditions

It is important to recognize toxic–metabolic encephalopathy as a cause of seizures, as the appropriate treatment is correction of the underlying metabolic defect rather than antiepileptic medication. Seizures occur most commonly with hypoglycemia, hyponatremia, hypocalcemia, hypomagnesemia, hypokalemia, and hyperkalemia. Many metabolic disturbances may be drug induced. Chemotherapy-related seizures are most commonly associated with cisplatin, busulfan, chlorambucil, 5-fluorouracil, methotrexate, interferon, and cyclosporin A. Most drug-induced seizures occur within hours or days of drug administration. However, they may occur after several days when the half-life of the drug is prolonged as a result of impaired hepatic or renal clearance. For instance, both cyclophosphamide and ifosfamide cause inappropriate vasopressin secretion and, consequently, hyponatremic seizures; bisphosphonates cause hypocalcemic seizures; and cisplatin may result in hypomagnesemia and seizures. Ten percent of patients with severe renal failure have seizures caused by metabolic disturbance, dialysis encephalopathy, or dialysis disequilibrium syndrome. Seizures are also a common symptom in hepatic failure, with or without hyperammonemia (Table 3.8).

### ⚜ CAUTION!

Even in patients with structural lesions that could potentially cause epilepsy, seizures can have a toxic-metabolic or other preventable cause. These should be excluded before assuming that epilepsy has developed.

### Seizures from drugs and toxins

Common chemicals that can produce seizures include alcohol, cocaine and other drugs, heavy metals, and carbon monoxide. Alcohol abuse is a relatively common cause of seizures in adolescents and adults. Seizures, nearly always generalized tonic-clonic, occur in about 10% of adults during alcohol withdrawal, with multiple seizures in about 60%. The first seizure occurs 7 h to 2 days after the last drink, and the time between the first and last seizure is usually 6 h or less. Sudden withdrawal from certain antianxiety or antidepressant drugs such as benzodiazepines, barbiturates, and tricyclic antidepressants can also provoke seizures.

### Conclusion

The epilepsies have diverse causes. A thorough assessment is essential, but the differential diagnosis and the details of this evaluation depend on the presumed epilepsy syndrome and the age of the patient. Correct determination of epilepsy etiology is a prerequisite for determining prognosis and selecting the correct treatment.

### Bibliography

Barkovich AJ, Guerrini R, Kuzniecky RI, Jackson GD, Dobyns WB. A developmental and genetic classification for malformations of cortical development: Update 2012. *Brain* 2012; **135**:1348–1369.

Battaglia A, Guerrini R. Chromosomal disorders associated with epilepsy. *Epileptic Disord* 2005; **7**:181–192.

Bindoff LA, Engelsen BA. Mitochondrial diseases and epilepsy. *Epilepsia* 2012; **53**(Suppl. 4):92–97.

Brust JC. Seizures and substance abuse: Treatment considerations. *Neurology* 2006; **67**(12 Suppl. 4): S45–S48.

Chang BS, Lowenstein DH. Mechanism of disease: Epilepsy. *New Engl J Med* 2003; **349**:1257–1266.

Chauvel PY. Seizure disorders. *Curr Opin Neurol* 2004; **17**:139–178.

Guerrini R. Epilepsy in children. *Lancet* 2006; **367**(9509):499–524.

Kharatishvili I, Pitkänen A. Posttraumatic epilepsy. *Curr Opin Neurol* 2010; **23**:183–188.

Shorvon S, Anderman F, Guerrini R. *The Causes of Epilepsy: Common and Uncommon Causes in Adults and Children*. Cambridge, UK: Cambridge University Press, 2011.

Silverman IE, Restrepo L, Mathews GC. Poststroke seizures. *Arch Neurol* 2002; **59**:195–201.

Weller M, Stupp R, Wick W. Epilepsy meets cancer: When, why, and what to do about it? *Lancet Oncol* 2012; **13**(9):e375–e382.

# Epidemiology of Seizures and Epilepsy

Aidan Neligan[1,2] and Josemir W. Sander[1,2,3]

[1] Department of Clinical & Experimental Epilepsy, UCL Institute of Neurology, London, UK
[2] Epilepsy Society, Chalfont St Peter, Buckinghamshire, UK
[3] SEIN-Epilepsy Institute in The Netherlands Foundation, Heemstede, The Netherlands

Epilepsy is the most common serious neurological condition, affecting over 60 million people worldwide; the majority of these people live in countries where they have limited access to treatment.

Epidemiology is concerned with the natural history and distribution of disease and determinants of health in populations. Epidemiological studies can be characterized into three broad categories: descriptive, analytical, and experimental (Table 4.1). In epilepsy, epidemiological research tends to be primarily descriptive (frequencies) and analytical (risk factors), with little experimental research.

It was long believed that epilepsy was a chronic progressive condition with little chance of recovery. Such a view was succinctly expressed by 19th-century neurological luminary William Gowers, who wrote that "The spontaneous cessation of the disease is an event too rare to be reasonably anticipated in any given case." Such a pessimistic viewpoint was routinely upheld until the early 1980s, when studies from sources other than tertiary referral centers challenged it.

Basic requirements in epidemiology include diagnostic accuracy, complete case ascertainment, and the need to control or minimize selection bias in the population under review. For instance, the fact that a negative understanding of the prognosis of epilepsy (where 70–80% of people in a cohort can be reasonably expected to achieve long remission) was maintained for so long underlies the importance of controlling for selection bias in study populations.

Many epidemiological studies from both developed and resource-poor countries have been published, but methodical differences, lack of standardized classifications, difficulties with case ascertainment, and diagnostic uncertainty have led to disparities in study findings. The International League Against Epilepsy (ILAE) has published several reports, most recently in 2011, attempting to standardize research definitions so that direct comparison of results from different studies can be made.

Case ascertainment and diagnostic accuracy are particular issues in epilepsy, as seizures can be a manifestation or symptoms of multiple etiologies, emphasizing the heterogeneous nature of the condition. Nevertheless, the majority of people with epilepsy will not have any overt physical manifestations between seizures. Ultimately, the diagnosis of epilepsy, which is normally made after two or more unprovoked seizures, is dependent on the clinical history, detailed eye-witness accounts (which can be notoriously

*Epilepsy*, First Edition. Edited by John W. Miller and Howard P. Goodkin.
© 2014 John Wiley & Sons, Ltd. Published 2014 by John Wiley & Sons, Ltd.

**Table 4.1.** Different streams of epidemiological research.[a]

| |
|---|
| *Descriptive epidemiology*: Observational studies of distribution and vital statistics (incidence and prevalence) of a condition in a population, without regard to causation |
| *Analytical epidemiology*: Hypothesis testing, typically with regard to ascertaining risk factors for the development of a condition, using cohort and case–control studies |
| *Experimental epidemiology*: Analysis of different outcomes after controlling for relevant risk factors for developing a condition |

[a]Epilepsy epidemiological research is predominantly descriptive or analytical.

**Table 4.2.** Different epidemiological terms to measure disease frequency.

| |
|---|
| *Incidence* is defined as the number of new cases of a condition in a well-defined population during a specified time period (typically 1 year) and is normally expressed as the number of cases per 100,000 people in the population per year. Incidence studies can be further subdivided by gender and age. |
| *Cumulative incidence* is the proportion of a fixed population that will develop the condition over a certain amount of time. |
| *Prevalence* is defined as the number of people with the condition in a defined population of the total population and is typically expressed as the number of cases per 1000 people. |
| The *period prevalence* (or simply *prevalence*) is the prevalence of the condition over a defined period of time (usually 1 year), while the *point prevalence* (used in most prevalence studies) is the prevalence of the condition at a defined moment of time. |

**Table 4.3.** Reported incidence rates by region.

| Incidence studies (age-adjusted incidence rate per 100,000) |
|---|
| Europe/USA 32.4–68.8 (all ages) |
| Asia 28.8–60.0 |
| Africa 49.0–156.0 |
| South America 113.0–190.0 |

unreliable), the chance witnessing or recording of an event, and the diagnostic skill and experience of the clinician. Given these difficulties, it is not surprising that a significant proportion of people referred to tertiary centers with chronic epilepsy do not, in fact, have epilepsy (the most common alternative diagnoses being psychogenic nonepileptic attacks and syncopal episodes). Many people with epilepsy do not seek medical attention; this may be due to ignorance, lack of awareness of the symptoms, or fear of stigmatization. Indeed, in many cases absence and complex partial seizures are only recognized in retrospect following presentation with a generalized seizure. Some people with a confirmed diagnosis of epilepsy may deny the fact for fear of the social and legal implications of such a diagnosis. For these reasons, door-to-door surveys in large populations, using standardized screening tools, are considered the gold-standard methodology for epidemiological research. For logistical reasons, these are, however, easier in theory than in practice.

## Incidence and prevalence

There are two main types of disease frequency that are used in epidemiological studies: the incidence and the prevalence (Table 4.2).

Incidence refers to the number of new cases in the population and is estimated using cohort or closed population studies, where a defined population (e.g., the population of a region) is followed up over a year and the number of new cases in the population is identified. Prevalence refers to the number of people with the condition in a population at one time; prevalence studies are carried out using cross-sectional studies that are much easier and less expensive to perform than incidence studies. Consequently, there are many more epilepsy prevalence studies than incidence studies from both developed and resource-poor countries. Prevalence studies are important for healthcare planning and service provision (Table 4.3).

## Incidence studies

Most incidence epilepsy studies have been retrospective and carried out in developed countries, although more recently, prospective community-based incidence studies have been performed.

The incidence of epilepsy in the developed world is remarkably consistent across different countries, with a median incidence rate of around 50 (range 40–70) per 100,000 per year. In a recent systematic review of 33 studies, 9 of which were from low-or low-middle–income counties, the median annual incidence was 50.4 per 100,000. The median incidence was 45.0 per 100,000 in high-income countries and 81.7 per 100,000 in low- and low-middle–income countries. In contrast, the incidence for single unprovoked seizures is probably between 50 and 70 per 100,000 per year; however, this figure is likely to be much higher in resource-poor countries.

Incidence studies from resource-poor countries are far less common, with much greater variation in reported rates between regions and countries. In the systematic review, the median incidence rate from the seven studies from resource-poor countries was 68.7 per 100,000 (compared to 43.4 per 100,000 for developed countries). Reported incidence rates are highest in South America and Sub-Saharan Africa (where there is great variation in rates between and even within countries). In contrast, reported incidence rates in Asia (India and China) are more in line with figures from developed countries.

Most incidence studies demonstrate a slighter higher rate in males, although this difference is rarely statistically significant. In the systematic review, no significant differences were seen between males and females. In a US study, the cumulative incidence of epilepsy was 1.2% by age 24 years, 3% by age 75, and 4.4% by age 80. Later studies from Scandinavia have corroborated these findings.

Most studies have not demonstrated any significant difference in ethnicity-specific incidence rates; any differences seen are largely attributable to differences in socioeconomic circumstances. Indeed, there is a strong association between age-adjusted incidence rates and socioeconomic deprivation, which was demonstrated in a study from London, where the age-adjusted incidence rate of epilepsy was 2.3 times as high in the most socially deprived fifth of the population as in the least deprived fifth.

Incidence studies from developed countries typically show a bimodal age distribution, with a very high incidence in infancy and early childhood and a subsequent decrease in adolescence and earlier adulthood, then a steady increase after the age of 50. While most studies have shown that the overall incidence of epilepsy has not changed appreciably over the past 20–30 years, there has been a decrease in the incidence in children, with a corresponding increase in the elderly (particularly those aged above 80) to the point that the elderly are now the most common age group with newly diagnosed epilepsy.

One area where there is a dearth of studies is in the incidence of epileptic syndromes, in part due to the difficulty in utilizing such a classification in epidemiological field studies. One of the few studies published is a population study from Iceland, where localization-related epilepsy predominated (18.6 per 100,000 person-years), with essentially equal figures for symptomatic and cryptogenic epilepsies. The incidence of isolated unprovoked seizures or status epilepticus was 22.8 per 100,000 person-years. Much more work is needed to accurately determine the epidemiology of the epileptic syndromes.

## Prevalence studies

Studies from developed countries typically give a prevalence of active epilepsy of between 4 and 10 per 1000, with most having a prevalence of 4–7 per 1000. Findings from prevalence studies reinforce those from incidence studies with respect to gender, ethnicity, the impact of socioeconomic factors, and age-specific variations. Some of the reported variation in prevalence rates, particularly with regard to active epilepsy, relates to the heterogeneous range of definitions employed and underlines the need for the use of standardized definitions in epidemiological research.

### ✋ CAUTION!

Prevalence studies are important in determining the impact of a disease within a community and for planning service provisions. Prevalence studies are not suitable for the investigation of causal relationships (risk factors), as they do not allow distinction between factors that cause the condition and factors caused by the condition in the population.
Incidence studies, which are typically prospective cohort studies, can be used to study cause and effect.

## Prognosis

Prognosis in epilepsy can have different connotations: it can relate to the risk of further seizures after a single unprovoked seizure; the risk of an unprovoked seizure or epilepsy following a provoked seizure or a childhood febrile seizure; the risk of further seizures after a second or third seizure; the short-, medium-, and long-term probability of seizure remission; identification of factors determining prognosis; the impact of treatment (both medical and surgical) on prognosis; prognosis following antiepileptic drug (AED) withdrawal; and the prognosis of people with chronic epilepsy.

The risk of further seizures increases with the number of seizures, with the probability increasing with the more seizures experienced. Presentation with multiple seizures within a 24 h period does not, however, imply a higher risk of recurrence compared to a single seizure. Nevertheless, the number of pretreatment seizures is recognized as one of the most important prognostic factors. Other identified prognostic factors include the epilepsy syndrome, with symptomatic focal epilepsies having a poorer prognosis than nonlesional focal epilepsies, which have, in general, a worse prognosis than the idiopathic generalized epilepsies (which have differing prognoses according to the individual syndromes). Similarly, people with multiple seizure types (typical of the childhood encephalopathies) tend to have a worse prognosis. Prognosis is also influenced by associated comorbidities; in particular, people with learning disability and epilepsy have a poorer seizure prognosis. Indeed, prognosis for people with epilepsy can be broadly stratified into four main prognostic categories (excellent, good, uncertain or AED-dependent, and bad) based on etiology and epileptic syndrome.

Most studies examining the prognosis of epilepsy and of the factors that influence it have been of relatively short duration of followup, Indeed, there are very few long-term studies, with only nine having a reported followup of 10 years or more (the majority of which were retrospective pediatric studies). The overall reported rates of terminal remission (typically defined as seizure freedom on or off treatment for the previous 5 years or more at the time of last followup) are of 60–80%, with studies with longer followup reporting more favorable outcomes. While it is recognized that the likelihood of seizure remission decreases with the number of failed AED trials, a concept central to the recently proposed ILAE definition of refractory epilepsy, few studies have looked at prognosis in people with established chronic epilepsy (ongoing seizures despite two or more appropriate AED trials). One study did show that a significant proportion with apparently drug-resistant or refractory epilepsy will become seizure-free (or have a significant reduction in seizure frequency) with further AED changes, although ultimately about half will subsequently relapse with more prolonged followup.

While it is known that a large proportion of people with epilepsy (60–70%) will be rendered seizure free with the introduction of the first or second AED, it is less clear long-term what proportion of people in remission will relapse (excluding those who relapse following intentional AED withdrawal) and what factors influence this. Further long-term prospective cohort studies of people with incident epilepsy and people with established drug-resistant epilepsy are needed better to elucidate the "natural history" of the condition.

## Mortality

It has consistently been shown that people with epilepsy are at increased risk of premature mortality and that this risk changes over the course of the condition. The most commonly reported measure of mortality employed in epilepsy studies is the standardized mortality ratio (SMR), which is defined as the ratio of observed deaths in a cohort divided by the expected number of deaths if the age-specific and sex-specific rates were the same as those of the general population. The SMR of people with epilepsy is two to three times that of the general population, being highest in the initial years following diagnosis and subsequently decreasing thereafter but remaining significantly elevated throughout. Causes of death in people with epilepsy can be divided into epilepsy-related and non-epilepsy–related causes. Epilepsy-related causes of death include status epilepticus and epilepsy-related accidents such as drowning and sudden unexpected death in epilepsy (SUDEP). Important non-epilepsy-related causes of death include pneumonia, cerebrovascular disease, ischemic heart disease, suicide (possibly epilepsy-related), and cancer.

Mortality in the early years after diagnosis is typically due to non-epilepsy-related causes but may be due to the underlying etiology of the epilepsy (for example, CNS tumors). Thereafter, epilepsy-related causes of death (particularly SUDEP) become more important, especially in children with refractory epilepsy. The risk of premature mortality remains persistently elevated more than 20 years after diagnosis in people with epilepsy (most in long-term remission), with the majority dying from non-epilepsy-related causes. The underlying mechanisms of premature mortality in people with epilepsy are poorly understood, although the risk is decreased but probably not eliminated by rendering a person completely seizure-free.

## The future

Epidemiological studies have provided some insight into the incidence, prevalence, associated comorbidities and risk factors, and prognosis of epilepsy, but further work is needed. In particular, further prospective community-based incident cohort studies are required for accurate ascertainment of temporal trends in age-specific incidence rates, definition of long-term seizure patterns and prognosis, and greater understanding of the mechanisms underlying the risk of premature mortality and the means of preventing it.

One area in which there is a significant gap in knowledge is the epidemiology of specific epilepsy syndromes. To date only three studies have attempted to estimate the incidence of individual epilepsy syndromes, with the numbers for many individual syndromes too small to estimate. The primary purpose of diagnosing someone with a specific epilepsy syndrome is to guide treatment strategy and provide a more accurate prognosis; without the epidemiological data to provide clinical insight, this approach lacks rigor. In particular, prospective cohorts of individual epilepsy syndromes (for example, juvenile myoclonic epilepsy) are almost completely lacking. Until this issue is addressed, it is difficult to envisage how the full potential of the syndromic classification can be utilized.

## Bibliography

Benn EK, Hauser WA, Shih T, et al. Estimating the incidence of first unprovoked seizure and newly diagnosed epilepsy in the low-income urban community of Northern Manhattan, New York City. *Epilepsia* 2008; **49**:1431–1439.

Christensen J, Vestergaard M, Pedersen MG, Pedersen CB, Olsen J, Sidenius P. Incidence and prevalence of epilepsy in Denmark. *Epilepsy Res* 2007; **76**:60–65.

Hauser WA, Annegers JF, Kurland LT. Incidence of epilepsy and unprovoked seizures in Rochester, Minnesota: 1935–1984. *Epilepsia* 1993; **34**: 453–468.

Heaney DC, MacDonald BK, Everitt A, et al. Socioeconomic variation in incidence of epilepsy: Prospective community based study in south east England. *BMJ* 2002; **325**:1013–1016.

Kwan P, Arzimanoglou A, Berg AT, et al. Definition of drug resistant epilepsy: Consensus proposal by the ad hoc Task Force of the ILAE Commission on Therapeutic Strategies. *Epilepsia* 2010; **51**: 1069–1077.

Neligan A, Bell GS, Shorvon SD, Sander JW. Temporal trends in the mortality of people with epilepsy: A review. *Epilepsia* 2010; **51**: 2241–2246.

Neligan A, Bell GS, Johnson AL, Goodridge DM, Shorvon SD, Sander JW. The long-term risk of premature mortality in people with epilepsy. *Brain* 2011; **134**:388–395.

Neligan A, Hauser WA, Sander JW. The epidemiology of the epilepsies. *Handb Clin Neurol* 2012; **107**:113–133.

Ngugi AK, Bottomley C, Kleinschmidt I, Sander JW, Newton CR. Estimation of the burden of active and life-time epilepsy: A meta-analytic approach. *Epilepsia* 2010; **51**:883–890.

Ngugi AK, Kariuki SM, Bottomley C, Kleinschmidt I, Sander JW, Newton CR. Incidence of epilepsy: A systematic review and meta-analysis. *Neurology* 2011; **77**:1005–1012.

Olafsson E, Ludvigsson P, Gudmundsson G, Hesdorffer D, Kjartansson O, Hauser WA. Incidence of unprovoked seizures and epilepsy in Iceland and assessment of the epilepsy syndrome classification: A prospective study. *Lancet Neurol* 2005; **4**:627–634.

Sander JW. Some aspect of prognosis in the epilepsies: A review. *Epilepsia* 1993; **34**:1007–1016.

Schiller Y, Najjar Y. Quantifying the response to antiepileptic drugs: Effect of past treatment history. *Neurology* 2008; **70**:54–65.

Thurman DJ, Beghi E, Begley CE, et al. Standards for epidemiologic studies and surveillance of epilepsy. *Epilepsia* 2011; **52**(Suppl. 7):2–26.

# Part II

# Working Up Seizures and Epilepsy

5

# Diagnosing and Localizing Seizures at the Bedside and in Clinic

**Joseph I. Sirven**

Department of Neurology, Mayo Clinic, Phoenix, AZ, USA

Despite the availability of sophisticated neurodiagnostic tests, identification of seizures and epilepsy is predicated on clinical evaluation. There is no substitute for a comprehensive history and physical for diagnosis and localization of seizures at the bedside. Oftentimes when a patient presents with a seizure, the first step is computed tomography (CT) of the head or routine electroencephalography (EEG), with little time spent obtaining detailed descriptions of how the spell occurred and the circumstances surrounding its presentation. Diagnosing and localizing seizures is based upon a thorough and comprehensive clinical history, with the physical examination and supporting laboratory, imaging, and neurophysiologic studies used only to confirm that a seizure occurred and investigate the etiology.

In this chapter, we focus on diagnosis and localization of seizures without using any supporting laboratory evaluation, dealing with the essential issues to be addressed when a patient presents with an episode. Fundamental questions need to be asked to arrive at an appropriate diagnosis which, in turn, leads to the correct therapeutic choices and, ultimately, improved quality of life. One cannot stress too greatly the importance of a comprehensive history and physical, because once a patient is diagnosed with seizures and treatment is initiated, very few physicians will ever refute or question the label of

epilepsy. This is why getting the diagnosis right from the onset is such an important issue. This chapter is organized around three important diagnostic questions addressed at the bedside that provide a logical, stepwise approach to making the appropriate diagnosis and guiding management of any patient presenting with a spell.

> ★ **TIPS AND TRICKS**
>
> Three important diagnostic questions to ask when a patient presents with a spell:
> - Is it a seizure?
> - What are the surrounding circumstances?
> - What kind of seizure is it?

## Is it a seizure?

The most important question is whether the episode is actually a seizure or one of its mimics. Inquiry about the duration of the event, the description of what the patient felt or did, the postictal characteristics, and the frequency of the events is essential. Getting the diagnosis right from the onset is important because treatment to prevent future spells depends upon their etiology.

*Epilepsy*, First Edition. Edited by John W. Miller and Howard P. Goodkin.
© 2014 John Wiley & Sons, Ltd. Published 2014 by John Wiley & Sons, Ltd.

**Table 5.1.** Distinguishing between seizures and their common mimics at bedside.

| Characteristic | Psychogenic nonepileptic event | Seizure | Syncope |
| --- | --- | --- | --- |
| Aura | Variable | Yes or nothing | None |
| Onset | Acute/gradual | Acute | Acute |
| Duration | Several minutes to hours | 1–2 min | Seconds to a minute |
| Movements | Variable, reprise phenomenon, asynchronous, eye closure, pelvic thrusting | Variable, tonic/clonic | Loss of tone, myoclonus |
| Incontinence | Variable | Variable | Variable |
| Trauma/injury | Rare | Occasional | Occasional |
| Posture | No impact | No impact | Patient is erect or standing |
| Occurs out of sleep | No | Yes | No |
| Post-spell characteristics | Rapid return to baseline, emotional | Confusion | Rapid return to baseline |

A number of differential diagnoses should be considered when a patient presents with an event. The three most common possibilities are an epileptic seizure, syncope, and a psychogenic nonepileptic event. In addition, several other conditions can also present in a paroxysmal manner, including panic attacks, hyperventilation episodes, transient ischemic attacks, migraines and migraine equivalents, narcolepsy, cataplexy, parasomnias, paroxysmal dyskinesias or dystonias, hyperekplexia, paroxysmal vertigo, and hypoglycemic events. For further information on the differential diagnosis of spells, see Chapters 1, 2, and 6. The present chapter will focus on the aspects of the clinical history suggesting seizures and epilepsy.

An epileptic seizure is a hypersynchronous, self-limited activity of neurons in the brain, occurring either as a symptom of an underlying condition or without clear provocation. Seizures last from seconds to a few minutes. There can be a prodrome or warning prior to an event, followed by a distinct warning known as an aura, followed by the actual seizure itself, followed ultimately by the postictal period – the time after a seizure. In the attempt to confirm that a seizure has occurred, initial questions must center on what occurred throughout these phases. Oftentimes, patients are amnestic for the event, so one has to rely on witnesses. It is critically important to record a detailed description of the attack in the patient's own words so that this account can be compared with descriptions of any subsequent episodes.

Epileptic seizures are stereotyped in their clinical presentation and duration, whereas psychogenic, nonepileptic events are often variable. Individuals with epilepsy often are amnestic for their events, so obtaining as much additional information from other family members, caregivers, and coworkers is important. In many ways, the diagnosis of seizures is like a classic detective novel in which the neurologist must interview all involved parties to get an accurate portrayal of what occurred. Table 5.1 provides an overview of the semiology of various paroxysmal event types, useful for distinguishing between epileptic seizures and psychogenic nonepileptic events. No diagnosis should ever depend on any single feature. When considering the onset of an episode, it is important to establish its clinical characteristics (semiology) and its progression, making certain that they are consistent with the overall findings of the physical examination and the rest of the history.

The onset of a seizure provides important diagnostic information. Myoclonic jerks may precede generalized tonic–clonic seizures in juvenile myoclonic epilepsy. There may be déjà vu or an aura of gastrointestinal distress that occurs prior to a temporal lobe seizure. The features of the onset of an attack are useful for distinguishing among various seizure types. A sensation of feeling hot, sweating, pallor, tunnel vision, vision closing in, and tinnitus are more common at the onset of syncope. Episodes in which the patient simply drops without warning or experiences drop attacks and returns rapidly to full conscious on the ground suggest circulatory disturbances such as syncope or arrhythmia as opposed to a seizure. Obtaining a history with those characteristics will be particularly helpful to diagnosing syncope if the episodes are also associated with orthostatic posture changes.

Psychogenic nonepileptic events can start suddenly or be preceded by a prodrome such as vague anxiety complaints. An important distinguishing feature is that seizures can occur out of sleep, but psychogenic events do not. However, many patients describe events that occur at night, yet on confirmatory video–EEG monitoring they are shown to be awake. Investigating this detail is important because events that awaken the patient out of sleep suggest a pathophysiological etiology rather than a psychiatric one.

## ☆ TIPS AND TRICKS

Of the three most common spells, syncope, seizure, and psychogenic nonepileptic spells, only epileptic seizures can arise directly out of sleep.

The manifestations of a seizure depend on the location of its onset and the regions to which the epileptic discharge spreads. Motor activity during a generalized tonic-clonic seizure, the most common seizure type, consists of vigorous, forceful, and repetitive movements persisting for more than 30 s. The frequency of muscle contractions in the clonic phase declines gradually in epileptic seizures, whereas it does not tend to change during a psychogenic nonepileptic event. Syncopal events are usually brief unless the patient is maintained in an upright posture. Myoclonic jerks during syncope are common, as is vocalization, brief limb posturing, upward and lateral deviation of the eyes, and eyelid flickering.

The duration of an event helps to differentiate spells. Syncopal attacks tend to last for a few seconds to a minute as opposed to epileptic seizures, which often last about a minute or more. Psychogenic nonepileptic events can last for more than 2 min to several hours. The eyes are typically closed in psychogenic nonepileptic events and open during epileptic seizures. Motor activity in psychogenic episodes commonly shows a reprise phenomenon in which activity either starts or stops without apparent pattern, with limb movements often more asynchronous or purposeful than in an epileptic seizure (for example, pushing away the examiner). Prolonged episodes of immobility with eyes closed, of looking around without responding, or of fixed dystonic posturing are unlikely to be epileptic events. Psychogenic nonepileptic events can also manifest as limpness with rapid recovery, which can easily be confused with syncope. Patients with psychogenic nonepileptic event may "foam at the mouth" during attacks. Reports of a bitten tongue without characterization of the severity of the injury do not reliably distinguish between patients with epilepsy and psychogenic nonepileptic events, nor does urinary incontinence. Both can occur in syncope. However, severe injuries to the tongue resulting in lateral bruising, taking days to heal, are more consistent with epilepsy than psychogenic events.

## ✋ CAUTION!

Incontinence and tongue biting do not distinguish between seizures and other events. However, lateral bruising of the tongue that takes days to heal may be more suggestive of epileptic seizures.

Descriptions of the ending of a seizure provide helpful diagnostic information. Postictal confusion is common in epileptic seizures. However, confusion is often reported in almost all spell types, especially following loss of consciousness, so it may not be a sensitive differentiator between epilepsy and other events. Amnesia for events during a seizure during which the patient had been alert and communicating suggests epilepsy. Soreness, rashes, conjunctival hemorrhage, lacerations and bruising of the tongue, and dislocation of the shoulders are very strong indicators of epilepsy. However, rapid recovery of consciousness suggests a syncopal attack. A syncopal episode that was prolonged because the patient was maintained in an upright posture may be followed by a prolonged period of confusion. With syncope, individuals may report feeling normal, as if they have awoken from sleep, or they may report having heard people talking but not having been able to respond. Recurrence of blackouts on rapid resumption of the upright position is typical for syncope.

After psychogenic nonepileptic events, patients may feel very emotional or weepy. Patients' descriptions of the period after seizure can vary dramatically. Some may report minor injury such as carpet burns and minor bruising but no other injuries. A history of injuries or urinary incontinence does not effectively distinguish psychogenic nonepileptic events from epileptic seizures. Postictal headache has been suggested to be more common in epilepsy, but it has not been proven to be a reliable distinguishing feature.

## What are the surrounding circumstances? Past medical history, provoking factors, and the neurological examination

The history must include assessment of the context in which the event occurred. For instance, an attack provoked by pain, dehydration, or micturition is more likely to be due to syncope, even when convulsive symptoms are described. Particular attention needs to be paid to the association between seizures and alcohol and illicit drug use. Seizures may be provoked by alcohol withdrawal in alcohol-dependent patients. Some patients with idiopathic generalized epilepsy have seizures provoked by sleep deprivation or occurring the morning after imbibing small amounts of alcohol if this is combined with sleep deprivation.

Several historical factors distinguish between epilepsy, syncope, and psychogenic nonepileptic events. It is important to ask about current life stressors, sleep hygiene, and whether new medications (prescription or over-the-counter) have recently been initiated. In those with a history of epilepsy, it is important to ask about recent anti-epileptic medication changes or substitutions and whether the patient has been adherent to their medication regimen. It is also important that one ask regarding herbals and botanical use. A careful history of infectious exposure such as by insect bites or travel is important for etiologies such as neurocysticercosis or encephalitis. It is also important to ask about changes in neurological function to assess whether underlying cerebrovascular disease, neoplasm, or neurodegenerative conditions are present.

### ★ TIPS AND TRICKS

Specific inquiries need to be made about new medications, herbal and botanical use, illicit drugs, medication adherence, over-the-counter drugs, and any recent antiepileptic medication regimen changes or substitutions.

The neurologic examination is often described by many general neurologists as unhelpful in patients presenting with spells. However, observation and examination during a seizure, although rarely possible, can be quite useful. The observation of closed eyes during a seizure, resisted eye opening, gaze avoidance, retained pupillary light reflex, semipurposeful movements, responsiveness to corneal reflex, and normal plantar responses would help support a diagnosis of psychogenic nonepileptic seizures. Clinical signs during a faint or syncopal event may include heart rhythm abnormalities and orthostatic hypotension. The examination of a patient after generalized tonic–clonic seizure should include looking for lateral tongue biting, bruising, skeletal injury, and petechial hemorrhages of the skin or conjunctiva. Interictal examination findings in patients with epilepsy may provide a clue to the underlying cause—for example, neurocutaneous syndromes, intracranial lesions, or other cortical problems.

### ★ TIPS AND TRICKS

Although psychiatric morbidity rates in patients with epilepsy and syncope are higher than those in the general population, a greater proportion of those with psychogenic nonepileptic events have evidence of mood disorder or other abnormalities on psychiatric examination.

Recently, there has been a critical appraisal of the clinical predictors of psychogenic nonepileptic seizures. Ictal stuttering, pelvic thrusting, and ictal eye closures are not reliable indicators of psychogenic nonepileptic events. In order to make the diagnosis, other semiologic aspects need to be considered, as well as the full context of the situation in which the event occurred. In women, it is important to ask whether the spells occurred in relationship to their menstrual cycles. In older patients, it is important to ask about newer medications and whether symptoms of other conditions are occurring. It is only by combing through all of the variables that one can determine whether an event represents a seizure.

### What kind of seizure is this? Focal (partial) versus generalized

Once an event is identified as a seizure, the next question is whether it represents a focal (partial) event or a generalized one. The classification of seizures will depend often upon whether a patient has lost consciousness during the event. Other important features that can help localize the event include the presence and characterization of motor symptoms, subjective sensory symptoms, and/or language changes. Chapter 2 describes the classification of seizures. Focal seizures localize to a discrete population of neurons within one or both cerebral hemispheres, whereas generalized seizures begin in both hemispheres.

Focal seizures are subcategorized as simple partial seizures and complex partial seizures based on whether there is impairment of consciousness. If it is not impaired, the seizure is simple partial. However, consciousness can be difficult to accurately assess. Simple partial seizures are easier to assess by clinical history because the patient's memory of the event is typically preserved. Auras are simple partial seizures and should be distinguished from another premonitory symptom, prodromes, which are a preictal phenomenon with

an unknown physiological basis. Prodromes may occur several hours prior to a seizure and have an insidious onset and a long duration. The most common manifestations are irritability, emotionality, and a bad temper. Cognitive changes can include slowing, inattention, apathy, insomnia, and insomnolence. Prodromes may last 30 min to several hours and are diagnostically useful because they are not commonly reported in conditions other than epilepsy.

★ TIPS AND TRICKS

Close to one-third of patients report prodromes more often with focal and partial epilepsies versus generalized. Prodrome symptoms are different than auras in their long duration and nonspecific constellations of complaints.

**Table 5.2.** Common focal epilepsies and their seizure behaviors.

| Location | Ictal behavior |
| --- | --- |
| Primary motor or perirolandic frontal lobe | Focal motor seizures with or without Jacksonian march, speech arrest, or dysphasia vocalization |
| Supplementary sensory motor | Focal tonic, asymmetric tonic posturing, versive movements of head and eyes, speech arrest, and vocalization |
| Dorsal lateral frontal lobe | Focal tonic or clonic activity, versive movements of head and eyes, speech arrest, or dysphasia |
| Orbital frontal lobe | Complex motor automatisms, olfactory hallucinations, and autonomic features |
| Anterior frontal polar | Versive movements of head and eyes, forced thinking, initial loss of contact or absence-like speech, or motor arrest |
| Opercular frontal | Mastication, salivation, swallowing, laryngeal symptoms, speech arrest, epigastric aura, fear, autonomic features, facial clonic activity, gustatory hallucinations |
| Cingulate frontal | Fear, vocalization, emotion or mood changes, complex motor automatisms, or autonomic features |
| Parietal lobe | Bilateral, cephalic, somatosensory aura, numbness or tingling in the contralateral upper extremity, sense of pulling, hot or cold feelings, tonic or clonic activity, versive head or eye movements, impaired consciousness, negative motor activity |
| Occipital lobe | Elementary visual hallucinations, flashing or colored lights, lights are often white and spherical, amaurosis, blindness, visual blurring, sensation of eye pulling, ictal eye deviation |
| Temporal lobe | Abrupt cessation or alteration of the patient's preictal behavior consisting of staring, oroalimentary automatisms such as chewing, simple manual automatisms consisting of picking or fumbling of hands. In mesial temporal regions, there may be an aura consisting of a rising sensation. |

**Table 5.3.** Common ictal behaviors and anatomic localization.

| Ictal behavior | Localization |
|---|---|
| Head turning | |
|   Early nonforced | Ipsilateral temporal lobe |
|   Early forced | Frontal lobe |
|   Late forced | Contralateral temporal lobe |
| Ocular version | Contralateral occipital lobe |
| Focal clonic | Contralateral temporal or frontal lobes |
| Dystonic limb | Contralateral temporal or frontal lobes |
| Unilateral tonic limb | Contralateral hemisphere |
| Fencing posture | Contralateral frontal and temporal lobes |
| Figure of 4 | Contralateral hemisphere to extended arm |
| Ictal paresis | Contralateral hemisphere |
| Todd's paresis | Contralateral hemisphere |
| Unilateral blinking | Ipsilateral hemisphere |
| Unilateral limb automatism | Ipsilateral hemisphere |
| Postictal nose rubbing | Ipsilateral temporal and frontal lobes |
| Postictal cough | Temporal lobe |
| Bipedal automastisms | Frontal and temporal lobes |
| Hypermotor | Supplementary motor area |
| Ictal spitting | Right temporal lobe |
| Gelastic | Mesial temporal or hypothalamus |
| Ictal vomiting | Right temporal |
| Ictal urinary urge | Nondominant temporal |
| Loud vocalization | Frontal and temporal lobes |
| Ictal speech arrest | Temporal lobe |
| Ictal speech preservation | Nondominant hemisphere |
| Preictal aphasia | Language-dominant hemisphere |

Reprinted with permission from Rudzinski LA, Shih JJ. The classification of seizures and epilepsy syndromes. *Continuum* 2010; **16**(3):15–35.

Auras, on the other hand, are simple partial seizures that suggest an electrical abnormality within a circumscribed cerebral region. Auras can occur with a myriad of presentations; however a striking number of patients with temporal lobe epilepsy report them. Frontal lobe epilepsy is the focal epilepsy that is next most likely to be associated with reports of auras. However, an aura can arise from any focal epilepsy arising anywhere in the cerebral cortex.

It was once rare to witness a live seizure. However, recent advances in video technology and the rampant use of cell phone cameras have markedly increased the likelihood that a seizure will be captured for a physician to view. Even without EEG recording, this video data provides important diagnostic and localizing information. Table 5.2 lists common focal epilepsies and their associated behaviors. Table 5.3 lists common ictal behaviors and their associated localizations. Observation of specific stereotyped behaviors provides a treasure trove of important localizing information. Awareness of these important semiological signs is essential for correlating clinical information with imaging and EEG data to determine where a patient's seizures begin.

## Summary

This chapter emphasizes the fact that the history and physical examination performed at the bedside is the single most important tool for diagnosing epilepsy. There is no single feature that will precisely localize a seizure. Moreover, no diagnostic studies can eliminate the need for a thorough history and physical. It is important to synthesize the history and physical with other supporting studies to make valid conclusions. Getting the diagnosis right is important because it ensures that appropriate treatment can be instituted. Only with stalwart commitment to the history and physical examination can we ever hope to improve outcomes for patients with spells.

## Bibliography

Berg A, Berkovic S, Brodie M, Buchhalter J, Cross H, and ILAE Commission on Classification and terminology, 2005–2009. Revised Terminology and concepts for organization of seizures and epilepsies. Epilepsia 2010; **51**(4):676–685.

Committee on the Public Health Dimensions of the Epilepsies. Epilepsy across the Spectrum: Institute of Medicine report. National Academies Press: Washington DC, 2012.

Devinsky O, Gazzola D, LaFrance W. Differentiating between nonepileptic and epileptic seizures. *Nat Rev Neurosci* 2011; **7**:210–220.

Hoerth MT, Wellik KE, Demaerschalk BM et al. Clinical predictors of psychogenic nonepileptic seizures: A critically appraised topic. *Neurologist* 2008 July; **14**(4):266–270.

Rudzinski LA, Shih JJ. The classification of seizures and epilepsy syndromes. *Continuum* 2010; **16**(3): 15–35.

Sirven JI, Stern J (eds). *Atlas of Video-EEG Monitoring*. New York: McGraw-Hill, 2011.

Sirven J (ed). Epilepsy. *American Academy of Neurology Continuum* 2010; **16**(3).

# Psychogenic Nonepileptic Episodes

**Vaishali S. Phatak**

Department of Neurology, UW Regional Epilepsy Center, University of Washington, Seattle, WA, USA

## Introduction: Clinical features

Psychogenic nonepileptic episodes (PNEE) are characterized by paroxysmal episodes of behavioral, sensory, motor, or psychic dyscontrol without the electrographic abnormalities seen with epileptic seizures. Symptoms are (1) involuntary and (2) of psychological origin. Although it is common practice to call these events "nonepileptic seizures," in fact, they are not seizures at all, so they are sometimes alternately referred to as "nonepileptic episodes" or "nonepileptic events."

Psychogenic nonepileptic episode semiology is diverse. No single sign or symptom is pathognomonic of the condition. However, signs that are more commonly observed during a PNEE include a fluctuating course, asynchronous movements, side-to-side head movements, pelvic thrusting, closing of the eyes, and an ictal cry. Suspicion of a nonepileptic event should also be raised if the event lasts longer than 2 min or there is forced eye closure when the patient is examined during the event.

### ✋ CAUTION!

Although pelvic thrusting, asynchronous movements, and side-to-side head movements can occur in PNEE, they are also seen with frontal lobe seizures.

Risk factors for PNEE in adults include female gender and a history of abuse. There are some conflicting reports on which type of abuse (i.e., emotional, physical, or sexual) is the strongest predictor of PNEE. Environmental stress underlying PNEE is typically more evident in children compared to adults. Risk factors for PNEE in children include difficulties in school or with family and other social relationship dysfunction such as bullying. Unexpectedly, physical and sexual abuse is not as highly associated with PNEE in children as in adults.

Psychogenic nonepileptic episodes tend to have a delayed diagnosis. Patients are, on average, diagnosed 7 years after the initial onset of seizures. PNEE is often a functionally debilitating condition that correlates with low employment rates.

Approximately 38% of individuals achieve complete PNEE remission. However, a sizeable minority of patients (19%) have an increase in the frequency of PNEE at followup. Predictors of better outcomes include younger age, positive reactions, such as relief or acceptance, on receiving the diagnosis of PNEE, and events characterized by unresponsiveness rather than dramatic motor activity. Predictors of poor outcomes are co-occurrence of epilepsy; comorbid psychiatric conditions; and anger, denial, or confusion after receiving PNEE diagnosis.

*Epilepsy*, First Edition. Edited by John W. Miller and Howard P. Goodkin.

## Epidemiology

Psychogenic nonepileptic episodes most commonly occur between the ages of 15 and 35. They are more common in women than men. There is no predilection to specific ethnic groups. The true incidence and prevalence of nonepileptic seizures has not been well identified. Extrapolation modeling suggests a 0.03% annual incidence in the general population. However, presentation of PNEEs in electroencephalogram (EEG) monitoring units is significantly higher at 20–40%.

## Diagnosis

Psychogenic nonepileptic seizures are classified in the *Diagnostic and Statistical Manual-IV (DSM-IV)* taxonomy under the larger category of somatoform disorders and more specifically under conversion disorders.

Video–EEG monitoring is the gold standard for diagnosis of PNEE. Representative events in the absence of epileptiform activity are considered indicative of a PNEE diagnosis, although it must be recognized that most simple partial seizures and some frontal lobe complex partial seizures may not have visible ictal EEG discharges on scalp EEG recording. Video–EEG monitoring is superior to standard EEG in part because of the existence of these seizure types that are not associated with EEG change.

Personality testing can help identify somatizing tendencies, poor social support, or other coping vulnerabilities as well as presence of other psychiatric disorders; however, it cannot be used as a stand-alone diagnostic test of PNEE. Neither cognitive nor effort testing has been found to be reliable in diagnosing PNEE.

A serum prolactin level test taken within 10–20 min after an event is a useful adjunct for distinguishing PNEE from generalized epileptic seizures or complex partial seizures. However, prolactin levels are not reliably useful in distinguishing between epileptic seizures and syncope.

Provocative testing is a controversial topic in diagnosis of PNEE. Provocative testing consists of a variety of methods used to induce a representative nonepileptic event. The most commonly used provocative method has been a placebo injection, although other methods including hypnosis, photic stimulation, hyperventilation, and placement of dermal alcohol patch have also been used. All these methods are intended to produce a PNEE. The ethics of using deception in diagnostic testing raises concerns about provocative testing. There is a serious risk of damaging the doctor–patient relationship because of the intentional deception. There is also the possibility of inducing a PNEE that is not a representative event in suggestible patients with epilepsy.

## Differential diagnosis

Although both epileptic seizures and PNEEs are paroxysmal, epileptic seizures are discrete stereotyped events that most often are associated with electrophysiological abnormalities that can be detected on video–EEG. PNEE are more likely to be longer in duration and have more variable behavior manifestations.

> ### ✋ CAUTION!
>
> Five to twenty-five percent of patients with PNEE are misdiagnosed as having epilepsy. Sixty-nine to eighty-three percent of individuals with PNEE are prescribed antiepileptic drugs (AEDs). AEDs are not effective in treating PNEE.

There are heterogenous psychiatric mechanisms underlying PNEE. As such, several psychiatric disorders should be considered in the differential diagnosis. The first consideration is an anxiety disorder such as panic disorder (PD) and post-traumatic stress disorder (PTSD) that can have involuntary or uncontrolled movements. Feelings of fear and anxiety are a prominent symptom of PD and PTSD. Anxiety is not that commonly associated with PNEE. The second is dissociative disorder, which is characterized by episodes of altered awareness. Dissociative episodes typically tend to be subjective feelings of depersonalization, amnesia, or dissociation and are more directly linked to trauma. PNEEs often have outward signs such as shaking, closed eyes, and convulsive movements. While trauma history is common, a direct link is not always evident in the natural history of PNEE symptoms. The third and last consideration is malingering, which is characterized by exaggeration or fabrication of symptoms for secondary gain. Malingering is difficult to diagnose because the episodes may be less likely to occur during a video–EEG monitoring study.

## Treatment

Psychotherapy is the main form of treatment for PNEE. Psychotherapy approaches, such as cognitive-behavioral therapy, have been shown to be effective in treating nonepileptic events.

Therapy can also help with management of stressful/traumatic life events, depression, anxiety, or difficult relationship problems.

Psychotherapy approaches typically involve educating the patient about PNEE and teaching coping mechanisms. Patients with PNEE who have comorbid mood or anxiety disorders should be evaluated for psychotropic medications.

The delivery and explanation of the PNEE diagnosis is a critical time point. The patient's reaction to the diagnosis can help improve prognosis. Patients typically report a variety of emotional reactions to the diagnosis including relief, frustration, anger, depression, confusion, embarrassment, and guilt. A patient can be conceptualized as going through grief stages (i.e., denial, anger, bargaining, depression, acceptance) on hearing the PNEE diagnosis. Providing the diagnosis so that it is cognitively understandable and emotionally accepted by patients optimizes the likelihood that they will reach the acceptance phase of the grief stages and improve their prognosis.

malfunction, whereas PNEE is a disease of the brain similar to a computer software malfunction. Brain "software" allows programs such as emotions to run successfully, but it is not visible on tests such as EEG or magnetic resonance imaging (MRI). We do not fully understand why the software malfunction has occurred, but often in times of overwhelming stress, there are unpredictable bugs.

## Conclusion

While PNEE can be suspected from descriptions of events and the presence of risk factors, its diagnosis rests upon capturing typical events with video–EEG monitoring. Establishment of a definitive diagnosis leads to improved utilization of medical resources and an opportunity to treat the condition through a constructive explanation of its nature to the patient, family, and caregivers, followed by psychotherapy.

## Bibliography

Benbadis SR, Hauser WA. An estimate of the prevalence of psychogenic non-epileptic seizures. *Seizure* 2000; **9**(4): 280–281.

Devinsky O, Gazzola D, LaFrance WC. Differentiating between nonepileptic and epileptic seizures. *Nat Rev Neurol* 2011; **7**(4):210–220.

Dickinson P, Looper KJ. Psychogenic nonepileptic seizures: A current overview. *Epilepsia* 2012; **53**(10):1679–1689.

Durrant J, Rickards H, Cavanna AE. Prognosis and outcome predictors in psychogenic nonepileptic seizures. *Epilepsy Res Treat* 2011; **2011**:274736.

Goldstein LH, Mellers JD. Recent developments in our understanding of the semiology and treatment of psychogenic nonepileptic seizures. *Curr Neurol Neurosci Rep* 2012; **12**(4):436–444.

Hall-Patch L, Brown R, House A, et al. Acceptability and effectiveness of a strategy for the communication of the diagnosis of psychogenic nonepileptic seizures. *Epilepsia* 2010; **51**(1):70–78.

LaFrance WC Jr, Miller IW, Ryan CE, et al. Cognitive behavioral therapy for psychogenic nonepileptic seizures. *Epilepsy Behav* 2009; **14**(4):591–596.

### ☆ TIPS AND TRICKS

***ABCs of Delivering PNEE Diagnosis***

<u>Assure</u> the patient that events are "real" and are a phenomenon of a recognized condition known as PNEE. Reassure the patient that feelings of confusion, anger, or worry are common when receiving the diagnosis, and provide hope that understanding their diagnosis will help improve their prognosis.

<u>Be</u> clear that nonepileptic seizures are not epilepsy. Providing the patient's other healthcare providers including his or her psychotherapist with a description of the spells and an appropriate course of action can help reduce the patient's emergency room visits. Some clinicians find it useful to call PNEEs events, spells, or episodes to distinguish them from (epileptic) seizures.

<u>Conceptualize</u> PNEE for the patient with an analogy. For example, epilepsy is a disease of the brain similar to a computer hardware

# What Can the EEG Tell Us?

## Mark Quigg

Department of Neurology, University of Virginia, Charlottesville, VA, USA

## Introduction

The electroencephalogram (EEG) measures the difference in voltage between pairs of electrodes placed in an array across the scalp (and, in some cases, directly upon or within the brain). During the long history of EEG – the first animal recording was performed by Canton in 1874 and the first human recording by Berger in 1924 – its role has evolved along with clinical and technical changes in neurology.

Electroencephalography has two general purposes. The first is the evaluation and treatment of epileptic seizures. The second is the assessment of encephalopathy. In these roles, the sensitivity and specificity of EEG diverges.

Electroencephalography carries a high specificity in epilepsy; the cardinal findings in the epileptic patient are difficult to mistake for others and are seldom seen in conditions outside of epilepsy. However, the sensitivity of EEG (technically, its positive predictive value) – its ability to confirm epilepsy in those who have it – is limited. Therefore, many techniques and technologies have arisen in EEG to help elicit epileptic abnormalities to help clinicians sort through the differential diagnosis of epilepsy.

Conversely, in encephalopathy, the EEG has high sensitivity and low specificity. The EEG is exquisitely sensitive in both detecting and reflecting the severity of encephalopathy but has little ability to distinguish among the myriad causes of encephalopathy.

The purpose of this chapter is to focus on the current clinical utility of the EEG applied to epilepsy (and its mimics) and encephalopathy.

### SCIENCE REVISITED

The physiology of the EEG can be summarized as follows, working from the neuronal level upwards:

- The primary source of the EEG lies in voltage fluctuations triggered by receptor-gated changes in the postsynaptic membrane of neurons. In other words, EEG voltage is the summation of excitatory and inhibitory postsynaptic potentials.
- The neurons most likely to be "seen" by the scalp EEG are large, radially oriented neurons in cortex close to the scalp.
- A large group of neurons is necessary to general potentials visible at the scalp; one estimate is that $10\,cm^2$ of cortex must act simultaneously to generate findings important in epilepsy.

*Epilepsy*, First Edition. Edited by John W. Miller and Howard P. Goodkin.

- Activities of groups of cortical neurons are organized by interactions with relay neurons of the thalamus; thalamocortical interactions create characteristic patterns denoting vigilance states (wakefulness, light/deep sleep).

The basic engineering principles of the EEG:

- Each pair of electrodes on the scalp forms a channel; each channel represents the difference in voltage between the pair.
- The arrangement of channels on the EEG page is the montage. The two basic montage types are bipolar montages, in which adjacent electrodes are joined in longitudinal or transverse chains (analogous to sagittal or coronal slices of a brain MRI), and referential montages, in which each electrode on the scalp is paired with a common reference electrode(s), yielding what is analogous to an axial view of the brain.
- Ohm's law dictates that in a simple electrical circuit, voltage is the product of electrical current and resistance. *Impedance* (the term used when resistance is encountered in a fluctuating current generated from a biological source) must be close among electrode pairs so that the same voltage recorded from the scalp is not artificially enhanced or diminished by virtue of a poor connection – high impedance – to the scalp (a practice called *impedance matching*). Good electrode care enables accurate EEG recording.

## Epilepsy

Findings in EEG important in epilepsy can be divided into those that occur in between epileptic seizures – interictal discharges – and those that happen as part of an epileptic seizure – ictal discharges.

### The interictal epileptiform discharge

The *interictal epileptiform discharge* (IED), otherwise known as the *spike* or *sharp wave*, is the critical finding in EEG in the evaluation of possible epilepsy. The colloquial definition of an IED is also the most memorable: an IED is any waveform that would hurt if sat upon. A more official definition is that an IED is a waveform that has a duration of 20–200 ms, has a "field" (meaning its distribution across different EEG channels indicates a cerebral rather than artifact or non-brain origin), interrupts rather than forms ongoing activities, and frequently features an aftercoming slow wave with the same polarity (Figure 7.1A). IEDs can occur singly (Figure 7.1A), in a burst of polyspike–wave discharges (Figure 7.1B), or in more than one location (independent multifocal spikes, Figure 7.1C).

Not all waveforms with sharp morphology are associated with epilepsy. Some artifacts, such as electrical pops and patient movements, can appear sharp (Figure 7.2A). *Benign epileptiform transients* are a group of findings, typically occurring during drowsiness or light sleep, that appear epileptiform but have no clinical significance. *Rhythmic midtemporal theta activities of drowsiness* (RMTD, Figure 7.2B), sometimes called *psychomotor variant*, are one of the more common. These discharges appear in the midtemporal region. Unlike spikes seen in temporal lobe epilepsy, these appear V-shaped (rather than with the sharp upslope and following slow-wave discharge of the spike), do not necessarily interrupt ongoing activities but often appear in conjunction with ongoing activities, usually appear more or less equally on both sides, and are exquisitely state dependent, meaning that they disappear with awakening or with deeper sleep. *Wickets* are a related pattern, consisting of sharply contoured midtemporal theta activity that may be mistaken for epileptiform discharges, particularly when occurring as single isolated waves. *Benign epileptiform transients of sleep* (BETS, or *small sharp spikes*, Figure 7.2C) similarly appear limited to drowsiness or light sleep. These consist of very small–amplitude, short duration waveforms that have broad, difficult-to-localize distributions, and like other benign epileptiform findings, these lack the typical morphology and "interruptiveness" of true spikes. Six- and fourteen-hertz positive bursts are waveforms featuring sharply contoured fast activities often superimposed upon or commingled with slower, sharply contoured theta activities (Figure 7.2D).

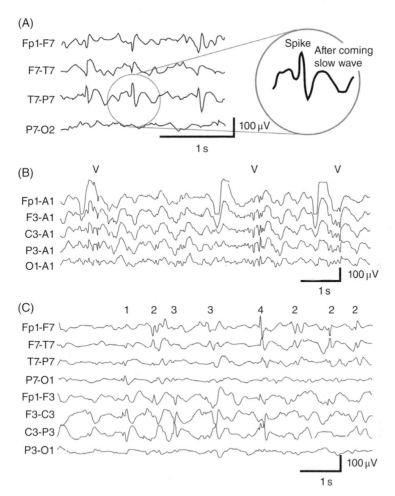

**Figure 7.1.** Examples of IEDs. (A) A train of spikes in the left temporal region. (B) Bursts (at marks) of generalized polyspike–wave discharges. (C) Independent multifocal spikes over the left (1) posterior temporal region, (2) anterior temporal region, (3) central region, and (4) frontopolar region.

## The ictal discharge

The *ictal discharge*, in its broadest definition, is any paroxysmal burst of activity that (1) interrupts ongoing EEG activity, (2) evolves (gradually changing in morphology, spatial distribution, or frequency), and (3) involves activity that is often but not obligately sharp. *Focal seizures* arise from one specific region (Figure 7.3A), and *generalized seizures* from the entire head (Figure 7.3B). When the ictal discharge accompanies clinical behaviors such as staring, behavioral interruption, confusion, or falling and shaking, then the EEG and behavior are together diagnostic of an epileptic seizure.

## Specificity and sensitivity in epilepsy

Unlike the capture of an epileptic seizure that confers diagnostic surety, IEDs provide diagnostic inference only on the evaluation of a patient with spells. Evaluating the specificity and sensitivity of the scalp EEG in the diagnosis of epilepsy is difficult because findings depend on the sample, the population from which it was selected, and technical details of the recordings.

Nevertheless, the probability of finding an IED during a single routine EEG in patients with known epilepsy is approximately 50%. Repeating routine studies increases sensitivity but with gradually diminishing returns, eventually attaining a ceiling

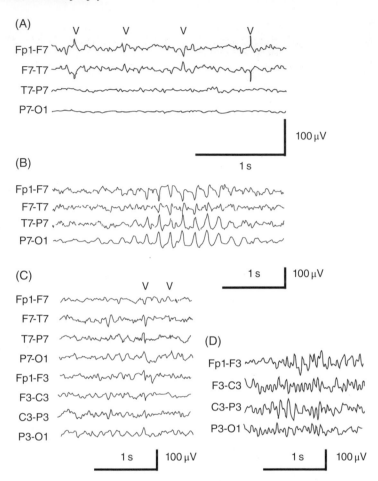

**Figure 7.2.** Examples of artifacts or other sharply contoured discharges that may mimic epileptiform activity. (A) Electrical artifacts from a poorly adherent F7 electrode (marks). (B) A burst of rhythmic, midtemporal sharp discharges occurring during drowsiness (RMTD), one of the more frequent benign sharp findings seen during drowsiness or light sleep. (C) BETS or small sharp spikes (marks). (D) Six- and fourteen-hertz spikes. Note that most benign epileptiform discharges usually occur during drowsiness or light sleep, and one of the tests is to observe whether the putative abnormalities persist into wakefulness or deeper sleep.

of 80–85% after the fourth recording. At this point, even more prolonged recordings, such as overnight video–EEGs, may not be of further utility. This means that about one-fifth of patients with epilepsy will lack interictal evidence of epilepsy. The variable sensitivity of IEDs in patients indicates that a lack of IEDs should not be taken as definitive evidence against seizures.

The specificity of IED depends on the surveyed population. For example, in "enhanced" populations – adults with transient loss of consciousness from either syncope or seizure – the presence of IEDs is specific for seizure in 95%. On the other hand, IEDs are rare in subjects without epilepsy or neurological disease; IEDs appear in 0.4–0.5% of normal adults and 1.5–3.5% of normal children.

The clinical importance of finding IEDs in asymptomatic individuals is controversial, especially in determining work-related risks. For example, in studies of military aircrew who underwent screening EEG as part of their training process, subjects with IED developed epilepsy at an incidence not much different from that of the base population (~2%). On the other hand, other studies calculate risks of developing epilepsy in this supernormal population at approximately 25%.

The clinical significance of IEDs in patients with suspected seizure, however, is much clearer. EEG

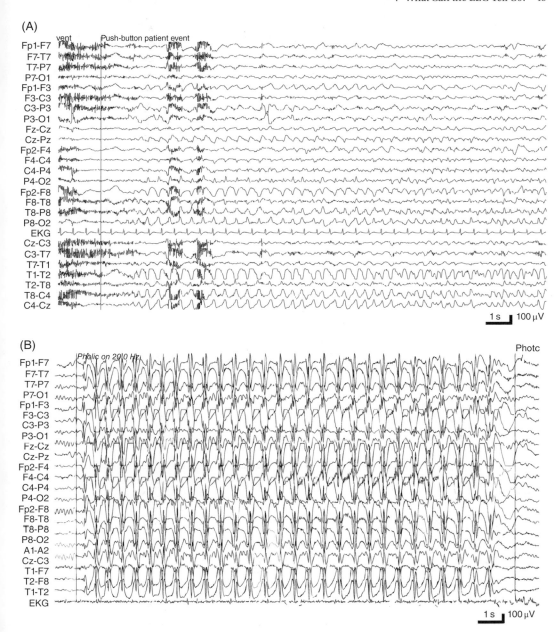

**Figure 7.3.** Two examples of ictal discharges (epileptic seizures). (A) A focal seizure arising across the right temporal region. The notation "Push-button patient event" indicates when the patient felt warning symptoms of nausea and activated a call button. (B) A generalized seizure consisting of rhythmic 3-Hz spike–wave discharges accompanied by behavioral arrest and staring. This particular seizure is activated by photic stimulation.

helps establish the type of seizure and epilepsy syndrome, which are important for prognosis and treatment. Seizure etiology and EEG findings are the strongest predictors of seizure recurrence in adults. Meta-analyses across many studies show that for all adults, risk of recurrent seizures following an initial, unprovoked seizure is 43%. The risk is highest, 65%, for those with a presumptive symptomatic cause and EEG findings consistent with focal abnormalities.

## Activation procedures

Activation procedures are intended to provoke latent IED or seizures in order to increase the sensitivity of the routine EEG.

### Sleep deprivation and sleep

Depending on age, some patients may be asked to stay awake for some of (children) or all of (adults) the night. Sleep deprivation provides stress, which in turn promotes the appearance of IED in susceptible individuals.

Sleep deprivation is also useful because it increases the likelihood of falling asleep during the study. Sleep itself (more accurately, non-REM sleep) is an independent activator of IED. In some epilepsy syndromes, IEDs appear almost exclusively during sleep, so the clinician, faced with a normal EEG in one suspected with epilepsy, should check the EEG report to make sure both wakefulness and sleep were recorded in the particular patient. Sleep and sleep deprivation have cumulative effects on activation of IED.

---

### ☆ TIPS AND TRICKS

Sleep deprivation probably shouldn't be ordered routinely for EEG recordings because of the impact on patient and family schedules. Be mindful that the sleep-deprived patient is usually accompanied by a family member who, in all likelihood, is also sleep deprived and that driving to the EEG lab in a sleep-deprived state in the morning may be dangerous for both patient and driver. Sleep deprivation can also serve as an effective "sedative" in the uncooperative child who may put up a fuss during electrode application but who will subsequently fall asleep promptly when unstimulated. Take care to warn the parent to not allow the sleep-deprived child to fall asleep during the trip to the EEG lab, as the child will arrive fully "recharged" and at maximal uncooperativeness.

---

### Hyperventilation

Hyperventilation induces transient hypocapnea, which in turn causes mild vasospasm and diminished cerebral perfusion. In patients without epilepsy, mild diffuse slowing is often elicited (a finding of mild encephalopathy as will be discussed in "Encephalopathy") and is termed normal *buildup*. In patients with epilepsy, hyperventilation may trigger seizures. For example, hyperventilation provokes spike-wave bursts in about 80% of patients with childhood absence epilepsy. Another response to hyperventilation may be no change at all, which is normal.

### Intermittent photic stimulation

*Intermittent photic stimulation* is a standard activation procedure. Although a variety of protocols are used, usually patients are exposed to a series of 10-s blocks of strobe-light stimulation at frequencies starting at 2 Hz and increasing to 20 Hz before decreasing again. Many centers repeat stimulation with eyes open and closed. Other labs expose patients to blocks of gradually and continuously increasing or decreasing flash frequencies.

The normal response to photic stimulation is a symmetric driving response, a rhythmic occipital or posteriorly dominant activity that occurs locked to the rate of flashes. Sometimes a brief burst of sharp activity with onset or offset of stimulation occurs, a normal "on-response" or "off-response." An abnormal finding associated with epilepsy is the photoparoxysmal response, a burst of generalized multiple spike-wave discharges. Photosensitivity provokes photoparoxysmal responses in about 50% of females with juvenile myoclonic epilepsy and in about 25% of males with this syndrome. Other responses may be flash-evoked spikes that may evolve to form occipital onset seizures or other generalized seizures (Figure 7.3B).

The absence of responses is not abnormal, but absence on only one side may indicate either poor fixation by the subject or focal pathology along the retrochiasmatic optic tract.

## Extended recordings/EEG monitoring

Beyond activation procedures, the main way to help improve the specificity and sensitivity of EEG is to extend the duration of the EEG study. Most modern EEG systems come with simultaneous video, so this procedure is usually called *continuous video–EEG monitoring* (CV–EEG, intensive monitoring, or long-term recording). There are four traditional reasons for which long durations of recordings may be useful.

The first is to help capture IED in the diagnosis of epilepsy. As discussed earlier, however, the duration of recording does not correlate well with successful documentation of IED, having a "ceiling function" in that about one-fifth of patients with epilepsy will remain without clear IED on scalp recordings no matter how long recorded. Nevertheless, extended recordings may aid in capturing IED because they increase the chance of recording different sleep–wake states, and non-REM sleep, for example, is a well-documented facilitator of IED.

The second is to increase the probability of capturing a diagnostic event, whether that event is an epileptic seizure or a nonepileptic event.

For both previously mentioned functions, what makes the EEG useful in diagnosis of epilepsy also makes it useful, once that diagnosis is achieved, in assigning the patient to a particular epilepsy syndrome. The diagnosis of epilepsy arises from a gestalt of clinical history, neurological examination, neuroimaging, and EEG. As discussed in other chapters, the goal of epilepsy evaluation should center on an attempt to place the patient within a well-defined epileptic syndrome from which treatment can be rationally arrived at and from which prognosis can most accurately be judged.

Chronic, recurrent spells that mimic epileptic seizures can also occur from nonepileptic, physiological events – syncope, for example – or from psychogenic nonepileptic episodes, sometimes called "pseudoseizures." The typical course for these patients is that previous evaluations have been inconclusive and that trials of anticonvulsant medications have been ineffective. In these cases, after routine EEG has been inconclusive, admission to an inpatient unit for CV–EEG is typically necessary to determine the nature of a captured spell. Some institutions prefer to use *ambulatory EEG*, a form of continuous EEG configured for home use that in some cases comes with a small video camera (which requires the patient to sit in range) or without video (in which the patient or family fills out an event diary)

Third, CV–EEG is the main method of localization of seizures as part of epilepsy surgery evaluation for patients with medically intractable focal epilepsy.

Finally, CV–EEG is useful in continued clinical–electrographic correlation in treatment of status epilepticus or other epileptic conditions, allowing direct confirmation of whether treatment methods are sufficient to extinguish ongoing electrographic seizures.

## Encephalopathy

**Clinical–electrographic correlations: The electroencephalogram spectrum of encephalopathy**

*Encephalopathy* denotes any alteration from normal consciousness. The EEG is exquisitely sensitive in detecting encephalopathy. Changes in the EEG correlate strongly with the severity of cerebral dysfunction, and EEG can be an invaluable tool in the evaluation of altered mental status or delirium.

Before we review the changes in EEG that denote the presence and severity of encephalopathy, there are several limitations to consider. First, because EEG can record only cortical activity, the EEG in cases of coma that do not involve the hemispheres, such as locked-in syndrome, psychogenic coma, or severe catatonia, may be normal. In these cases, the normal EEG excludes bihemispheric dysfunction as a cause of the patient's altered mental state. Second, with a few important exceptions, the EEG, although sensitive in evaluating the severity of encephalopathy, is relatively unhelpful in providing a specific diagnosis as to the cause of encephalopathy. For example, drug intoxication, hypoglycemia, hepatic dysfunction, and anoxia can all result in similar changes to the predominant EEG findings, provided that the metabolic disarray or toxicity results in an overall similar level of consciousness. Accordingly, the severity of encephalopathy can result in characteristic changes in terms of predominant EEG frequency, amplitude, reactivity, and morphology (Figure 7.4).

| Alert | Sleep | Lethargic | Stupor | Coma |
|---|---|---|---|---|
| | | **Frequency** | | |
| Alpha 8–12 Hz | | Theta 4–8 Hz Intermittent slowing | Delta 1–4 Hz Continuous slowing | |
| | | **Amplitude** | | |
| Normal | | | | Suppression |
| | | **Reactivity** | | |
| Reactive | | | Unreactive | |
| | | **Morphology** | | |
| Alpha rhythm | Loss of alpha rhythm | Triphasic waves Periodic discharges | Suppression/burst | |

**Figure 7.4.** The spectrum of EEG changes with severity of encephalopathy.

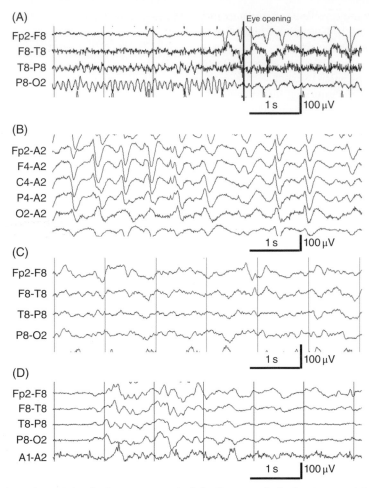

**Figure 7.5.** (A) The waking alpha rhythm in a normal adult. The posteriorly dominant activity attenuates with eye opening. (B) Triphasic waves in a lethargic patient. (C) Unreactive arrhythmic delta activity in a stuporous patient. (D) Burst–suppression in a comatose patient.

The predominant EEG activity of a healthy, relaxed, and awake adult is the *alpha rhythm* (Figure 7.5A). Whereas alpha activity simply describes a frequency band, alpha rhythm denotes a pattern of EEG findings that, in the awake patient, is the main feature of a normal tracing.

**EVIDENCE AT A GLANCE**

- Features of the alpha rhythm, sometimes referred to as the posterior waking rhythm (PWR), vary with age; deviations from expected patterns can be a clue to encephalopathy or epileptic lesions.
- The PWR first appears at age 3–4 months.
- The frequency at onset is approximately 3–4 cps, should be around 6 cps at 6 months and 7 cps at 24 months, and should attain the minimum adult frequency of 8 cps by 3 years.
- Posterior slow waves of youth are sporadic delta activities that appear within the PWR typically within late childhood and early adolescence. They can be distinguished from pathological slowing by the finding that they react to eye opening and appear during wakefulness along with the PWR.

*Frequency*

In general, worsening encephalopathy correlates with decreasing frequency. In lighter stages of encephalopathy, the alpha rhythm may be slow in frequency. Worsening to delirium or lethargy may cause the alpha rhythm to be replaced altogether by theta or delta activity. The persistence of theta or delta activity increases with worsening consciousness, appearing in brief bursts in mild lethargy and in continuous runs in stupor.

*Amplitude*

During mild encephalopathies the overall amplitude of activity may increase, corresponding to normal waking activities being replaced by predominant theta or delta activities. However, as neuronal dysfunction worsens, the number of neurons able to contribute to EEG activity decreases. Suppression, therefore, corresponds to a severe encephalopathy in which underlying neurons have become inactive or are lost. The loss of all cerebral activity is termed electrocerebral silence (ECS) and is one of the criteria of death due to brain injury.

*Reactivity*

Because the EEG is exquisitely responsive to state, the loss of the ability of the EEG to change either with endogenously mediated states (sleep or wake, eye opening or closure) or with responses to environmental stimuli (such as responses to mild painful stimuli) indicates worse bihemispheric dysfunction. These responses to stimuli are termed *reactivity*.

*Morphology*

Certain patterns of waveforms correspond with severity of encephalopathy. Lethargic patients may have intermittent bursts of rhythmic delta activity (intermittent rhythmic delta activity [IRDA]). Patients in the transition to stupor may show triphasic waves (Figure 7.5B). Alpha coma, or unreactive, diffuse low-amplitude alpha activity, corresponds to stupor or coma (Figure 7.5C), as does bursts of high-amplitude activities separated by periods of suppression (Figure 7.5D, burst–suppression).

Some patterns occur with more specific disorders. Periodic epileptiform discharges (PEDs) are associated with spongiform encephalopathies such as Creutzfeldt-Jakob disease. Ictal discharges in the form of rhythmic or periodic discharges may be present in patients with nonconvulsive status epilepticus (NCSE).

**Prognosis of encephalopathy**

In parallel with the lack of specificity to etiology, EEG patterns lack specificity in the evaluation of the prognosis of stupor and coma. For example, although a burst–suppression pattern in a comatose patient denotes severe encephalopathy, burst–suppression can arise from reversible (anesthesia, for one) as well as irreversible, potentially fatal causes (severe anoxia, for another). However, EEG is still useful in the evaluation of altered mental status if ongoing seizure activity – a potentially treatable cause or contribution to altered consciousness – is present.

**Summary**

The EEG is a neurological diagnostic and correlative tool that is important in the (1) evaluation and characterization of epileptic seizures and their mimics and (2) in the evaluation and examination correlate of states of impairment of consciousness. Subsequent chapters will describe specific findings important in particular epilepsies.

# What Can Neuroimaging Tell Us?

**Edward J. Novotny**

Pediatric Epilepsy Program | Child Neurology, University of Washington, Seattle Children's Hospital, Seattle, WA, USA

## Introduction

Brain imaging of patients with epilepsy relies heavily on methods that detail normal brain structure and pathology. Magnetic resonance imaging (MRI) is the modality of choice in both new-onset seizures and chronic epilepsy. Unique MRI imaging techniques and functional brain imaging with both nuclear medicine and fMRI methods are important when considering epilepsy surgery.

## Imaging in the initial evaluation of epilepsy

Structural imaging is important for evaluation, management, and treatment of the person with epilepsy. MRI is the imaging modality of choice because of superior anatomic resolution, excellent characterization of pathological processes, and lack of ionizing radiation. Imaging is indicated in most but not all patients with epilepsy. The indications for imaging include clinical or electroneurodiagnostic findings consistent with focal or secondarily generalized seizures, abnormal neurological examination or physical findings, and epilepsy onset in children under 2 years of age. Imaging is not indicated in patients with a normal neurological exam and electroneurodiagnostic findings of certain epilepsy syndromes. These include benign epilepsy of childhood with centrotemporal spikes, childhood absence epilepsy, juvenile absence epilepsy, and juvenile myoclonic epilepsy. Multispecialty practice parameters for obtaining neuroimaging in patients presenting emergently with seizures are presented in Table 8.1.

The role of structural neuroimaging is to detect an underlying cerebral abnormality that may be causally related to the epilepsy or comorbid cognitive, neurological, or psychological impairment. In the pediatric age group, nearly 50% of patients with new-onset focal seizures have abnormal imaging; in 15–20% of the total, the apparent cause of the epilepsy is found. In series of adults with chronic epilepsy, high-resolution MRI enables the apparent cause to be found in more than 50%. By contrast, past studies of CT imaging of patients presenting with first-time seizures in the emergency department have shown that this procedure will demonstrate findings that change acute management in 9–17% of adults and in 3–8% of children. MRI is now recommended as the first-line imaging study in new-onset seizures in children and most adults because of increased availability, better resolution and sensitivity, and increasing concern about the risks of ionizing radiation.

Imaging early in the evaluation of epilepsy is directed at detecting a cause that might require urgent medical or surgical treatment. That is, certain acute or subacute processes such as tumor, acute

**Table 8.1.**  Guidelines for neuroimaging in patient presenting with emergent seizures.

| Category | First-time seizure | Recurrent seizures |
|---|---|---|
| *Emergent*<br><br>*Serious structural lesion suspected*<br><br>Immediate imaging | New focal deficits, persistent altered mental status (with or without intoxication), fever, recent trauma, persistent headache, history of cancer, history of anticoagulation, or suspicion of AIDS<br><br>Also considered if age > 40 years or focal-onset seizure | New focal deficits, persistent altered mental status (with or without intoxication), fever, recent trauma, persistent headache, history of cancer, history of anticoagulation, or suspicion of AIDS<br><br>Also considered if new seizure pattern or seizure type or prolonged postictal confusion or worsening mental status |
| *Urgent*<br><br>*Possible structural lesion*<br><br>Imaging appointment included in disposition or before disposition when followup not assured | No clear-cut cause identified (e.g., hypoglycemia, hyponatremia, tricyclic overdose) | No clear-cut cause has been identified (e.g., hypoglycemia, hyponatremia, tricyclic overdose) |
| *Not indicated*<br><br>Imaging not performed or scheduled | Typical febrile seizures | Typical febrile seizures or typical recurrent seizures related to previously treated epilepsy |

Reproduced with permission from Quality Standards Subcommittee of the American Academy of Neurology in cooperation with American College of Emergency Physicians, American Association of Neurological Surgeons, American Society of Neuroradiology. Practice parameter: Neuroimaging in the emergency patient presenting with seizure – summary statement. *Neurology* 1996; **47**(1):288–291.

stroke or hemorrhage, encephalitis, leukodystrophy, hydrocephalus, or findings suggesting a metabolic or neurogenetic disorder will direct further diagnostic evaluations and acute treatments. Central nervous system (CNS) infections from parasitic disorders such as cysticercosis are a common cause of epilepsy in many areas of the world and require concomitant treatment of the infection and epilepsy.

Imaging can also identify chronic symptomatic lesions such as encephalomalacia, porencephalic cysts, and atrophy, which are due to remote traumatic brain injury, stroke, perinatal injury, or CNS infections (Figure 8.1). Other chronic pathologies (Figure 8.1) include malformations of cortical development (MCD), focal cortical dysplasias (FCD), vascular malformations, and mesial temporal sclerosis. More severe malformations such as holoprosencephaly, lissencephaly, schizencephaly (Figure 8.1), and hemimegalencephaly (Chapter 3) often present with severe

epilepsy in early childhood. New knowledge about the molecular neurobiology of brain development has resulted in modification of the classification of MCD (Chapter 3) and new molecular diagnostic tests. FCD is secondary to abnormal postmigrational development and can result from injury during later stages of brain development, and it is potentially amenable to epilepsy surgery (Chapter 27). It can also be associated with other vascular lesions and neoplasms, such as gangliogliomas or dysembryoplastic neuroepithelial tumors, and with genetic disorders such as tuberous sclerosis.

Hippocampal sclerosis (HS, Figure 1, Chapter 3) is one of the most important structural abnormalities associated with chronic epilepsy in older children and adults. The MRI shows decreased hippocampal volume with loss of internal architecture and increased signal intensity on T2-weighted images. There is often additional atrophy of adjacent temporal structures

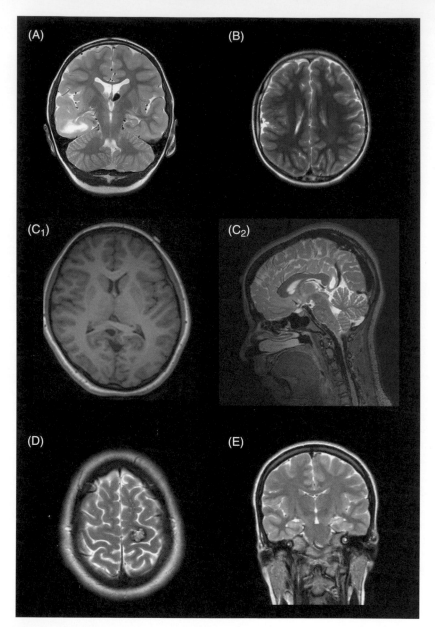

**Figure 8.1.** Imaging abnormalities associated with epilepsy. (A) Patient with right temporal lobe epilepsy due to tuberous sclerosis. Coronal T2-weighted image showing large cortical tuber with increase in T2 signal in white matter and distortion of gyral and sulcal pattern of anterior temporal lobe. Also a calcified, subependymal nodule is noted near the foramen of left lateral ventricle. (B) Patient with symptomatic focal motor and secondarily generalized seizures with schizencephaly of right frontoparietal region with polymicrogyria involving region near central sulcus observed on T2-weighted axial image. (C1 and C2) Patient with pharmacoresistant focal seizures with semiology suggestive of temporal lobe seizures showing a cystic lesion in medial parietooccipital region. C1 is a sagittal T2-weighted image demonstrating the cystic lesion arising from the posterior cingulate gyrus and posterior to the splenium of the corpus callosum. C2 is an axial T1-weighted image showing lesion arising from the right hemisphere. The lesion was identified as an oligodendroglioma on pathology following surgical removal. (D) Patient with focal motor seizures due to cavernous vascular malformation seen on axial T2-weighted image. Hemosiderin is observed surrounding the lesion. (E) Patient with focal seizures with oromotor automatisms, behavioral arrest, and irregular motor movements. Image demonstrates mesial temporal sclerosis in left temporal lobe on coronal T2-weighted image demonstrating increase in T2 signal and smaller hippocampus compared to the opposite side.

(mesial temporal sclerosis). Detection of these findings often requires thin-slice coronal images of the temporal lobes and is important because the epilepsy associated with HS is most often pharmacoresistant but has an excellent chance of control with neurosurgery (Chapter 27).

> ★ **TIPS AND TRICKS**
>
> When evaluating patients with HS, it is also important to look for additional lesions in the same hemisphere ("dual pathology"). HS may also be bilateral.

There is no consensus on specific MRI protocols for epilepsy, but appropriate imaging sequences for children or adults are summarized in Table 8.2. Maximal slice thickness should not exceed 4–5 mm. When metabolic disorders are suspected, magnetic resonance spectroscopy (MRS) may be helpful. A subset of the imaging sequences in Table 8.2 is used for many patients with new-onset epilepsy. Appropriate alterations for developmental age in the imaging sequences are needed in children under 2 years of age. An MRI field strength of 3 T and above permits a better anatomic resolution and a shorter acquisition time. This is improved even further with use of phased array coils combined with image reconstruction.

The previously described imaging protocol includes pulse sequences optimized to detect certain pathologies. The thin-slice volumetric T1-weighted gradient-recalled echo sequence provides high resolution to look for the subtle anatomic changes of

**Table 8.2.** An imaging protocol for evaluation of epilepsy.

| |
| --- |
| Anatomic, thin-slice volumetric T1-weighted gradient-recalled echo sequence |
| Axial and coronal T2-weighted sequence |
| Fluid-attenuated inversion recovery (FLAIR) sequence (axial, and coronal if possible) |
| High-resolution oblique coronal T2-weighted imaging of the hippocampus (fast or turbo spin echo-weighted sequence) |
| Thinner slices (2 or 3 mm) or else 3D volume acquisitions (with thickness of 1–2 mm) if subtle cortical malformations are a consideration |

FCDs. The fluid-attenuated inversion recovery (FLAIR) and T2-weighted sequences permit identification of pathology associated with brain edema. MRS permits measurement of chemicals such as lactate, creatine, and glycine in the brain to provide further information on the underlying cause of epilepsy. Imaging protocols for epilepsy patients should be developed by radiologists with input from neurologists, epileptologists, and neurosurgeons based on the patient populations seen at the facility and the specific capability and specifications of the MR equipment. The imaging protocols should be updated and reviewed at regular intervals and compared to published procedures.

> ★ **TIPS AND TRICKS**
>
> Both children with onset of epilepsy before age 2 years and older patients who develop pharmacoresistant epilepsy should have repeat MRI studies. Optimally, these studies should be done using more advanced imaging sequences and hardware.

## Advanced neuroimaging in pharmacoresistant epilepsy

### Structural MRI

Patients with pharmacoresistant epilepsy who are being evaluated for surgical treatment (Chapter 27) should be rescanned with more advanced equipment and structural imaging methods. In 5–20% of patients with unremarkable 1.5 T MRI studies, reimaging at 3 T with the correct sequences will identify focal abnormalities, such as MCDs, or provide useful clarification of uncertain findings. Some FCD is identified only by small differences in cortical thickness, indistinct borders between cortical gray and white matter, or minor changes in signal characteristics of the white matter that can be observed only with specific pulse sequences.

Manual hippocampal volumetry has been long available to identify HS by looking for unilateral and bilateral hippocampal atrophy and local changes, but it is time-consuming and is not widely used in clinical practice. A different method, which can be automated, is voxel-based morphometry (VBM), an image analysis technique that uses statistical parametric methods to identify quantitative differences in the gray and white matter content of brain structures. With temporal lobe epilepsy, VBM has shown widespread gray matter loss in the thalamus, limbic system, and cerebellum.

Diffusion tensor imaging (DTI) is sensitive to spatial displacement of water molecules, enabling inferences about microstructural integrity of axons and myelin sheaths. DTI tractography allows three-dimensional (3D) depiction of white matter tracts, which can help localize epileptogenic pathology, which often has abnormal connections. It can also help explain comorbid cognitive and neurological disorders.

## Functional imaging

The roster of noninvasive functional imaging tests useful for epilepsy localization is constantly advancing. Nuclear medicine procedures used in epilepsy presurgical evaluation include [18F]-2-fluoro-2-deoxy-D-glucose positron emission tomography (FDG-PET) and single-photon emission computed tomography (SPECT) acquired after injection of radioactive tracer during a seizure ("ictal SPECT"). Functional MRI (fMRI) outlines cerebral networks mediating language, motor, sensory, and other functions by localizing changes in blood-oxygen-level-dependent (BOLD) signal during performance of tasks. Functional MRI during the resting state (no task performance), known as rs-fMRI, also can identify functional brain networks. These fMRI methods are used not only in presurgical evaluation but also in the characterization of comorbid cognitive and neuropsychological disorders.

FDG-PET can locate regions of decreased cerebral metabolism, often corresponding to the site of seizure origination. It is often not required in the presurgical workup of temporal lobe epilepsy patients with concordant MRI lesion and clinical neurophysiological data. However, in some patients with refractory focal epilepsy and unremarkable MRI, the finding of focal hypometabolism on FDG-PET can lead to a decision to pursue surgery and perform invasive intracranial EEG recording. It is also particularly useful for diagnosis and surgical planning in epilepsy due to tuberous sclerosis, FCD, and Rasmussen's syndrome. The sensitivity and specificity of FDG-PET is improved by quantitative analysis using parametric mapping and other statistical methods.

Single-photon emission computed tomography can image brain perfusion changes during an actual clinical seizure. Successful ictal SPECT requires

> ⚠ **CAUTION!**
>
> It is important to perform concurrent recording of EEG with FDG-PET to establish that the study was obtained in the interictal period. The presence of active interictal discharges or clinical and subclinical seizures during the study significantly influences the results.

injection within 30 s of the onset of the clinical seizure as determined by simultaneous video–EEG recording. The sensitivity, specificity, and inter-rater reliability of SPECT imaging is markedly improved by digital subtraction of an interictal scan from the ictal study and then coregistration to MRI anatomic images. This allows patients to serve as their own controls through comparison with individual baseline states. Coregistration to MRI provides more precise anatomic localization. The logistics of successfully injecting the isotope as early as possible after seizure onset remain a practical challenge. The very patients most likely to benefit from ictal SPECT are those with seizures that arise in extratemporal neocortex and spread rapidly, but this often results in difficult-to-interpret ictal blood flow changes. Nonetheless, SPECT can identify the side for temporal lobe resection in patients whose findings on structural MRI are equivocal or bilateral.

Functional MRI is a noninvasive technique that in the context of epilepsy is used primarily to locate eloquent brain functions to spare during brain resection. Language-processing areas in frontal and temporal regions, primary sensorimotor cortex, and primary visual cortex can be identified reliably by having the patient perform tasks during imaging—for example, finger tapping for motor activation. Preliminary studies have suggested that fMRI lateralization of language may be comparable to the older Wada (invasive intracarotid amobarbital) test, but fMRI cannot be used alone to confidently assess the risk of postsurgical amnesia syndrome. An alternative approach is rs-fMRI or functional connectivity MR imaging, which can be performed on patients unable to cooperate with task-based paradigms, such as young children and patients who are encephalopathic, sedated, paretic, or aphasic. Early investigations have indicated that rs-fMRI data may localize epileptogenic regions, identify functional networks for presurgical planning, and predict surgical outcome.

## Multimodal imaging

To maximize the value of structural and functional information obtained from imaging data, it is useful to co-register the imaging data with clinical neurophysiological studies such as magnetoencephalography or surface and intracranial EEG studies (Figure 8.2), which is then used for neurosurgical planning and to implement image-guided neurosurgery. Image registration transforms images acquired at different time points, or with different imaging

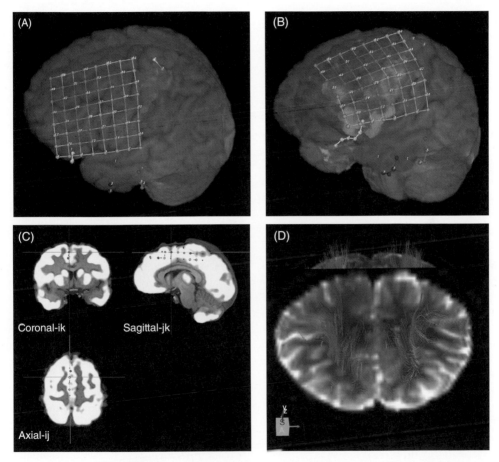

**Figure 8.2.** Multimodal imaging for intracranial EEG planning in a patient with nonlesional epilepsy originating from the language-dominant left frontal lobe. The images were obtained both preoperatively and postoperatively after intracranial electrode placement and registered to the same coordinate system. The preoperative co-registered images were used with an image-guided surgical system for electrode placement. (A) Task-based fMRI of right-hand sensorimotor activation registered to 3D T1-weighted MRI with left frontotemporal grid (from postoperative CT scan); (B) task-based fMRI of language activation registered to 3D T1-weighted MRI with left frontotemporal grid and lateral frontal, frontopolar, anterior, and midtemporal strips (from postoperative CT scan); (C) FDG-PET registered to 3D T1-weighted MRI with location of left frontal interhemispheric, 16-contact strip (from postoperative CT scan); (D) diffusion tractography of major tracts in frontal regions in same subject. (*See plate section for color version of this figure.*)

modalities, into the same coordinate system. Modern image-guided surgical systems primarily use structural imaging for surgery, but increasingly, it is important to integrate data from co-registered functional and structural imaging to guide placement of intracranial electrodes and define the resection target to decrease morbidity (Figure 8.2). This permits investigations of relationships among the various imaging modalities and clinical neurophysiological data with respect to both function and pathology, as well as longitudinal studies tracking this data in the same subject over time.

## Conclusions

Brain imaging has an important role in the diagnosis and management of patients with epilepsy. In the acute setting, imaging with MRI can identify the cause of a patient's seizures and epilepsy, alter treatment, and provide important prognostic information. In the greater than 30% of patients that fail to respond to medical treatment, imaging using both structural and functional methods is critical to determining what patients may be surgical candidates and to guiding the surgical procedure.

## Bibliography

Blumenfeld H, McNally KA, Vanderhill SD, et al. Positive and negative network correlations in temporal lobe epilepsy. *Cereb Cortex* 2004 August; **14**(8):892–902.

Bonilha L, Halford JJ, Rorden C, Roberts DR, Rumboldt Z, Eckert MA. Automated MRI analysis for identification of hippocampal atrophy in temporal lobe epilepsy. *Epilepsia* 2009 February; **50**(2):228–233.

Concha L, Kim H, Bernasconi A, Bernhardt BC, Bernasconi N. Spatial patterns of water diffusion along white matter tracts in temporal lobe epilepsy. *Neurology* 2012; **79**(5):455–462.

Desai A, Bekelis K, Thadani VM, et al. Interictal PET and ictal subtraction SPECT: Sensitivity in the detection of seizure foci in patients with medically intractable epilepsy. *Epilepsia* 2012; **54**(2):341–350.

Gaillard WD, Chiron C, Cross JH, et al. Guidelines for imaging infants and children with recent-onset epilepsy. *Epilepsia* 2009 September; **50**(9):2147–2153.

Goense JB, Logothetis NK. Neurophysiology of BOLD fMRI signal in awake monkeys. *Curr Biol* 2008 May; **18**(9):631–640.

Joshi A, Scheinost D, Vives KP, Spencer DD, Staib LH, Papademetris X. Novel interaction techniques for neurosurgical planning and stereotactic navigation. *IEEE Trans Vis Comput Graph* 2008 November–December; **14**(6):1587–1594.

Lee MH, Smyser CD, Shimony JS. Resting-state fMRI: A review of methods and clinical applications. *Am J Neuroradiol* 2013 Oct; **34**(10):1866–1872.

McNally KA, Paige AL, Varghese G, et al. Localizing value of ictal-interictal SPECT analyzed by SPM (ISAS). *Epilepsia* 2005; **46**(9):1450–1464.

Negishi M, Martuzzi R, Novotny EJ, Spencer DD, Constable RT. Functional MRI connectivity as a predictor of the surgical outcome of epilepsy. *Epilepsia* 2011; **52**(9):1733–1740.

Nguyen DK, Rochette E, Leroux JM, et al. Value of 3.0 T MR imaging in refractory partial epilepsy and negative 1.5 T MRI. *Seizure* 2010; **19**(8):475–478.

Quality Standards Subcommittee of the American Academy of Neurology in cooperation with American College of Emergency Physicians, American Association of Neurological Surgeons, American Society of Neuroradiology. Practice parameter: Neuroimaging in the emergency patient presenting with seizure – summary statement. *Neurology* 1996; **47**(1):288–291.

Risholm P, Golby AJ, Wells W, 3rd. Multimodal image registration for preoperative planning and image-guided neurosurgical procedures. *Neurosurg Clin N Am* 2011; **22**(2):197–206, viii.

Strandberg M, Larsson EM, Backman S, Kallen K. Presurgical epilepsy evaluation using 3 T MRI. Do surface coils provide additional information? *Epileptic Disord* 2008; **10**:83–92.

Willmann O, Wennberg R, May T, Woermann FG, Pohlmann-Eden B. The contribution of 18F-FDG PET in preoperative epilepsy surgery evaluation for patients with temporal lobe epilepsy: A meta-analysis. *Seizure* 2007; **16**:509–520.

# Workup of New-Onset Seizures

**Jennifer Langer**

Department of Neurology, University of Virginia, Charlottesville, VA, USA

## Introduction

Seizures are one of the most common complaints in neurological practice. The estimated incidence of a single unprovoked seizure is 23–61 per 100,000 person-years. Approximately 30% will recur in the first 5 years and meet the diagnostic criterion for epilepsy, specifically, two or more unprovoked seizures.

The initial evaluation of the first seizure is critical in establishing the correct diagnosis and etiology and determining the likelihood of recurrent events. It is the likelihood of recurrent events that helps to frame the decision of whether or not to initiate treatment after a single event. With the evaluation also comes an educational opportunity with the patient and family regarding seizure first aid and seizure precautions.

## Differential diagnosis

Not everything that looks and acts like a seizure is in fact an epileptic seizure (Chapter 5). The differential diagnosis of paroxysmal spells is quite broad, including seizure, syncope, psychogenic nonepileptic spells, migraine, movement disorders, transient ischemic attack (TIA), and toxic–metabolic disturbance. Pediatric populations have additional considerations including breath-holding spells, febrile seizure, and self-stimulating behaviors typically in developmentally delayed children. Nocturnal spells may also represent parasomnias. A good history can narrow down the differential diagnosis, although video–EEG recording of a typical event may be required for definitive diagnosis. Three of the more common seizure mimics seen in practice are highlighted in the succeeding text. Psychogenic nonepileptic events are covered in Chapter 6.

Syncope is defined as a loss of consciousness and postural tone caused by cerebral hypoperfusion with spontaneous recovery. Twelve percent of patients with syncope have an associated convulsion termed a post-syncopal convulsion that can be confused with an epileptic seizure. In a video study of clinical features of induced syncope, the most common finding was myoclonus, and less frequent findings were automatisms and head turn. Features of the history suggesting syncope include preceding pallor, sweating, light-headedness, diminution of hearing and vision, and chest pain. Postural triggers and changes in blood pressure or heart rate preceding or during the event also are suggestive.

*Epilepsy*, First Edition. Edited by John W. Miller and Howard P. Goodkin.
© 2014 John Wiley & Sons, Ltd. Published 2014 by John Wiley & Sons, Ltd.

Migraine headaches may have associated visual or sensory auras that can overlap with symptomatology seen in focal seizures. Migraine auras are more prolonged than epileptic auras and can last minutes to hours in comparison with epileptic auras, which are usually seconds in duration. Visual auras tend to be flickering, black and white zigzags in migraine, whereas in focal seizures involving visual cortex, visual phenomena are usually bright and multicolored. Sensory auras, including tingling or numbness, can be present in both but typically spread more slowly in migraine compared with seizure, which generally has a fast, marching anatomic spread.

Transient ischemic attacks (TIA) usually present with negative symptoms that vary depending on the vascular territory involved. Although seizures are typically associated with positive symptoms, there are specific seizure semiologies that may clinically overlap with a TIA, including isolated intermittent aphasia, which can represent focal ischemia or a focal seizure of the dominant hemisphere. Todd's paresis, consisting of focal weakness following a seizure, can often be confused for a stroke if the preceding seizure is not witnessed.

## Clinical history and examination

One of the most important initial steps in the evaluation of new-onset seizures is a detailed clinical history and examination. Obtaining a clinical description of the events is the first step in determining the etiology of events. Information should be obtained from the patient when possible as well as from other individuals who have observed the event of interest. The patient's recollection may be limited by alteration in consciousness or postictal confusion, and observer reports can be unreliable. Chapter 5 details the process by which the history and examination can be used at the bedside to establish whether an individual's events are seizures.

> ☆ **TIPS AND TRICKS**
>
> When available, a video recording of the event will provide helpful information and eliminate the need to rely either on second-hand information or on an eyewitness who may not have full recall of the events.

> ☆ **TIPS AND TRICKS**
>
> Seizure risk factors should be assessed in any evaluation of a patient with a new-onset spell. These risk factors increase the patient's likelihood of having a seizure above that of the general population.
>
> These risk factors include:
>
> 1. History of central nervous system (CNS) infection
> 2. History of CNS trauma with loss of consciousness (there is debate as to the extent of trauma required to increase risk of seizure)
> 3. History of febrile seizure as a child
> 4. Family history of seizures or epilepsy
> 5. Abnormal birth or developmental history

The clinical background in which the seizure occurred can help determine etiology. A history of prodromal fever may suggest an infectious etiology. Care must be taken not to overinterpret fever at the time of acute seizure presentation, as a seizure itself may cause transient hyperthermia. A history of alcohol or drug use can raise suspicion for alcohol withdrawal or drug overdose, respectively.

A detailed medical, family, and social history may clarify the likelihood that the index event is a seizure by discerning whether the patient has any seizure risk factors, which may increase the individual's likelihood of seizure above that of the general population.

Depending on how soon the clinical examination is performed after the index event, the patient may still experience postictal confusion or fatigue, limiting the ability to perform a thorough neurological examination. In this setting, focus should be placed on the presence or absence of focal or lateralizing findings such as focal motor weakness, reflex asymmetry, or plantar responses that can provide evidence for a focal onset.

## Neurodiagnostic evaluation

No single test can replace history taking and physical examination in diagnosis and evaluation of a first seizure; however, diagnostic procedures such as neuroimaging or electroencephalogrphy (EEG) can provide supportive data for diagnosis and prognosis.

## EEG

There has been ongoing debate regarding the necessity of EEG for evaluation of a first seizure, although the 2007 American Academy of Neurology (AAN) practice parameter for adults and 2000 AAN practice parameter for children both recommend routine EEG in this setting. Specifically, the value of EEG is largely twofold: (1) it allows individual prediction of seizure recurrence and (2) it identifies patterns consistent with specific epilepsy syndromes. Approximately 30% of EEGs obtained to evaluate initial seizure are abnormal. Consistently, an abnormal EEG and an identified etiology are associated with an increased risk of seizure recurrence. More specifically, the abnormal findings of generalized or focal epileptiform discharges are associated with an approximately two times greater risk of seizure recurrence. Therefore, the presence of these discharges may prompt initiation of antiepileptic medication even after the first event. Chapter 7 further discusses EEG procedures and indications and common findings seen in patients with epilepsy.

> ### ✋ CAUTION!
>
> While an EEG with focal or generalized epileptiform discharges is predictive of seizure recurrence, a normal EEG does not exclude the possibility of subsequent seizures, as patients with epilepsy may have a normal EEG.

An EEG may also demonstrate characteristics of specific epilepsy syndromes such as juvenile myoclonic epilepsy or childhood absence epilepsy, which may influence antiepileptic choice. King and colleagues prospectively identified 300 consecutive patients 5 years old or older who presented with an initial seizure. An epilepsy syndrome was diagnosed based on clinical history and examination in 47% of patients. The addition of EEG data allowed for diagnosis of an epilepsy syndrome in 77% of patients. If the EEG demonstrates changes associated with idiopathic generalized epilepsy, it may negate the need for neuroimaging. EEG findings associated with syndromes such as childhood absence epilepsy, benign rolandic epilepsy, or benign occipital epilepsy of childhood, all of which typically remit during childhood, may alleviate parental concerns in the high-anxiety state following a first seizure.

> ### ★ TIPS AND TRICKS
>
> There are a few specific situations in which an EEG may not be required. An EEG is not necessary after a first simple febrile seizure. It is also probably not necessary when the etiology is obvious, for example, as in brain tumor or stroke.

## Neuroimaging

Compared with EEG, less systematic data is available to assess the utility of neuroimaging in the diagnostic evaluation of first seizure, with most literature involving the use of CT. The AAN practice parameter for adults suggests neuroimaging using CT or MRI should be considered as part of the evaluation. The AAN practice parameter for children suggests that there is insufficient evidence to support a recommendation for use of routine imaging, although if imaging is obtained, MRI is recommended. Neuroimaging is specifically recommended in these situations: a postictal focal deficit not quickly resolving and a slow return to baseline following seizure. Nonurgent imaging is recommended in any child with cognitive or motor impairment of unclear etiology, unexplained abnormal neurological examination, focal onset seizure, or EEG pattern not consistent with benign epilepsy, or in children under 1 year of age. Chapter 8 details neuroimaging procedures, particularly MRI, that are used for the evaluation of new-onset and chronic epilepsy and describes common MRI findings that may cause epilepsy.

The theoretical value of neuroimaging is twofold: (1) identification of an abnormality requiring acute intervention and (2) support for a diagnosis of a specific epilepsy syndrome. MRI is more sensitive for determining etiology than CT, so MRI is recommended for evaluation of first seizure. However, there is still a role for CT in the acute emergency room setting to evaluate patients for causes requiring emergency interventions. In King's evaluation of 300 consecutive patients with epilepsy, 92% had neuroimaging with MRI, making it the most common imaging modality. All patients with generalized epilepsy and EEG findings of generalized discharges had normal MRI. Among 154 patients with focal epilepsy, MRI revealed epileptogenic lesions in 17%. Among 59 patients with unclassified epilepsy based on clinical history and EEG, MRI had a diagnostic yield of 15% and resulted in reclassification of the epilepsy syndrome.

A recommended approach to the use of EEG and neuroimaging in the evaluation of first seizure is presented in Figure 9.1. In this approach, EEG is recommended in all patients, with the use of MRI hinging largely on EEG findings in the appropriate clinical setting. This algorithm is helpful in an outpatient setting; however, in some emergency room settings, MRI and EEG are not quickly available, and in those cases clinical history and examination should guide the use of more easily obtainable neuroimaging such as CT.

**Laboratory studies**

Blood glucose, blood counts, and electrolyte panels are often part of the evaluation for first seizure. In this setting, the yield of laboratory testing is typically low, on the range of 0–15%, with none reported as significant. It is recommended that decision making regarding the need for routine lab work be guided by history and physical examination, as they often predict which patients will demonstrate significantly abnormal results. A patient with persisting altered mental status, fever, or focal neurological deficits warrants a more extensive laboratory evaluation.

Drug intoxication is in the differential diagnosis for first seizure, with some studies of emergency room visits suggesting it is the cause of 3% of all first seizures. No studies have looked at systematic screening of all first-time seizure patients; therefore, there is not sufficient data to recommend its routine

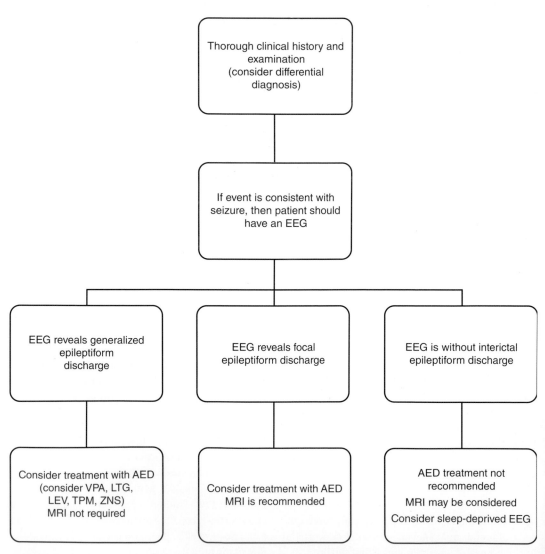

**Figure 9.1.** Suggested algorithm for evaluation of first, unprovoked seizure. LEV, levetiracetam; LTG, lamotrigine; TPM, topiramate; VPA, valproate; ZNS, zonisamide.

use in all patients. Instead, toxicology including urine drug screen or blood testing should be used if suggested by the clinical history.

Lumbar punctures are performed to evaluate for CNS infection as a cause of a first seizure. Studies suggest that approximately 8% of lumbar punctures done in the setting of a first seizure evaluation are significantly abnormal. Lumbar puncture should be considered in the febrile patient, particularly if there is no identified cause for fever. With that said, fever can often accompany a seizure, but in this setting it should not be persistent. A persistent fever following an isolated seizure requires further evaluation.

## Treatment after a first seizure

As only 30% of patients with a single seizure will have a second seizure within 5 years of the index event, treatment is not required or indicated for all patients presenting with their first seizure. The goal of the aforementioned evaluation is to determine which of these patients is at higher risk for recurrence and therefore should be considered for treatment with antiepileptic medication. Predictors of seizure recurrence include focal or generalized epileptiform abnormalities on EEG and known structural etiology. If a medication is started after a first seizure, medication selection should be based on the presumed type of epilepsy, focal or generalized. Additional information on choosing and initiating antiepileptic medications can be found in Chapter 11.

### ★ TIPS AND TRICKS

If the EEG obtained after a first seizure is abnormal due to the presence of focal epileptiform discharges (especially if located in the temporal or frontal regions), generalized epileptiform discharges, or changes that are pathognomonic of a specific epilepsy syndrome (e.g., juvenile myoclonic epilepsy), it is appropriate to discuss initiating treatment, as these EEG findings are associated with an increased risk of subsequent seizures.

## Patient education

A key component of the evaluation of a first seizure is patient education, which is largely threefold: review (1) seizure first aid, (2) seizure precautions, and (3) driving regulations, if age appropriate. Chapter 34 further outlines the risks of different types of accidents that can occur with epilepsy.

Education regarding seizure first aid is aimed largely at the family or caregivers of the patient. It is often helpful to provide the patient with written material if family or caregivers are not present. It is important to stress that during a convulsive seizure, caregivers should focus on maintaining patient safety during the event; this involves lowering the patient to safe ground and positioning the patient on his/her side to minimize risk of aspiration. To minimize the risk of choking/biting, nothing should be placed in the patient's mouth. During nonconvulsive seizures, the patient should be supported in a safe environment. Often, attempting to constrain the patient during a seizure may increase risk of agitation in the ictal or postictal setting. Emergency services are generally not required for seizures lasting less than 3 min; however, for more prolonged seizures greater than 4–5 min, it is advisable to obtain emergency medical care.

Seizure precautions are aimed at reducing the risk of injury in the setting of subsequent seizures. Baths are not recommended due to risk of drowning. If a bath is necessary, the environment should be continuously visually supervised. Similar caution is advisable for swimming. Activities including operating heavy machinery, climbing ladders, and working around a stove should be avoided.

Driving regulations are state specific in the USA, typically ranging from 3 months to 1 year without driving following a seizure involving loss or alteration of consciousness. It is the responsibility of the physician seeing the patient at the time of the first seizure to make the patient and family aware of this issue. This is typically toughest for adult patients in nonurban settings who require transportation for employment.

### ☝ CAUTION!

The following states currently require the physician to report patients who experience a seizure to the Department of Motor Vehicles: California, Delaware, Nevada, New Jersey, Oregon, and Pennsylvania. It is important for neurologists to intermittently check the laws of the states in which they reside to ensure that they are aware of any changes in the driving laws.

## Conclusion

The evaluation of the first-time seizure is critical in early identification of those who will go on to develop epilepsy. As reviewed in this chapter, a detailed clinical history is the most important part of the evaluation; this is aided by a good physical examination and supporting data including EEG and MRI. This evaluation is also a critical point of contact for patient education regarding seizure first aid, appropriate age-specific precautions, and driving restrictions.

## Bibliography

Harden CL, Huff JS, Schwartz TH, et al. Reassessment: Neuroimaging in the emergency patient presenting with seizure (an evidence-based review): Report of the Therapeutics and Technology Assessment Subcommittee of the American Academy of Neurology. *Neurology* 2007; **69**:1772–1780.

Hauser WA, Rich SS, Lee JR, Annegers JF, Anderson VE. Risk of recurrent seizures after two unprovoked seizures. *N Engl J Med* 1998; **338**:429–434.

Hirtz D, Ashwal S, Berg A, et al. Practice parameter: Evaluating a first nonfebrile seizure in children: Report of the Quality Standards Subcommittee of the American Academy of Neurology, the Child Neurology Society, and the American Epilepsy Society. *Neurology* 2000; **55**:616–623.

King MA, Newton MR, Jackson GD, et al. Epileptology of the first-seizure presentation: A clinical, electroencephalographic, and magnetic resonance imaging study of 300 consecutive patients. *Lancet* 1998; **352**:1007–1011.

Krumholtz A, Wiebe S, Gronseth G, et al. Practice parameter: Evaluating an apparent unprovoked first seizure in adults (an evidence-based review): Report of the Quality Standards Subcommittee of the American Academy of Neurology and the American Epilepsy Society. *Neurology* 2007; **69**:1996–2007.

McKeon A, Vaughan C, Delanty N. Seizure versus syncope. *Lancet Neurol* 2006; **5**:171–180.

# Evaluation of the Patient with Medically Refractory Epilepsy

**Gregory L. Holmes**

Department of Neurological Sciences, University of Vermont, Burlington, VT, USA

## Introduction

Epilepsy treatment is directed towards preventing seizures and achieving control early in the illness. While most individuals with epilepsy respond well to antiepileptic drugs (AEDs), approximately one-third continue to have seizures, despite trying multiple medications, and are considered medically refractory, also termed medically intractable. The operational definition of refractory epilepsy requires failure to control seizures after trying two or three seizure medications (whether as monotherapies or in combination) appropriately chosen and used. The die is cast rather early in the course of the disorder; even failing the first AED results in a significantly increased risk of experiencing adverse health outcomes. Unfortunately, the mechanisms of refractory epilepsy remain uncertain.

> ### ⚙ SCIENCE REVISITED
>
> The biological basis of medically refractory epilepsy is unknown. Recent basic research has suggested two postulated mechanisms for refractory epilepsy. According to one postulated mechanism, plasticity of AED targets, with a concomitantly decreased sensitivity to AEDs, leads to medical intractability. The hypothesis proposes that pharmacoresistance involves an upregulation of multidrug transporters at the blood–brain barrier. Upregulation of these transporters limits the concentration of AEDs to the brain parenchyma, thus resulting in a reduced drug concentration at the respective drug target. The second postulated mechanism is that the molecular targets of AEDs are modified and thus are less sensitive to these drugs in chronic epilepsy.

Refractory epilepsy often has significant adverse effects on the physical, psychological, cognitive, social, educational, and vocational state of the patient. It results in a higher risk for a shortened life expectancy, injury, neuropsychological and mental health impairment, and social disability. Individuals with refractory epilepsy have high risks of comorbidities including attention deficit disorder, depression, and anxiety. Underachievement in school, unemployment, and underemployment are common in individuals with refractory epilepsy.

Refractory epilepsy is clearly an important public health issue, and clinicians need to make every attempt possible to control seizures. However, aggressive treatment of refractory epilepsy does not

*Epilepsy*, First Edition. Edited by John W. Miller and Howard P. Goodkin.

mean that medications should be used at any cost to suppress seizures. As discussed later in this chapter, overtreatment can actually result in increased seizures. In addition, using high doses or multiple AEDs increases the risk of side effects such as headache, fatigue, bone loss, irritability, and cognitive impairment and also increases monetary costs.

## Diagnosis of refractory epilepsy

An early step in evaluating individuals with refractory epilepsy is to be certain they have epilepsy. Misdiagnosis is common due to the myriad of signs or symptoms seen in this complex disorder. Accurately diagnosing epilepsy is challenging because clinicians rarely have the opportunity to observe seizures. Therefore, the diagnosis is typically based on the patient's self-report or the family member's description of seizures and the medical history. There are many conditions in children and adults that mimic epilepsy. Unfortunately, a significant number of patients with disorders such as REM sleep behavior disorder, night terrors, and psychogenic nonepileptic seizures are being misdiagnosed and then treated unsuccessfully with AEDs for months to years.

---

### ☆ TIPS AND TRICKS

Psychogenic nonepileptic seizures may present as chronic epilepsy. When eliciting history, ask if eyes were open or closed during the event. Most patients with epileptic seizures have their eyes open during an epileptic seizure, whereas in psychogenic nonepileptic events, the eyes are tightly closed. In addition, asynchronous movements, pelvic thrusting, side-to-side head or body movement, ictal crying, and memory recall and absence of postictal confusion are signs of psychogenic nonepileptic seizures rather than epileptic seizures. The presence of postictal stertorous breathing is indicative of an epileptic generalized tonic–clonic seizure and is rarely, if ever, seen following a nonepileptic seizure.

---

To avoid prolonged use of ineffective AEDs, the epilepsy diagnosis should be reconsidered for any patient who does not respond to therapy. This process begins with a detailed history in which the "seizures" are described in detail. While the patient's account of the event is important, it is critical that a parent, spouse, or caregiver who witnessed the event also provide a description. Details about time of occurrence, duration, and precipitating factors are important. As discussed in the following text, the history should include a description of the behavioral features of the seizure. This information should be obtained at every visit of a patient with refractory epilepsy.

Electroencephalography can be an important tool when diagnosing patients with epilepsy. While there are no legitimate reasons for repeating EEGs at every visit when the patient is doing well, repeating the EEG when the patient continues to have seizures can be helpful in assisting with seizure classification and syndrome identification. To gain the maximum amount of information, the EEG should be recorded during wakefulness, drowsiness, and sleep along with hyperventilation and photic stimulation. Recording an actual event is ideal, so continuous video–EEG monitoring, lasting from hours to days, should be done if questions about the diagnosis remain. If the individual has frequent events, ambulatory EEG may be helpful. However, if AEDs are withdrawn in the attempt to induce an event, it is usually safer to do the monitoring in the hospital. Video–EEG monitoring is particularly helpful in distinguishing epileptic from nonepileptic events.

With the ready availability of cell phone cameras, digital cameras with video capabilities, and video monitoring in home settings, family members can record events on video as they occur. This information can be invaluable in differentiating seizures from nonepileptic behaviors. With the patient's or family's permission, these video clips can be shared with colleagues to assist in diagnosis.

## Determining seizure type

One possible cause of refractory epilepsy is the use of the incorrect drug for the seizure type. Seizures are classified into two broad categories: (1) focal seizures (seizures beginning in a limited location in the brain) and (2) generalized seizures (seizures that are bilaterally symmetric and without focal onset). The pathophysiological mechanisms of focal seizures and generalized seizures are different, although the common endpoint, such as a generalized tonic–clonic seizure, can be quite similar. Similarly, AEDs are broken down into two categories: AEDs that are effective in focal seizures and those effective in generalized seizures. Certain AEDs that are effective in both seizure types are considered broad spectrum. Treating a patient with the wrong AED for his or her seizure type may not only not control the seizures but could actually exacerbate the condition. For example, treating a patient with a primary generalized epilepsy with carbamazepine could make seizures such as myoclonic, absence, and generalized tonic–clonic seizures worse. Likewise, ethosuximide, a highly effective drug for absence seizures, has limited efficacy against other seizure types.

The first step in determining the correct seizure type is to obtain a detailed description of seizure semiology. While the diagnosis of a generalized tonic–clonic (convulsive) seizure is rarely difficult, determining whether the seizure has a focal onset may be more difficult. Asking about auras and lateralized features at onset, such as eye or head deviation, may help identify a focal onset. Distinguishing between absence and focal seizures with altered awareness can be difficult but is essential in picking the correct AED. Compared to focal seizures with altered awareness (formerly termed complex partial seizures), absence seizures are shorter (<15 s) and have an abrupt onset and offset. Absence seizures result in a "blank" facial appearance with upward eye deviation and may be accompanied by eye blinking. Individuals with focal seizures with altered awareness often have an aura and appear confused and disoriented. Also, automatisms are common, and most patients have some degree of postictal impairment. In both children and adults, absences but not focal seizures are readily induced by hyperventilation.

The interictal EEG can be very helpful in distinguishing focal seizures from generalized seizures (Chapter 7). Typically, focal seizures have focal EEG abnormalities, whereas generalized seizures have generalized discharges. However, generalized discharges on the EEG may have a subtle focal onset followed by rapid generalization. In addition, seeing occasional focal spikes in a patient with generalized epilepsy is not uncommon.

Capturing the patient's seizures using long-term EEG video monitoring can be quite helpful in correctly classifying seizure type (Chapter 7). The use of this technique allows correlation of behavior with EEG changes and is very useful in determining if the seizure has a focal or generalized onset, which has major implications in drug treatment.

## ⚠ CAUTION!

Antiepileptic medications that can make seizures worse:

Carbamazepine/oxcarbazepine – absence, myoclonic, and generalized tonic–clonic
Gabapentin – myoclonic
Lamotrigine – myoclonic
Phenytoin – myoclonic
Tiagabine – generalized seizures, particularly subclinical spike–wave
Vigabatrin – absence

## Pseudo-intractability

Pseudo-intractability refers to resistance to treatment that is, in fact, caused by clinical errors. Such errors include incorrect diagnosis (seizure type and/or syndrome) with inappropriate choice of medication, therapeutic errors such as overtreatment, issues with medication compliance, and failure to identify potential seizure-precipitating factors. These factors all should be considered when evaluating patients with refractory epilepsy.

Some individuals with epilepsy have triggers such as lack of sleep, stress, flashing lights, fever, menstruation, or excessive alcohol consumption that increase their susceptibility to seizures. Once these precipitants are identified and addressed, refractory epilepsy can be controlled.

Adhering to a medication regimen is a significant challenge for many people with epilepsy, and non-adherence frequently contributes to refractory epilepsy. Reviews of claims data of adults with epilepsy find a high rate of nonadherence, with almost 40% of patients not able to adhere to their prescribed regimen at some point during a 27-month period. AED nonadherence was associated with increased likelihood of hospitalization and emergency room visits. Reasons for nonadherence are multiple and include concern about side effects and costs. Forgetting to take the medication and forgetting to reorder the prescription also are factors. Managing medications requires critical self-management skills that include monitoring pill taking and use of pill boxes, reminders, and alarms. Nonadherence should be considered in all patients with refractory epilepsy.

Finally, excessive drug load can lead to suboptimal outcomes, including greater incidence or severity of side effects or even increased seizure frequency. For example, with high serum concentrations, phenytoin may cause a paradoxical increase of seizures. An excessive drug load can occur when one or more seizure medications is not the right choice for the individual's seizure type or syndrome, when higher than necessary dosages are prescribed or used, or when medication interactions are not considered. Reducing drug load or identifying drugs that may be exacerbating seizures can reduce the likelihood of refractory epilepsy.

## Etiology

The etiology of the epilepsy is the most important factor in prognosis and has a major role in determining the therapeutic approach to the patient. In some cases targeting the underlying etiology will treat the epilepsy. For example, children with seizures secondary to pyridoxine dependency will respond to vitamin B6. Likewise, seizures in the glucose transporter type 1 deficiency, which results in low spinal fluid concentrations of glucose, respond well to the ketogenic diet. Clues to the etiology may come from the physical examination.

Many physical examination findings can be used to formulate a differential diagnosis. Even a simple measurement such as head circumference may provide clues to diagnosis. Macrocephaly may indicate disorders such as neurofibromatosis, fragile X syndrome, or Alexander or Canavan disease, whereas microcephaly can be seen in malformations of cerebral development and Rett and Angelman syndromes. Dysmorphic features can suggest such disorders as trisomy 21 and other chromosome abnormalities. A thorough skin examination is critical. Tuberous sclerosis has characteristic skin findings (hypopigmented macules, facial angiofibromas, shagreen patch). Sturge–Weber has a characteristic facial port-wine stain. Likewise, hypomelanosis of Ito, linear nevus sebaceous syndrome, incontinentia pigmenti, and neurofibromatosis type 1 have specific skin findings. Focal neurological findings on examination at any age, such as an asymmetric smile or unilateral weakness, would point to a structural cause of the patient's epilepsy.

All patients with refractory epilepsy should have a brain MRI (Chapter 8). Even patients with refractory absences should have an MRI to evaluate for a mesial

frontal lobe structural lesion that results in rapid secondary seizure generalization. Although there is no consensus regarding the ideal MRI sequences, the International League Against Epilepsy recommends that all epilepsy protocols include thin-slice (5 mm or less) volumetric T1-weighted gradient-recalled echo sequences, axial and coronal T2-weighted sequences, and high-resolution oblique coronal hippocampal, axial, and coronal fluid-attenuated inversion recovery sequences. When the MRI is normal, consideration should be given to repeating the study, particularly if the initial MRI was done during the first 5 years of life. Subtle disorders of cerebral development may be overlooked or remain undetected on the initial MRI in young children due to reduced myelination compared to older children and adults. In addition, if the prior MRI used a 1.5 T magnet, using a higher-tesla magnet, for example, 3 T, may increase the diagnostic yield.

Mesial temporal sclerosis is a common cause of refractory mesial temporal epilepsy in adults. It may not be apparent on MRI scans done early in the course of temporal lobe epilepsy, and repeating the MRI with attention to the hippocampus may detect hippocampal abnormalities. Repeating the MRI in adult patients with refractory epilepsy may detect previously undiagnosed structural abnormalities. Lesions that are particularly important causes of intractable focal epilepsy in adults include tumors, vascular anomalies, atrophic lesions, and focal cortical dysplasia. Benign or low-grade neoplasms, including meningiomas, dysplastic neuroepithelial tumors, gangliogliomas, oligodendrogliomas, and astrocytomas, may cause chronic epilepsy. The most common epileptogenic vascular anomalies are cavernous hemangiomas and arteriovenous malformations. Common atrophic lesions in both children and adults result from stroke or traumatic brain injury. Detecting any of these epileptogenic lesions on MRI could dramatically change management by raising the possibility of neurosurgical treatment for medically intractable epilepsy.

It is important to note that not all structural abnormalities observed on the MRI are necessarily the cause of the patient's seizures. It should not be assumed that abnormalities such as arachnoid cysts, venous anomalies, or even small areas of cerebral dysgenesis or encephalomalacia are always epileptogenic. Abnormal MRI findings should always be evaluated in the context of a patient's history, seizure semiology, and EEG findings.

There has been an explosion in neurogenetics over the last few decades (Chapter 22). Epilepsy is a major component of many genetic disorders that have other prominent neurological problems, namely intellectual disability. For example, trisomy 21, fragile X, tuberous sclerosis complex, Rett syndrome and Angelman syndrome, the progressive myoclonic epilepsies, and a host of other genetic conditions have epilepsy associated with various other neurological symptoms, most prominently intellectual impairment. More recently it has been shown that a gene mutation can result in epilepsy without other abnormalities. Mutations in ion channel-encoding genes have been found in a variety of inherited diseases associated with hyperexcitability or hypoexcitability of the affected tissue, the so-called channelopathies. An increasing number of epileptic syndromes belong to this group of rare disorders: generalized seizures with febrile seizures and Dravet syndrome caused by sodium channel mutations, autosomal dominant nocturnal frontal lobe epilepsy caused by mutations in a neuronal nicotinic acetylcholine receptor, benign familial neonatal convulsions caused by mutations in potassium channels, and episodic ataxia type 1 – which is associated with epilepsy in some and is caused by mutations within another voltage-gated potassium channel. In individuals without a diagnosis, it is reasonable to obtain genetic testing using the patient's examination findings, seizure type, and history to direct the specific tests ordered. In the absence of signs and symptoms pointing to a specific genetic syndrome, a DNA microarray and karyotype may be considered.

Diagnosing a genetic disorder can direct AED selection (Chapter 22). Lamotrigine is avoided in individuals with Dravet syndrome and phenytoin should not be given to patients with Unverricht–Lundborg disease because the AEDs can increase rather than decrease seizure frequency in both of these conditions. Determining a genetic cause for the epilepsy would eliminate consideration of surgical therapy in most patients. The one major exception is tuberous sclerosis complex, where surgery can be effective in some patients. It is important for individuals and their families to know the cause of seizures, as well as the prognosis and risk of the condition in other family members.

Patients with refractory epilepsy should be evaluated for neurometabolic conditions if this evaluation has not already been performed (Chapter 23). This is particularly important for conditions with specific treatments. Glucose levels of spinal fluid should be obtained because a glucose transporter deficiency can present with poorly controlled seizures. Spinal fluid neurotransmitter precursors and metabolites can also be measured to rule out disorders such as cerebral folate deficiency. Children with possible pyridoxine dependency should receive 100 mg of pyridoxine during an EEG to assess response. Pyridoxal phosphate, 10 mg/kg IV, can also be used instead of pyridoxine. Children with pyridoxine phosphate oxidase deficiency respond to pyridoxal phosphate but not to pyridoxine. Pipecolic acid in plasma and cerebrospinal fluid can be measured if pyridoxine dependency is a possibility. Children with other neurological or systemic symptoms besides epilepsy should have urine organic acids and plasma amino acids measured to rule out disorders such as phenylketonuria, homocystinuria, maple syrup urine disease, biotinidase deficiency, and glutaric aciduria.

Neurometabolic disorders resulting in epilepsy typically have signs and symptoms other than seizures and are symptomatic in early childhood. The diagnostic yield of extensive neurometabolic testing in a child over the age of 6 years or an adult with refractory epilepsy and no other concerning signs or symptoms is very low.

## Referral to a tertiary center

Patients with refractory epilepsy should be referred to epilepsy centers to determine whether the diagnosis is correct, which medications are appropriate, and whether surgery is a treatment option (Chapter 27). There have been significant advances in epilepsy surgery over the past few decades. Surgically remediable epilepsy syndromes are easier to recognize than they were previously, largely because of improvements in MRI and other imaging technologies, which allow noninvasive identification of areas in the brain with abnormal neural function.

Randomized controlled studies have shown that people with mesial temporal lobe epilepsy who receive epilepsy surgery have a significantly higher likelihood of becoming seizure-free by 1 year after the surgery when compared to a group receiving conventional medical therapy.

**EVIDENCE AT A GLANCE**

In the first randomized controlled study of medically intractable temporal lobe epilepsy, 40 patients were assigned to surgery and 40 were assigned treatment with AEDs. At 1 year, the cumulative proportion of patients free of seizures impairing awareness was 58% in the surgical group and 8% in the medical group ($p < 0.001$). Those in the surgical group had fewer seizures impairing awareness and a significantly better quality of life ($p < 0.001$ for both comparisons) than those in the medical group. No patients in the surgery group died, while one in the medical group did. This study showed that in temporal lobe epilepsy, surgery is superior to prolonged medical therapy.

An evidence review by the Quality Standards Subcommittee of the American Academy of Neurology, conducted to develop practice parameters for epilepsy surgery, found that surgery's benefits outweighed the benefits of continued medical therapy in people with mesial temporal lobe epilepsy, without posing greater risk. The subcommittee recommended consideration of referral to an epilepsy surgery center for individuals with refractory seizures. Currently there is not sufficient data to recommend surgery over medical therapy for non-temporal lobe epilepsy; however, it is clear that in selected patients with non-temporal lope epilepsy, surgery can eliminate or greatly reduce seizure frequency without causing neurological deficits. While not all those with refractory epilepsy are surgical candidates, it is recommended that they be evaluated at epilepsy centers where surgery is routinely conducted. These centers typically have the capability to perform high-quality neuroimaging including positron emission tomography (PET), single-photon emission computed tomography (SPECT), anatomic and functional MRI, long-term video–EEG monitoring, intracranial EEG monitoring, and neuropsychological evaluations. By incorporating multiple disciplines including neurology, neurosurgery, neuroscience nursing, psychiatry, neuropsychology, neuroradiology, and social work, specialized epilepsy centers can provide comprehensive evaluations of individuals with epilepsy and develop individualized treatment plans that may or may not include a surgical approach. These centers also are often studying new pharmaceutical agents in refractory epilepsy and may be able to offer therapies not available elsewhere. To this end, the Committee on the Public Health Dimensions of the Epilepsies of the Institute of Medicine recently published a report recommending that patients with medically intractable epilepsy be referred to a tertiary center.

## Conclusion and summary

The evaluation of the patient with medically refractory epilepsy consists of systematic use of the history, examination, laboratory tests, neuroimaging, and EEG to confirm that the patient has epileptic seizures, determine the seizure types, and investigate the etiology of the condition. Selecting the correct AED and optimizing compliance are important to optimizing seizure control. Those who remain uncontrolled despite these efforts should be referred to tertiary epilepsy centers for a comprehensive evaluation and consideration of possible surgical or experimental treatments.

## Acknowledgment

Supported by the Michael J. Pietroniro Research fund.

## Bibliography

Avbersek A, Sisodiya S. Does the primary literature provide support for clinical signs used to distinguish psychogenic nonepileptic seizures from epileptic seizures? *J Neurol Neurosurg Psychiatry* 2010; **81**:719–725.

Bajacek M, Hovorka J, Nezadal T, Nemcova I, Herman E. Is pseudo-intractability in population of patients with epilepsy still alive in the 21st century? Audit of 100 seizure-free patients, referred with the diagnosis of pharmacoresistant epilepsy. *Neuro Endocrinol Lett* 2010; **31**:818–822.

Berg AT, Langfitt J, Shinnar S, et al. How long does it take for partial epilepsy to become intractable? *Neurology* 2003; **60**:186–190.

Chemmanam T, Radhakrishnan A, Sarma SP, Radhakrishnan K. A prospective study on the cost-effective utilization of long-term inpatient video-EEG monitoring in a developing country. *J Clin Neurophysiol* 2009; **26**:123–128.

Committee on the Public Health Dimensions of the Epilepsies, Board on Health Sciences Policy, Institute of Medicine. *Epilepsy Across the*

*Spectrum: Promoting Health and Understanding.* Washington, DC: The National Academies Press, 2012.

Engel J, Jr, Wiebe S, French J, et al. Practice parameter: Temporal lobe and localized neocortical resections for epilepsy: Report of the Quality Standards Subcommittee of the American Academy of Neurology, in association with the American Epilepsy Society and the American Association of Neurological Surgeons. *Neurology* 2003; **60**:538–547.

Fisher RS, Vickrey BG, Gibson P, et al. The impact of epilepsy from the patient's perspective I. Descriptions and subjective perceptions. *Epilepsy Res* 2000; **41**:39–51.

Fisher RS, Vickrey BG, Gibson P, et al. The impact of epilepsy from the patient's perspective II. Views about therapy and health care. *Epilepsy Res* 2000; **41**:53–61.

Gaillard WD, Chiron C, Cross JH, et al. Guidelines for imaging infants and children with recent-onset epilepsy. *Epilepsia* 2009; **50**:2147–2153.

Kwan P, Brodie MJ. Early identification of refractory epilepsy. *N Engl J Med* 2000; **342**:314–319.

Pearl PL, Capp PK, Novotny EJ, Gibson KM. Inherited disorders of neurotransmitters in children and adults. *Clin Biochem* 2005; **38**:1051–1058.

Schmitt B, Baumgartner M, Mills PB, et al. Seizures and paroxysmal events: Symptoms pointing to the diagnosis of pyridoxine-dependent epilepsy and pyridoxine phosphate oxidase deficiency. *Dev Med Child Neurol* 2010; **52**:e133–e142.

Skjei KL, Dlugos DJ. The evaluation of treatment-resistant epilepsy. *Semin Pediatr Neurol* 2011; **18**:150–170.

Wiebe S, Blume WT, Girvin JP, Eliasziw M. A randomized, controlled trial of surgery for temporal-lobe epilepsy. *N Engl J Med* 2001; **345**:311–318.

# Part III

# Using Antiepileptic Medications

# Choosing, Initiating, Adjusting, and Changing Antiepileptic Medications

**John W. Miller**

Departments of Neurology and Neurological Surgery, University of Washington, Seattle, WA, USA

UW Regional Epilepsy Center, Harborview Medical Center, Seattle, WA, USA

Optimal use of antiepileptic drugs (AEDs) is one of the most challenging tasks in clinical neurology because the epilepsies are exceedingly heterogeneous as to etiology, natural history, and response to treatment. It is an advantage that many different agents are available, but this makes the clinician's task of choosing and using these drugs more complex. A rational, stepwise approach is required.

## When to start AEDs

After a first seizure, the decision to initiate medications is based on the risk of future seizures. This risk depends on the circumstances of the seizure and the results of diagnostic testing (Chapter 4). The 10-year risk of a subsequent spontaneous seizure is 19% after an acute symptomatic seizure due to traumatic brain injury, stroke, or CNS infection, but the risk is more than three times higher after a first spontaneous unprovoked seizure. Among those with a first unprovoked seizure, predictors of a higher risk of recurrence are evidence of a possible causal neurological condition (remote symptomatic seizure), status epilepticus, or generalized spike-and-wave activity on EEG. Risk of recurrence is even higher after multiple seizures, with about 75% of those with two or three unprovoked seizures having further seizures within 4 years. The most

common approach is not to start long-term AEDs after acute symptomatic seizures or a single unprovoked seizure in patients without status epilepticus and with normal MRI and EEG, but to do so after a remote symptomatic seizure or any recurrent unprovoked seizures.

## Choosing the AED

If AEDs are prescribed, the goal is a medication that is rapidly effective and without adverse effects, although this certainly cannot always be achieved in the initial medication trial. Available agents and their indications are given in Table 19.1 of Chapter 19.

---

### ☆ TIPS AND TRICKS

There are two key steps to choosing an AED to initiate:

1. Assembling a list of agents with the highest probability of efficacy for the patient's epilepsy syndrome
2. Choosing the safest agent on this list with the lowest chance of adverse effects concerning for the patient's situation and medical comorbidity

---

*Epilepsy*, First Edition. Edited by John W. Miller and Howard P. Goodkin.
© 2014 John Wiley & Sons, Ltd. Published 2014 by John Wiley & Sons, Ltd.

**Table 11.1.** The author's suggested lists of preferred AEDs for focal and generalized epilepsy, current in 2014.

| Focal and secondarily generalized epilepsy | Generalized epilepsy |
| --- | --- |
| Carbamazepine | Acetazolamide (adjunctive) |
| Eslicarbazepine acetate | Clonazepam[a] |
| Lacosamide | Clobazam (adjunctive) |
| Lamotrigine[a] | Ethosuximide (absence seizures only) |
| Levetiracetam | Lamotrigine[a,b] |
| Oxcarbazepine[a] | Levetiracetam[b] |
| Phenytoin | Topiramate[a,b] |
| Pregabalin | Valproate[a,b] |
| Topiramate[a] | Zonisamide |
| Zonisamide | |

[a]FDA approved specifically for monotherapy in at least some situations.
[b]FDA approved for at least some seizure types in generalized epilepsy.

## Identifying potentially effective agents

The list of possibly effective AEDs is determined by the epilepsy syndrome. It is important to determine whether the patient has a focal epilepsy, with focal seizures and secondarily generalized convulsions, or a generalized epilepsy, with seizures that are bilateral (generalized) at their onset, such as absence, myoclonic, and some generalized convulsions. This distinction is important primarily because certain AEDs are known to exacerbate some generalized seizure types, especially myoclonic or absence seizures, and so are typically avoided in generalized epilepsy. This phenomenon is best documented for carbamazepine, oxcarbazepine, gabapentin, pregabalin, tiagabine, and, in occasional cases, lamotrigine and phenytoin. There is inadequate information on use in generalized epilepsy of the most recently released agents – lacosamide, ezogabine, and perampanel. On the other hand, there is evidence from a randomized study that valproate may be less effective than carbamazepine for complex partial seizures. These points, taken together with safety and adverse effect considerations, lead to preferred (but not exhaustive) lists of AEDs for focal and generalized epilepsy available at

the time of publication of this book (Table 11.1). The most recently approved agents, ezogabine and perampanel, are not included, as their role in clinical practice is still being determined. It should be noted that the US FDA has not specifically approved the generalized epilepsy indication for many AEDs. Also, many agents commonly used in monotherapy are not specifically FDA approved for this purpose, although older agents may be "grandfathered in."

Treatment differs in special pediatric syndromes and situations. The most common initial agent for neonatal seizures is phenobarbital (Chapter 20), while infantile spasms in West syndrome are often treated with ACTH, high-dose corticosteroids, or vigabatrin (Chapter 21). Lennox–Gastaut syndrome is most commonly treated with valproate, lamotrigine, topiramate, rufinamide, clobazam, or felbamate (Chapter 21).

## Comparing efficacy

Table 11.1 is based on clinical experience and opinion, but is there objective evidence that individual agents from the lists in Table 11.1 are more effective? Because of the difficulty and expense of designing and carrying out meaningful blinded randomized controlled trials comparing efficacy, level 1 evidence is sparse. Two VA cooperative studies found carbamazepine and phenytoin more effective than pyrimidine and phenobarbital, likely due to tolerance issues, and carbamazepine more effective than valproate for controlling complex partial seizures. The combined results of several randomized trials comparing carbamazepine and lamotrigine suggest that lamotrigine is better tolerated but similar in efficacy. A recent prospective trial comparing valproate, lamotrigine, and ethosuximide for new-onset childhood absence epilepsy demonstrated that lamotrigine is less efficacious than the other two but that ethosuximide is better tolerated than valproate. Therefore, in most situations, the choice among medications on the lists in Table 11.1 will not be based on comparative efficacy, but on other issues.

## Safety and adverse effect concerns determine the final choice

Safety (Chapter 12) trumps all other concerns. Since felbamate is associated with risk of aplastic anemia or liver failure and vigabatrin with irreversible retinopathy, these agents are at the bottom of the medication choice list. Recently, an association between chronic ezogabine exposure and blue discoloration of lips, nail beds, and skin, as well as retinal pigmentary changes, has also been reported. The most common safety issue with AEDs is allergy (Table 11.2). Lamotrigine, carbamazepine, phenytoin, and phenobarbital are agents associated with higher risk of allergy, and a history of allergy to one of these increases the risk of a reaction to the others. Patients with a history of sulfa allergy may be at higher risk of allergy to zonisamide. Rapid introduction of lamotrigine and phenytoin has been demonstrated to increase the risk of allergic reaction. Possible allergic reactions to AEDs include maculopapular eruption and hypersensitivity syndrome, defined as a rash accompanied by multiorgan involvement, such as hepatitis and nephritis, fever, and arthralgias. The most serious reactions are

Stevens–Johnson syndrome and toxic epidermal necrolysis, which are characterized by a blistering exanthema with mucosal involvement and skin detachment and have potential mortality.

### SCIENCE REVISITED

The *HLA-B\*1502* allele, present in some Asian populations, particularly Han Chinese, is associated with a higher risk of Stevens–Johnson syndrome and toxic epidermal necrolysis on exposure to carbamazepine and likely structurally related AEDs such as phenytoin, oxcarbazepine, and lamotrigine. Screening for this allele should be done before starting these agents in patients at risk.

**Table 11.2.** Choice of AEDs as a function of comorbidity and circumstances.

| Comorbidity or situation | Preferred AEDs | AEDs to avoid if possible |
|---|---|---|
| Depression | Lamotrigine | Levetiracetam, phenobarbital, topiramate, zonisamide |
| Bipolar disorder | Carbamazepine,[a] lamotrigine,[a] oxcarbazepine, valproate[a] | |
| Migraine | Topiramate,[a] valproate[a] | |
| Obesity/metabolic syndrome | Felbamate, topiramate, zonisamide | Gabapentin, pregabalin, valproate |
| Pediatric population | | Phenytoin, valproate |
| Women of childbearing age | Lamotrigine | Phenobarbital, phenytoin, topiramate, valproate |
| Use of oral contraceptives | Gabapentin, lacosamide, levetiracetam, pregabalin, tiagabine, zonisamide | Carbamazepine, felbamate, lamotrigine, oxcarbazepine, perampanel, phenobarbital, phenytoin, primidone, topiramate |
| Geriatric populations | Lacosamide, lamotrigine, pregabalin | Carbamazepine, oxcarbazepine, phenobarbital, topiramate |
| History of nephrolithiasis | | Acetazolamide, topiramate, zonisamide |
| History of allergy | Lacosamide, levetiracetam, pregabalin, topiramate | Carbamazepine, lamotrigine, phenytoin, zonisamide (depending on prior allergy history) |
| Chronic pain | Carbamazepine,[a] gabapentin, lacosamide, oxcarbazepine, pregabalin,[a] topiramate | |
| Use of warfarin | | Carbamazepine, phenobarbital, phenytoin, primidone |

[a]FDA approved for treatment of listed comorbidity.

Antiepileptic drugs that are carbonic anhydrase inhibitors (Table 11.2) have a risk of nephrolithiasis, particularly calcium phosphate stones, and should be used with caution in patients with a history of renal stones.

Antiepileptic drug safety during pregnancy is an important issue, discussed in detail in Chapter 25. Since pregnancy may be unplanned, and most serious fetal malformations develop in the first trimester, often before pregnancy is reported, drugs with serious teratogenic risk should be avoided in women of childbearing age whenever possible. Higher-risk agents (pregnancy class D) to be avoided if possible include phenobarbital, phenytoin, topiramate, and especially valproate. Lamotrigine has the best current evidence for safety in pregnancy, although concern about increased risk of cleft palate has been raised.

> ⚠ **CAUTION!**
>
> Valproate and divalproex should be avoided in woman of childbearing age because fetal exposure to these agents is associated with a 21% risk of major malformations and a lower mean IQ of the child.

Consideration of possible adverse effects (Chapters 12 and 19) usually determines final choice. The most common adverse effects of concern are mood changes, impaired concentration, and sedation. AEDs are associated with depression, and the US FDA has issued a warning of an increased risk of suicide with all of them. However, clinical experience is that risk of depression varies considerably among agents. Lamotrigine generally has the lowest risk of depression, as well as less sedation and cognitive impairment. However, its value as initial therapy is limited because it must be introduced slowly over 8 weeks or longer to reduce the risk of rash.

Concerns about particular adverse effects are greatly affected by the specific situation and the presence of other medical problems (Table 11.2). For example, an overweight patient with type 2 diabetes mellitus might do better on an AED associated with weight loss. If topiramate or valproate is an appropriate agent for an individual's epilepsy, it might also provide prophylaxis for migraine. Age is also important. Valproate has a risk of hepatic failure in infants, but this is very rare in adults. Children and adolescents are particularly prone to cosmetic adverse effects from phenytoin. Geriatric patients may be less tolerant of cognitive adverse effects from agents such as phenobarbital and topiramate and have a higher risk of developing hyponatremia with carbamazepine and especially oxcarbazepine. All of these issues (Table 11.2) must be taken into account when choosing the AED with the lowest chance of unacceptable adverse effects for a particular patient.

## Other factors influencing drug choice

Drug interactions are varied (Chapter 13) but can occasionally be a major concern. The most common culprits are AEDs causing induction of the hepatic cytochrome P450 enzymes, such as carbamazepine, phenytoin, and phenobarbital, which not only can lower the level of other AEDs that are metabolized by these enzymes but can also reduce the efficacy of anticoagulation with warfarin and increase the risk of failure of oral contraceptives. Other drugs such as omeprazole or rifampin also induce this hepatic system and affect AED levels.

> ⚠ **CAUTION!**
>
> Many oral contraceptives result in lowering of lamotrigine levels and an increased risk of seizures.

When patients present with new-onset acute repetitive or prolonged seizures in the emergency department or hospital, rapid control is imperative. This situation requires the use of AEDs that can be loaded to a therapeutic serum level, especially those that can be given intravenously, such as phenobarbital, phenytoin, valproate, levetiracetam, or lacosamide. Parenteral administration of AEDs is discussed in Chapter 18.

Ease of use is not just a matter of convenience for the provider but an aid to compliance. Simple instructions, shorter titration schedules, and a lower risk of safety issues or severe adverse effects all increase the chance that the planned regimen will be achieved. Cost is an even more important factor. It is important to be familiar with the approximate cost of drugs you prescribe. Patients may not volunteer their financial situation, so particularly in the USA, it is important to inquire about their prescription drug insurance coverage. After all, if

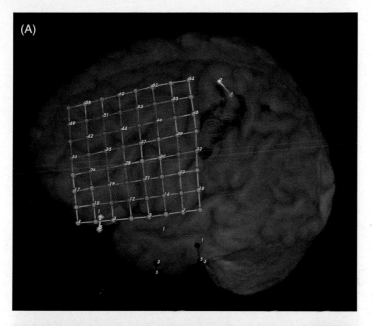

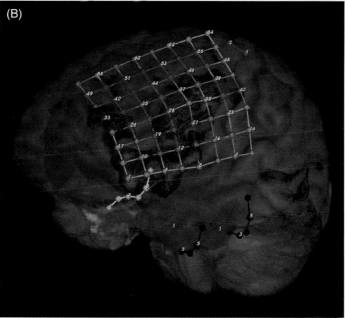

**Figure 8.2.** Multimodal imaging for intracranial EEG planning in a patient with nonlesional epilepsy originating from the language-dominant left frontal lobe. The images were obtained both preoperatively and postoperatively after intracranial electrode placement and registered to the same coordinate system. The preoperative co-registered images were used with an image-guided surgical system for electrode placement. (A) Task-based fMRI of right-hand sensorimotor activation registered to 3D T1-weighted MRI with left frontotemporal grid (from postoperative CT scan); (B) task-based fMRI of language activation registered to 3D T1-weighted MRI with left frontotemporal grid and lateral frontal, frontopolar, anterior, and midtemporal strips (from postoperative CT scan).

*Epilepsy*, First Edition. Edited by John W. Miller and Howard P. Goodkin.
© 2014 John Wiley & Sons, Ltd. Published 2014 by John Wiley & Sons, Ltd.

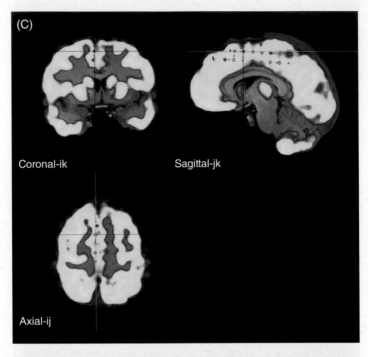

Coronal-ik    Sagittal-jk

Axial-ij

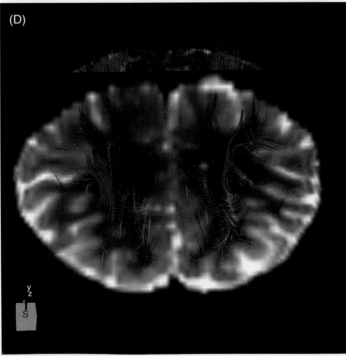

**Figure 8.2.** (*Continued*) (C) FDG-PET registered to 3D T1-weighted MRI with location of left frontal interhemispheric, 16-contact strip (from postoperative CT scan); (D) diffusion tractography of major tracts in frontal regions in same subject.

the drug regimen is tolerated and controls seizures, the patient will likely need to be able to obtain the drug – without interruption – for years to come.

> ✋ **CAUTION!**
>
> Don't expect patients to take medications that they cannot afford.

The issue of generic substitution is critically relevant to these financial issues because generic products often are much less expensive than the brand-name ones. However, it has been questioned whether generics produce results in clinical practice similar to those of brand-name agents. Although this subject is controversial, there are no adequate randomized studies that demonstrate a meaningful difference in clinical response between brand-name and generic products. This absence of trials is not surprising, because generics are not really a class of medications at all, but rather a collection of different products that might potentially differ somewhat in their bioavailability and absorption properties from each other and from the brand-name product. The best information on this issue comes from assessment of the US FDA's own bioequivalence data on approved generic and brand AEDs. The overall drug delivered per dose differed between brand and generic formulations by less than 10% in 83% of comparisons and by more than 15% in only 1 of 595 comparisons. There was more variability in the rate of absorption and the peak concentrations after dosing these agents. Peak concentrations differed by 15–25% in 11% of comparisons. These data suggest that transitions between different generic products, rather than brand to generic substitutions, are more likely to cause greater changes in AED level and that the most common problem to look out for with substitutions would be the emergence of adverse effects at times of peak concentrations in patients that already have high AED levels. The variation was highest for oxcarbazepine, and indeed, formulation of products with consistent bioavailability would be expected to be most challenging for AEDs that have poor water solubility, such as oxcarbazepine, carbamazepine, and phenytoin. It would be expected that highly water-soluble agents, such as levetiracetam, lamotrigine, topiramate, valproate, zonisamide, and pregabalin, would be easier to formulate consistently.

A rational approach would be to use generic products initially and change to brand-name preparations only if problems arise that might be attributable to substitution. The author's clinical experience with this approach is that it is actually uncommon for a change to brand-name formulation to lead to seizure control when the generic product has failed. An alternative in this situation would be for patients to work with their pharmacists to ensure that they receive a specific generic product to avoid generic-to-generic substitution.

## Initiating the AED

While it is sometimes necessary to give a loading dose of AEDs for acute seizures, when treatment is less urgent, it is preferable to gradually titrate the dose so that it will be better tolerated. One should establish a target goal of a moderate dose of the agent, one that has a reasonable possibility of being tolerated and effective. The titration schedule should be given in writing and involve simple steps at weekly intervals. Common adverse effects should be explained and the patient, family, and/or caregivers instructed how to keep a log recording occurrence of seizures or troublesome adverse effects. They should be encouraged to call your office should these occur. A follow-up visit to assess medication response and plan any needed further dose adjustments should be scheduled.

> ☆ **TIPS AND TRICKS**
>
> Rapid initiation of AEDs increases early adverse effects. This may decrease the chance the patient will comply with the prescribed regimen.

An example of how an AED is started would be introduction of an agent currently in common use, levetiracetam, in an adult patient with new-onset epilepsy. The risk of sedation with this agent is reduced with a titration schedule of 250 mg at night for the first week, then 250 mg twice a day for the second week, then 250 mg in the morning and 500 mg at night for the third week, followed by 500 mg twice a week. This moderate dose is often effective and more likely to be tolerated. The patient should be warned of the more common adverse effects, particularly mood changes such as depression or irritability. If the patient calls because of seizures or adverse effects, the dose can be adjusted over the phone, and this can also occur at a follow-up visit in 8–12 weeks.

## Optimizing compliance

Successful medical treatment of epilepsy involves not only finding the right AED but also ensuring that it is taken faithfully, because even an occasional missed dose may lead to seizures. The first step in increasing compliance is enlisting the trust and cooperation of the patient, family, and/or caregivers with a frank and clear discussion about the consequences of uncontrolled seizures, including activity limitations and risks of disability, morbidity, and mortality (Chapters 33 and 34). The proposed medication trial should be reviewed; this conversation should include why the agent was chosen, safety issues, possible adverse effects, and the possibility that it might not control the seizures. Future treatment options if the medication doesn't work out should also be discussed.

Instructions should be in writing and as simple as possible. Agents with once or twice daily dosing (Chapter 19) should be used whenever possible, as noncompliance is higher with more frequent dosing. Dosing times can be cued to consistent daily activities such as meals. Cell phone or wristwatch alarms are also useful reminders. For patients without adequate caregiver support that are unable to follow the dosing regimen, the pharmacist should be enlisted to organize the doses in blister packs.

### ☆ TIPS AND TRICKS

The use of a weekly pill holder for all medication doses allows detection of missed doses and nearly eliminates the risk of double dosing.

Despite such measures, some patients will nonetheless have seizures related to noncompliance. AED serum levels may not detect this, because individuals may be more compliant when they know that a level will be drawn. The clinician needs to calmly discuss and rediscuss the consequences of missed medications in a non-accusatory fashion in the hope that recurrent seizures will eventually persuade the patient of the benefits of taking medication correctly.

## Adjusting the dose

Dose adjustment is needed when adverse effects occur or when seizures happen that are not explained by missed doses or precipitating factors such as ethanol abuse. If adverse effects are mild and dose related, small dose adjustments may be sufficient. On the other hand, if seizures are the issue, repeated small increases in dose may lead to a prolonged period of inadequate seizure control. In that situation, it is appropriate to implement a schedule to titrate the AED to a high dose, or to the maximal tolerated dose, defined as the highest dose that doesn't cause significant adverse effects.

Serum AED levels can be particularly useful for monitoring compliance, adjusting medication levels during pregnancy, dealing with drug interactions, and monitoring phenytoin, which has tricky nonlinear pharmacokinetics. However, AEDs must be assessed and adjusted primarily on their clinical effects – seizure control and adverse effects – not on levels. In a patient with good seizure control without adverse effects, it is inappropriate to adjust AED dosage solely based on serum levels.

## When and how to try other AEDs

If the first AED produces unacceptable adverse effects at low doses or is ineffective at high doses or doses with significant adverse effects, it is time to transition to another agent. One way to do this is the crossover, where the first agent is progressively tapered as the second is titrated so that after a number of weeks, the patient is on monotherapy with the second agent. The other approach is the add-on, where the second agent is titrated up while the first agent continues, perhaps with a slight reduction in its dose to reduce the possibility of adverse effects. This method leaves the tapering of the first agent to a later date, after the efficacy of the second drug has been assessed.

### ☆ TIPS AND TRICKS

When possible, change only one drug at a time in a medication trial. This makes it easier to judge the cause of adverse effects or changes in seizure control.

The process of changing medications ultimately requires a decision about whether to attempt monotherapy or to allow the patient to remain on a drug combination. There are real advantages to monotherapy, even though many AEDs are not approved for it by the FDA. Monotherapy reduces adverse effects and eliminates pharmacokinetic and pharmacodynamic drug interactions between AEDs. However, there are situations where patients remain on two drugs because of worsening seizure control with tapering of the initial agent. Nonetheless, there is little evidence that combinations of more than two AEDs improve seizure control.

## Drug-resistant epilepsy

Almost one-half of patients with new-onset epilepsy are controlled with the first AED tried, but only two-thirds are ultimately controlled by any AEDs. Furthermore, if the first two AEDs are tolerated but fail because of the lack of efficacy, the chances of achieving seizure freedom with further medication are low, so at that point the next step most often should be further diagnostic evaluation rather than additional medication trials (Chapter 10).

### ✴ TIPS AND TRICKS

Epilepsy is considered drug resistant after the failure of two tolerated, appropriately chosen and used antiepileptic medications to produce sustained seizure freedom. In this situation, consider referral to an epilepsy specialist and possible video–EEG monitoring to confirm the diagnosis and the epilepsy syndrome and determine candidacy for surgical treatment if appropriate.

## Conclusions

This chapter demonstrates the complexity of using AEDs. Although safety issues are limited, adverse effects are common and varied. The initial agent tried often is not adequately effective or tolerated, so multiple serial drug trials are not unusual. For clinicians who treat epilepsy, mastery of a single drug is inadequate. Rather, a systematic approach that utilizes different agents in different situations is necessary.

## References

Anderson, GD. Understanding the ramifications of switching among AEDS: What are the data? *Adv Stud Med* 2008; **8**:229–234.

Cramer JA. Optimizing long-term patient compliance. *Neurology* 1995; **45** (suppl. 1):S25–S28.

Gamble C, Williamson PR, Chadwick DW, Marson AG. A meta-analysis of individual patient responses to lamotrigine or carbamazepine monotherapy. *Neurology* 2006; **66**:1310–1317.

Glauser TA, Ben-Menachem E, Bourgeois B, et al. ILAE treatment guidelines: Evidence-based analysis of antiepileptic drug efficacy and effectiveness as initial monotherapy for epileptic seizures and syndromes. *Epilepsia* 2006; **47**:1094–1120.

Glauser TA, Cnaan A, Shinnar S, et al. Ethosuximide, valproic acid, and lamotrigine in childhood absence epilepsy. *N Engl J Med* 2010; **362**:790–799.

Hauser WA, Rich SS, Annegers JF, Anderson VE. Seizure recurrence after a 1st unprovoked seizure: An extended follow-up. *Neurology* 1990; **40**: 1163–1170.

Hauser WA, Rich SS, Lee JR, Annegers JF, Anderson VE. Risk of recurrent seizures after two unprovoked seizures. *N Engl J Med* 1998; **338**:429–434.

Hesdorffer DC, Benn EKT, Cascino GD, Hauser WA. Is a first acute symptomatic seizure epilepsy? Mortality and risk for recurrent seizure. *Epilepsia* 2009: **50**:1102–1108.

Krauss GL, Caffo B, Chang YT, Hendrix CW, Chuang K. Assessing bioequivalence of generic antiepilepsy drugs. *Ann Neurol* 201; **70**:221–228.

Kwan P, Brodie MJ. Early identification of refractory epilepsy. *N Engl J Med* 2000; **342**(5):314–319.

Mattson RH, Cramer JA, Collins JF, et al. Comparison of carbamazepine, phenobarbital, phenytoin, and primidone in partial and secondarily generalized tonic-clonic seizures. *N Engl J Med* 1985; **313**:145–151.

Mattson RH, Cramer JA, Collins JF. Prognosis for total control of complex partial and secondarily generalized tonic clonic seizures. Department of Veterans Affairs Epilepsy Cooperative Studies No. 118 and No. 264 Group. *Neurology* 1996; **47**:68–76.

Meador KJ, Baker GA, Browning N, et al. Cognitive function at 3 years of age after fetal exposure to antiepileptic drugs. *N Engl J Med* 2009; **360**:1597–1605.

# Antiepileptic Drug Adverse Effects: What to Watch Out For

**Jacquelyn L. Bainbridge[1] and Caleb Y. Oh[2]**

[1]Departments of Clinical Pharmacy and Neurology, University of Colorado Skaggs School of Pharmacy and Pharmaceutical Sciences and School of Medicine, Anschutz Medical Campus, Aurora, CO, USA
[2]Department of Clinical Pharmacy, University of Colorado Skaggs School of Pharmacy and Pharmaceutical Sciences, Anschutz Medical Campus, Aurora, CO, USA

## Introduction

Adverse effects can occur with any drug but are particularly common with antiepileptic drugs (AEDs). They occur in as many as 88% of surveyed patients. Most *pharmacological adverse reactions* are typically dose dependent and often occur during introduction of the medication. Pharmacological adverse reactions sometimes correlate with higher serum drug levels and resolve when the dose is reduced. *Idiosyncratic adverse reactions* to AEDs are rare, not related to the agent's pharmacology, do not show an obvious relationship with the dose, and may not resolve with removal of the drug. These idiosyncratic events cannot be prevented by monitoring serum levels or other blood tests. This chapter outlines the pharmacological and idiosyncratic adverse effects of AEDs (Table 12.1) that one must be familiar with to optimally manage these medications.

## Common adverse effects

### Neurological

The most common central nervous system (CNS) pharmacological adverse effects are sedation and fatigue. However, a few AEDs, particularly felbamate and lamotrigine, are associated with insomnia and disturbed sleep. Other common CNS side effects are dizziness, visual distortion, eye movement abnormalities, tremor, ataxia, cognitive impairment, and headaches. These effects can be bothersome and lead to poor medication compliance, discontinuation, or failure to reach effective dosing. Slow dose escalation when introducing an agent or lowering the dose and reescalating more slowly over time may reduce these complaints.

> **⚠ CAUTION!**
>
> Although many AEDs are thought to be sedating, some patients, especially young children and the elderly, will experience paradoxical hyperactivity.

Dizziness is particularly common in agents with a primary mechanism of sodium channel blockade. Often, this is a peak-dose effect, occurring an hour or two after the drug is taken. Visual distortions such as diplopia, trailing vision, and blurred vision are common complaints with carbamazepine, oxcarbazepine, and lamotrigine that also correlate with peak levels.

Common ocular side effects include nystagmus and saccadic intrusions during smooth pursuit. The saccadic intrusions are rarely perceived by the patients and can be used as a simple measure on examination to screen for adherence. On the other

**Table 12.1.** Pharmacological and idiosyncratic adverse effects of AEDs.

| Drug | Pregnancy category[a] | Common concentration-dependent adverse events | Less common adverse events |
|------|-----------|-----------------------------------|----------------------|
| Carbamazepine | D | Tremor, myoclonus, sexual dysfunction, diplopia, risk of osteopenia/osteoporosis, hyponatremia | Life-threatening rash, leukopenia, cardiotoxicity, agranulocytosis, aplastic anemia |
| Clobazam | C | Somnolence, lethargy, aggressive behavior | |
| Ethosuximide | C | Nightmares, sedation, hiccups, nausea, vomiting, headaches | Aplastic anemia, life-threatening rash, systemic lupus erythematosus-like syndrome |
| Ezogabine | C | Dizziness, somnolence, fatigue, confusion, vertigo, tremor, diplopia, attention/memory impairment | Urinary retention, QT prolongation, retinal pigmentary changes, blue discoloration of skin, lips, and nail beds |
| Felbamate | C | Insomnia, weight loss, headache, nausea | Aplastic anemia, hepatic failure, blood dyscrasias |
| Fosphenytoin | D | Same as phenytoin | Same as phenytoin |
| Gabapentin | C | Myoclonus, pedal edema, irritability, dizziness, weight gain | Life-threatening rash |
| Lacosamide | C | Dizziness, headache, nausea, diplopia, irritability | PR-interval increase (minimal), life-threatening rash |
| Lamotrigine | C | Diplopia, dizziness, insomnia, headache, nonspecific rash | Life-threatening rash |
| Levetiracetam | C | Sedation, behavioral changes, irritability, depression, aggression | Suicidal ideation |
| Oxcarbazepine | C | Dizziness, visual distortion, risk of osteopenia/osteoporosis, diplopia, hyponatremia | Life-threatening rash |
| Perampanel | C | Hostility, aggression, dizziness, sleepiness, fatigue | Suicidal ideation, homicidal ideation |
| Phenobarbital | D | Erectile dysfunction, sedation, risk of osteopenia/osteoporosis, cognitive impairment, hyperactivity | Connective tissue disorder, life-threatening rash |
| Phenytoin | D | Ataxia, nystagmus, risk of osteopenia/osteoporosis, dizziness, sedation, gingival hyperplasia | Systemic lupus erythematosus-like syndrome, life-threatening rash |
| Pregabalin | C | Same as gabapentin | Same as gabapentin |
| Primidone | D | Same as phenobarbital | Same as phenobarbital |
| Rufinamide | C | Headache, somnolence, rash | Shortened QT interval, drug hypersensitivity |

*(Continued)*

**Table 12.1.** (*Continued*)

| Drug | Pregnancy category[a] | Common concentration-dependent adverse events | Less common adverse events |
|---|---|---|---|
| Tiagabine | C | Myoclonus, decreased concentration, somnolence, weakness, tremor | Encephalopathy, status epilepticus |
| Topiramate | D | Somnolence, word-finding difficulties, anorexia, paresthesias, weight loss | Renal stones, glaucoma, metabolic acidosis, oligohidrosis |
| Valproic acid | D | Tremor, pedal edema, hair loss, weight gain, mood changes, confusion | Encephalopathy, hyperammonemia, pancreatitis, hepatotoxicity (highest in patients younger than 2 years on multiple AEDs), parkinsonism, middle ear dysfunction (elderly patients) |
| Vigabatrin | C | Drowsiness, fatigue, hyperactivity, nystagmus, tremor, blurred vision, weight gain | Irreversible visual field defects |
| Zonisamide | C | Somnolence, dizziness, anorexia, rash, paresthesias, weight loss | Renal stones, metabolic acidosis, oligohidrosis, psychosis, life-threatening rash |

[a] Pregnancy category C: risk cannot be ruled out because of inadequate well-controlled human studies. Animal studies have shown a risk to the fetus. Consideration of risks and benefits of therapy should be assessed before beginning therapy. Pregnancy category D: positive evidence of human fetal risk. FDA Drug Category Ratings. American Pregnancy Association. Last updated: June 2006. Available at www.americanpregnancy.org/pregnancyhealth/fdadrugratings.html.

hand, nystagmus may affect vision and require a dose reduction. Similarly, tremor and gait ataxia may interfere with activities of daily living and often lead to a decrease in dose.

Cognitive dysfunction can occur with any AED but is commonly associated with barbiturates, topiramate, and zonisamide. Polypharmacy can also increase the risk of cognitive dysfunction as well. Complaints often include difficulties with verbal expression or word finding, mental slowing, and poor concentration. These complaints are often dose related and can be more problematic in those over 60 years of age. AED overdose can lead to encephalopathy. Rarely, there may be specific AED-mediated mechanisms contributing to a stuporous state, such as valproate-induced hyperammonemia or tiagabine-related nonconvulsive status epilepticus.

★ **TIPS AND TRICKS**

When adding an AED to existing therapy, it is important to consider the total burden of all medications, because CNS adverse effects can be additive. When a new CNS adverse effect is precipitated, many practitioners will decrease or discontinue the most recently added drug. However, in some cases, the adverse effect will abate with reduction or removal of one of the original medications (e.g., when lacosamide has been added to sodium channel–blocking drugs).

**Psychiatric**

Adverse effects of AEDs on mood and behavior are major determinants of quality of life. These effects may range from mild irritability to psychosis, but the most common issue is depression. Levetiracetam is an agent currently in wide use that is more likely to have adverse effects on mood than other AEDs. On the other hand, euphoria has been seen with lacosamide and pregabalin. Homicidal ideation has been reported with higher doses of perampanel in clinical trials.

---

### ★ TIPS AND TRICKS

Valproate, carbamazepine, oxcarbazepine, and lamotrigine may have mood-stabilizing effects that can be beneficial in bipolar I disorder. Lamotrigine is less likely to cause depression and may reduce depression in some individuals.

---

Starting at high doses and escalating too quickly increases the risk of mood and behavioral adverse effects with several AEDs but is more of a concern with topiramate. Caution should be used in those with preexisting psychiatric disorders. Antidepressants may be helpful even when depressive adverse effects occur in those without preexisting mood disorders. Psychiatric disorders in epilepsy and their associations with AED use are discussed further in Chapter 37.

---

### ☟ CAUTION!

In 2008, the FDA issued an alert of increased risk of suicide in patients prescribed AEDs. However, the International League Against Epilepsy published an expert consensus stating that an increase in risk of suicidality with AEDs has not been adequately determined but appears to be very low. Providers should be cognizant that patients with epilepsy may be at risk for suicide, but this is multifactorial, and each case must be evaluated individually.

---

### Gastrointestinal

Nausea, vomiting, anorexia, and diarrhea are common adverse effects that sometimes require AED dose reduction or discontinuation. In addition, constipation may occur with several AEDs, such as carbamazepine. Nausea and vomiting may be peak-dose-related adverse effects. Taking AEDs with meals, changing to a time-release AED preparation, or rearranging the dosing regimen into smaller, more frequent doses might help reduce these symptoms.

### Weight change

While weight change is often classified as idiosyncratic, experience with this adverse effect is common with several AEDs and appears to be dose related. Weight gain is most common with valproate and pregabalin but can also occur with carbamazepine, oxcarbazepine, vigabatrin, gabapentin, and clonazepam. Pregabalin, valproate, and gabapentin are also known to cause peripheral edema, which may exacerbate weight gain. In contrast, felbamate, topiramate, and zonisamide are associated with weight loss. Weight change may affect medical comorbidities. The possibility of weight change is of great concern to many patients, and this may strongly influence medication selection.

### Hyponatremia

Hyponatremia may be regarded as idiosyncratic, but it is common with carbamazepine and oxcarbazepine, and in some instances it appears to be dose related. Possible mechanisms are increased sensitization of antidiuretic hormone (ADH) on the distal renal collecting tubules, an altered response by the hypothalamic osmoreceptors affecting serum osmolality, or inappropriate ADH secretion. Treatments may include fluid restriction, eliminating medications (e.g., diuretics) that exacerbate hyponatremia, maintaining adequate sodium intake, or discontinuing the drug. Though direct comparative studies do not exist, hyponatremia appears to be more common with oxcarbazepine than carbamazepine. The risk of hyponatremia increases with age, so many clinicians use oxcarbazepine with caution in elderly patients.

### Osteopenia/osteoporosis

The risk of fractures is increased in epilepsy, and decreased bone mineral density is associated with the use of enzyme-inducing AEDS (e.g., carbamazepine, phenytoin, and phenobarbital) and valproate. Newer AEDs may be more appropriate in patients with known osteopenia or osteoporosis. Screening of bone mineral density with a dual-energy X-ray absorptiometry (DEXA) scan should be considered in high-risk patients. Calcium and vitamin D supplementation is appropriate for patients using enzyme-inducing AEDs. Also, safe weight-bearing exercises should be encouraged.

## Other common adverse effects

Headache is a nonspecific adverse effect of all AEDs. It is most commonly encountered with felbamate, carbamazepine, and lamotrigine but can even occasionally occur with agents used to treat migraine, such as valproate, topiramate, gabapentin, and pregabalin.

Mild morbilliform rashes, distinct from severe allergic reactions, may occur in the first few weeks of treatment with carbamazepine, phenytoin, and lamotrigine and rapidly go away when the agent is stopped. However, these agents may also affect other skin conditions; for example, phenytoin may worsen acne and lamotrigine may exacerbate eczema.

Gingival hyperplasia is a common dose-related adverse effect of phenytoin and may sometimes be averted with proper oral hygiene.

Decreased libido and erectile dysfunction are associated with both epilepsy and AED use. Hepatic enzyme-inducing AEDs such as carbamazepine and phenytoin are associated with increased serum sex hormone-binding globulin and decreased free androgen levels, perhaps contributing to these adverse effects. In addition, enzyme-inducing AEDs are associated with amenorrhea. This can also occur with valproate, as there may be an increased risk of polycystic ovarian syndrome with its use.

## Uncommon and idiosyncratic adverse reactions

### Hypersensitivity reactions

A hypersensitivity reaction is a serious, T-cell-mediated idiosyncratic event that can be triggered by exposure to an AED and requires immediate withdrawal of the agent. This may result in a maculopapular eruption, which occasionally progresses to drug rash with eosinophilia and systemic symptoms (DRESS) with fever, arthralgia, and internal organ (e.g., liver) involvement. Another type of hypersensitivity reaction, Stevens–Johnson syndrome/toxic epidermal necrolysis (SJS/TEN), is characterized by a blistering exanthema with mucosal involvement and skin detachment, with mortality rates that may approach 25%. Its incidence ranges from 1 in 1000 to 1 in 10,000. Carbamazepine, phenytoin, lamotrigine, phenobarbital, oxcarbazepine, and zonisamide have a higher risk of hypersensitivity reactions than other AEDs. These serious allergic responses are most likely to occur within the first 60 days after drug introduction and with rapid initiation of the agent, although this can infrequently occur later in therapy. Slow introduction of lamotrigine over 6–10 weeks is particularly important to reduce the risk of hypersensitivity to that drug.

### ⚖ SCIENCE REVISITED

Idiosyncratic (type B) reactions are rare, unpredictable events. These can result from immune-mediated processes as in the case of hypersensitivity reactions, from reactive cytotoxic metabolites as in the case of the liver toxicity associated with carbamazepine, or from an off-target pharmacological effect such as the precipitation of an attack of acute intermittent porphyria. However, the pathophysiological mechanisms of some idiosyncratic effects are not known.

The risk of SJS/TEN with exposure to carbamazepine is two to three times higher in people of Han Chinese descent than Caucasians. This increased incidence correlates with the presence of the HLA-B*1502 allele, which is found in several Asian racial groups but not in Caucasians. An FDA advisory recommends screening Asians for this allele prior to starting carbamazepine. There is evidence suggesting that such a relationship may also exist for phenytoin, phenobarbital, and lamotrigine.

### ✋ CAUTION!

Patients who have experienced a hypersensitivity reaction to an AED containing an aromatic ring (carbamazepine, lamotrigine, oxcarbazepine, eslicarbazepine, phenytoin, primidone, phenobarbital, lacosamide, rufinamide, perampanel) should be changed to an AED that does not contain an aromatic ring (e.g., pregabalin, levetiracetam, topiramate, or valproate) because of the risk of cross-sensitivity.

### Blood dyscrasias

Serious blood dyscrasias occur in 3–4 out of 100,000 AED prescriptions but are more common in patients over 60 years of age. The most serious one is aplastic anemia, occurring in 1 of 4000 patients exposed to felbamate, rarely with carbamazepine and acetazolamide, and very rarely with phenytoin and valproate. Mild reversible leucopenia can be seen in a minority of patients taking carbamazepine; therefore, it is important to obtain a baseline serum white blood cell count prior to starting therapy. Life-threatening agranulocytosis is rare with carbamazepine and very rare with phenytoin and most other AEDs. Thrombocytopenia is most common and clinically significant with valproate; infrequently platelet counts may fall below 40,000/mm$^3$. Thrombocytopenia may also be seen with carbamazepine, phenytoin, lamotrigine, felbamate, tiagabine, and primidone.

## Hepatotoxicity

Hepatotoxicity may range from mild asymptomatic elevation of transaminases to acute liver failure. AEDs containing an aromatic ring may cause liver injury in the context of allergic hepatitis in DRESS. With valproate exposure, fulminant hepatic failure, which is due to a metabolic mechanism, occurs primarily in children under 2 years of age, with a risk as high as 1 in 500 exposures. The risk is also increased with inborn errors of metabolism or abnormal mitochondrial function. The risk of hepatic failure with felbamate is about 1 in 20,000 exposures. A metabolic or immunological mechanism has been proposed.

## Renal stones

Nephrolithiasis can infrequently occur with the carbonic anhydrase-inhibiting AEDs, topiramate, zonisamide, and acetazolamide, usually with calcium oxalate or calcium phosphate stones. The risk is likely dose dependent and related to systemic metabolic acidosis but may be 1–2% or higher. Avoiding these agents in those with a past history of renal stones and advising patients to maintain adequate fluid intake reduces risk.

## Pancreatitis

Acute pancreatitis is a rare, serious idiosyncratic effect of valproate, presenting with nausea, vomiting, abdominal pain, and elevated amylase. This may be hemorrhagic and occasionally fatal. Patients should not be rechallenged with valproate even after resolution of pancreatitis. A few cases of pancreatitis have also been reported with carbamazepine.

## Ophthalmologic

Vigabatrin has been associated with retinopathy with permanent loss of peripheral vision in about 40% of patients. The risk of peripheral vision loss correlates with cumulative exposure to vigabatrin; therefore, patients on this drug should have regular visual field assessments. Topiramate can occasionally cause reversible secondary angle-closure glaucoma. There is a recent FDA safety alert reporting pigmentary changes in the retina (as well as blue discoloration of the skin, lips, and nail beds) with chronic exposure to ezogabine. Effects on vision are still being assessed.

## Urinary retention

Ezogabine can be associated with urinary retention, possibly due to effects on bladder smooth muscle. Urinary retention usually manifests as hesitancy on urination.

## Cardiac conduction issues

A few AEDs can cause cardiac conduction changes. A mild asymptomatic prolongation of the PR interval may be seen with carbamazepine, lacosamide, eslicarbazepine, or pregabalin. Ezogabine is associated with QT interval prolongation, while QT shortening has been observed with rufinamide. An ECG should be reviewed prior to initiating these agents if there is a known cardiac conduction abnormality or a family history of a cardiac conduction abnormality, or if the patient is taking other agents that affect cardiac conduction.

## Teratogenicity and neurodevelopmental adverse effects

While no AED has been demonstrated to be free of risk of teratogenicity, the agent of gravest concern is valproate. It is associated with a 21% risk of major malformations and a reduction in the IQ of the offspring, as measured in childhood. If at all possible, this agent should be avoided in women of childbearing age. All women of this age on AEDs should receive supplemental folic acid because it decreases the risk of neural tube defects, although it has not been proven to reduce other birth defects. Please see Chapter 25 for an extensive review of the teratogenic effects of AEDs as well as other adverse effect issues specific to women.

## Conclusion

The choice of an AED is governed as much by potential adverse effects as by its chance of controlling seizures. Patients need to be informed of the common adverse effects of the agent they will take as well as any possible dangerous idiosyncratic reactions. Slow and careful dose escalation will reduce the risks of many pharmacological adverse effects. Nonetheless, adverse effects are a common pitfall on the path to a stable, effective, tolerated treatment regimen.

## Acknowledgements

The authors would like to acknowledge Lisa Hong, Pharm.D. candidate, and Karrine D. Roberts, Pharm.D. candidate, for their written and editorial contributions to this chapter. Additionally, the authors would like to acknowledge Jennifer M. Rother, Pharm.D. candidate, and John Shin, Pharm.D. candidate, for their editorial contributions.

## Bibliography

Baker GA, Jacoby A, Buck D, Stalgis C, Monnet D. Quality of life of people with epilepsy: A European study. *Epilepsia* 1997; **38**(3):353–362.

Blackburn SC, Oliart AD, García Rodríguez LA, Pérez Gutthann S. Antiepileptics and blood dyscrasias: A cohort study. *Pharmacotherapy* 1998; **18**(6):1277–1283.

Brent RL. Environmental causes of human congenital malformations: The pediatrician's role in dealing with these complex clinical problems caused by a multiplicity of environmental and genetic factors. *Pediatrics* 2004; **113**(4 Suppl.):957–968.

Eddy CM, Rickards HE, Cavanna AE. Behavioral adverse effects of antiepileptic drugs in epilepsy. *J Clin Psychopharmacol* 2012; **32**:362–375.

Ferrell PB Jr., McLeod HL. Carbamazepine, HLA-B*1502 and risk of Stevens-Johnson syndrome and toxic epidermal necrolysis: US FDA recommendations. *Pharmacogenomics* 2008; **9**(10):1543–1546.

Gidal BE. Antiepileptic drug formulation and treatment in the elderly: Biopharmaceutical considerations. *Int Rev Neurobiol* 2008; **81**:299–311.

Hernandez S, Smith CR, Shen A, et al. Comparative safety of antiepileptic drugs during pregnancy. *Neurology* 2012; **78**:1692–1699.

Knowles SR, Shapiro LE, Shear NH. Anticonvulsant hypersensitivity syndrome: Incidence, prevention and management. *Drug Saf* 1999; **21**:489–501.

Meador KJ, Baker GA, Browning N, et al. Effects of fetal antiepileptic drug exposure: Outcomes at age 4.5 years. *Neurology* 2012; **78**(16):1207–1214.

Pirmohamed M, Breckenridge AM, Kitteringham NR, Park BK. Adverse drug reactions. *BMJ* 1998; **316**(7140):1295–1298.

Wang XQ, Shi XB, Au R, Chen FS, Wang F, Lang SY. Influence of chemical structure on skin reactions induced by antiepileptic drugs – The role of the aromatic ring. *Epilepsy Res* 2011; **94**(3):213–217.

Wlodarczyk BJ, Palacios AM, George TM, Finnell RH. Epileptic drugs and pregnancy outcomes. *Am J Med Genet A* 2012; **158A**:2071–2090.

# Antiepileptic Drug Interactions

**Philip N. Patsalos**

Department of Clinical and Experimental Epilepsy, UCL-Institute of Neurology, London, UK
Epilepsy Society, Chalfont Centre for Epilepsy, Chalfont St Peter, Buckinghamshire, UK

## Introduction

Antiepileptic drug (AED) drug–drug interactions are commonly encountered in epilepsy treatment and represent a substantial challenge to physicians. There are various reasons for this: (1) although monotherapy AED is the therapeutic mainstay, AED combinations continue to be widely prescribed in patients who do not respond to monotherapy; (2) because of the chronic nature of epilepsy, the likelihood of AEDs being coadministered with other drugs for management of comorbidities is considerable; (3) many AEDs are potent inducers (e.g., carbamazepine, phenytoin, phenobarbital, primidone) or inhibitors (e.g., valproic acid, felbamate, stiripentol) of drug-metabolizing enzymes and are highly likely to modify pharmacokinetics of concurrently administered drugs; and (4) most AEDs have a narrow therapeutic index, with even modest changes in their plasma drug concentration resulting in seizure exacerbation or increased adverse effects.

> ### SCIENCE REVISITED
>
> Drug interactions can be divided into pharmacokinetic and pharmacodynamic types. Pharmacokinetic interactions are associated

with a change in drug plasma concentration and are readily detectable and quantifiable with a well-characterized time course. Pharmacokinetic interactions can be due to a change in the absorption, distribution, metabolism, or excretion of the affected drug. These effects comprise most reported interactions, with most being the consequence of changes in hepatic metabolism. Pharmacodynamic interactions occur at the site of drug action in the brain and consequently are less well recognized and are usually concluded by default when a change in the clinical status consequent to a drug interaction is not associated with a change in a drug's plasma concentration.

## Anticipating and predicting metabolic interactions

Databases listing substrates, inhibitors, and inducers of different cytochrome P450 (CYP) isoenzymes are invaluable for predicting and avoiding potential interactions. For example, knowledge that carbamazepine is an inducer of CYP3A4 allows prediction that it will reduce the plasma concentration of CYP3A4

*Epilepsy*, First Edition. Edited by John W. Miller and Howard P. Goodkin.
© 2014 John Wiley & Sons, Ltd. Published 2014 by John Wiley & Sons, Ltd.

substrates such as ethosuximide, tiagabine, steroid oral contraceptives, and cyclosporin A. However, it must be appreciated that not all theoretically possible interactions highlighted in such databases will be clinically important. The most powerful predictor that an AED will not be associated with a pharmacokinetic interaction is that it does not undergo hepatic metabolism.

### ☆ TIPS AND TRICKS

New steady-state blood concentrations are achieved by five half-lives of the drug that is inhibited, while enzyme induction completes by 3–4 weeks after introduction of the inducing drug. Only when these times have passed would the maximum therapeutic consequence of the interaction be observed clinically.

## Prevention and management of adverse antiepileptic drug interactions

Antiepileptic drug interactions are prevented by avoiding polytherapy and selecting drugs with lower or absent potential to interact. A few simple rules, highlighted in Table 13.1, can assist in minimizing potentially adverse consequences of AED interactions.

Management comprises understanding the underlying mechanism of putative interactions to anticipate therapeutic outcome and close clinical monitoring. Also, with the aid of therapeutic drug monitoring, it is possible to ascertain the time course of the interaction and to implement appropriate dosing strategies, thereby circumventing undesirable consequences (seizure breakthrough or presentation of adverse effects).

**Table 13.1.** How to minimize potentially adverse consequences of AED interactions.

| | |
|---|---|
| 1 | Only when there is a clear clinical indication should an additional AED be prescribed. Most patients with epilepsy (70%) are best managed with a carefully individualized dosage of a single AED. |
| 2 | Be aware of the most important pharmacokinetic interactions involving the drugs that you intend to prescribe and also their underlying mechanisms. Many interactions can be predicted based on knowledge of drug effects on specific liver isoenzymes. If appropriate, adjust dose to compensate for the predicted effects of the interaction. |
| 3 | Avoid combining AEDs with similar adverse effect profiles and whenever possible select combinations for which there is clinical evidence of a favorable pharmacodynamic interaction. |
| 4 | After adding/removing an AED, monitor the clinical response carefully and consider the possibility of an interaction if there is an unexpected change in response. Continue the observation for a period consistent with the pharmacokinetic and pharmacodynamic characteristics of the drugs involved. A dosage adjustment should be undertaken if necessary. |
| 5 | If a pharmacokinetic interaction is anticipated, monitor plasma concentration of the affected drug. Be aware that under certain circumstances (e.g., a displacement of drug from plasma proteins), routine total drug concentration measurements may be misleading and management may benefit from monitoring free drug concentration. Also, when a pharmacologically active metabolite is affected, it may be advantageous to monitor plasma concentration of the metabolite. In some cases, dosage adjustments may have to be implemented at the time the interacting drug is added or removed. |
| 6 | If a patient with epilepsy suffers from comorbidities that will require treatment with additional drugs, it is preferable to treat the epilepsy with an AED having a low interaction potential. Gabapentin, lacosamide, lamotrigine, oxcarbazepine, levetiracetam, pregabalin, topiramate, tiagabine, and vigabatrin have little or no ability to cause enzyme induction or inhibition. Among AEDs, the lowest interaction potential is associated with those that are renally eliminated (e.g., gabapentin, levetiracetam, pregabalin, and vigabatrin). |
| 7 | Likewise, when adding a drug to treat a comorbidity or an intercurrent condition, choose the drug from the needed therapeutic class that is least likely to cause problematic interactions. |
| 8 | Finally, ask patients to report any symptoms (e.g., seizure exacerbation or toxicity) that may suggest a drug interaction. |

Figure 13.1 highlights the impact of AED interactions on clinical outcome, while a therapeutic algorithm illustrating management options in response to such interactions is summarized in Figure 13.2.

## Pharmacokinetic interactions between antiepileptic drugs

A comprehensive summary of pharmacokinetic interactions between AEDs is given in Table 13.2. Those most relevant clinically are discussed briefly in the succeeding text.

### Interactions mediated by enzyme induction

Carbamazepine, phenytoin, phenobarbital, and primidone are potent inducers of various CYP isoenzymes and also induce uridine glucuronyl transferases (UGTs) and epoxide hydrolases. As a result, these AEDs stimulate the metabolism of other concurrently administered AEDs, most notably clobazam, clonazepam, ethosuximide, felbamate, lamotrigine, oxcarbazepine and its active monohydroxy metabolite, perampanel, rufinamide, stiripentol, tiagabine, topiramate, valproic acid, and zonisamide.

When AEDs are associated with pharmacologically active metabolites, the consequence of enzyme induction complicates the outcome of the interaction because, paradoxically, potentiation of the effects of the affected drug can occur. For example, with primidone, which is metabolized partly to phenobarbital, enhancement of metabolism in patients comedicated with phenytoin or carbamazepine may actually enhance the production of the latter metabolite and increase pharmacological effects. Although stimulation in valproic acid metabolism by enzyme-inducing AEDs typically results in decreased plasma levels and decreased effectiveness of valproic acid, this interaction may also lead to increased formation of hepatotoxic metabolites, which may explain why patients taking phenytoin, phenobarbital, or carbamazepine are more susceptible to valproate-induced liver toxicity. Other AEDs that are associated with pharmacologically active metabolites include carbamazepine, clobazam, oxcarbazepine, and eslicarbazepine acetate.

### Interactions mediated by enzyme inhibition

Valproic acid is a notable inhibitor of drug metabolism resulting in three major interactions (i.e., with carbamazepine, phenobarbital, and lamotrigine) and two potentially moderate interactions (i.e., with felbamate and rufinamide). On average, the increase

in plasma phenobarbital concentration after adding valproic acid is 30–50%, and a reduction in phenobarbital (or primidone) dosage by up to 80% may be required to avoid side effects, particularly sedation and cognitive impairment. The effect of valproic acid on lamotrigine metabolism involves inhibition of the UGT1A4 enzyme responsible for the glucuronide conjugation of lamotrigine, and inhibition of lamotrigine metabolism is already maximal at valproic acid doses within the usual target ranges (≥500 mg/day in adults).

Valproic acid can inhibit the enzyme epoxide hydrolase, which is responsible for metabolism of the pharmacologically active metabolite carbamazepine-10,11-epoxide. Thus, in patients co-prescribed carbamazepine and valproic acid, an increase in plasma carbamazepine-10,11-epoxide concentrations can occur without any marked changes in carbamazepine concentrations, resulting in toxicity.

> ### ✋ CAUTION!
>
> Typically, prolongation of lamotrigine half-life from 30 h to about 60 h occurs in patients co-prescribed lamotrigine with valproic acid, markedly reducing lamotrigine dosage requirements. Because lamotrigine administration can be associated with a cutaneous rash, particularly when a fast increment in plasma lamotrigine concentration occurs, introduction of lamotrigine in a patient already taking valproic acid should be undertaken with caution, using a low starting dose (in adults, 25 mg on alternate days) and a slow dose escalation rate. However, there is no risk of rash if valproic acid is introduced in a patient already stabilized on lamotrigine, although a reduction in the dosage of lamotrigine (as a rule of thumb, by about 50%) is advisable as soon as the dosage of valproate reaches about 250–500 mg/day in adults.

### Interactions mediated by displacement from plasma protein binding sites

The implications of plasma protein-binding displacement interactions are often misunderstood and are important primarily for AEDs that are over 90% bound (e.g., phenytoin, valproic acid, diazepam, and tiagabine). As a rule, displacement from

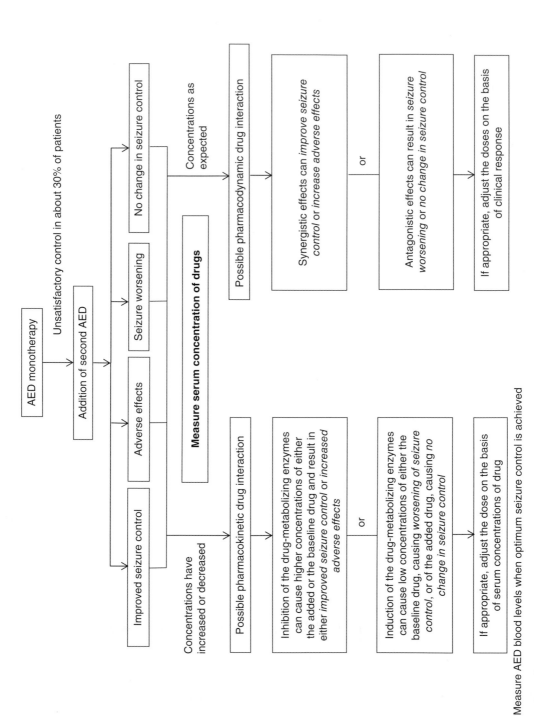

**Figure 13.1.** Effect of AED interactions on therapeutic outcome. Reprinted by permission from John Wiley & Sons from Patsalos PN, Froscher W, Pisani F, van Rijn CM. The importance of drug interactions in epilepsy therapy. *Epilepsia* 2002; **43**:365–385.

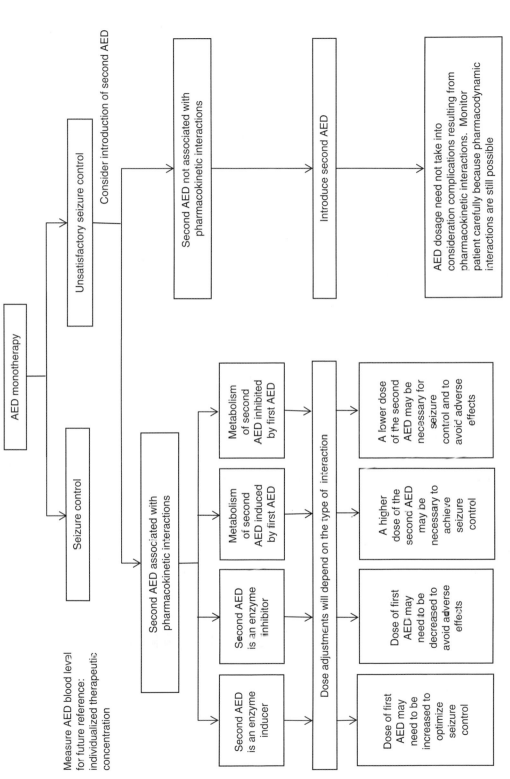

**Figure 13.2.** Strategies for managing interactions: dosage adjustment based on interaction mechanism. Reprinted by permission from John Wiley & Sons from Patsalos PN, Froscher W, Pisani F, van Rijn CM. The importance of drug interactions in epilepsy therapy. *Epilepsia* 2002; **43**:365–385.

Table 13.2. Interactions between AEDs: Expected changes in plasma concentrations (levels) when an AED is added to a preexisting AED regimen.

| AED added \ Preexisting AED | CBZ | CLB | CZP | ESL-a | ESM | FBM | GBP | LCM | LTG | LEV | OXC | PMP | PB | PHT | PGB | PRM | RTG | RFN | STP | TGB | TPM | VPA | VGB | ZNS |
|---|---|---|---|---|---|---|---|---|---|---|---|---|---|---|---|---|---|---|---|---|---|---|---|---|
| CBZ | AI | CLB⇓ DMCLB⇑ PB↑ | CZP⇓ | ESL↓ | ESM⇓ | FBM⇓ | ↔ | ↔ | LTG⇓ | LEV↓ | H-OXC↓ | PMP⇓ | ↔ | PHT↑↓ | ↔ | PRM↑ | RTG↓ | RFN↓ | STP⇓ | TGB⇓ | TPM⇓ | VPA⇓ | ↔ | ZNS⇓ |
| CLB | CBZ↑ CBZ-E↑ | – | NA | NA | NA | NA | NA | NA | ↔ | ↔ | ↔ | ↔ | ↔ | PHT↑ | NA | PRM↑ | NA | NA | STP↑ | ? | NA | VPA↑ | NA | NA |
| CZP | ↔ | NA | – | NA | NA | ↔ | NA | NA | ↔ | ↔ | NA | ↔ | ↔ | PHT↑↓ | NA | ↔ | NA | NA | NA | NA | NA | ↔ | ↔ | ↔ |
| ESL-a | ↔ | ↔ | NA | – | NA | NA | ↔ | ↔ | LTG↓ | ↔ | NCCP | ? | ↔ | PHT↑ | NA | NA | ? | ? | NA | NA | TPM↓ | VPA↓ | NA | ? |
| ESM | ↔ | NA | NA | NA | – | NA | NA | NA | ↔ | ↔ | NA | ? | ↔ | PHT↓ | NA | PRM↑ | ? | NA | NA | NA | TPM↓ | VPA↓ | NA | ↓ |
| FBM | CBZ↓ CBZ-E↑ | CLB⇑ DMCLB⇑ | CZP↑ | ? | – | – | NA | NA | LTG↑ | ↔ | ↔ | ? | PB⇑ | PHT⇑ | NA | PRM↑ | ? | ? | ? | ? | ? | VPA⇑ | VGB↓ | NA |
| GBP | ↔ | NA | NA | ↔ | NA | FBM↑ | – | NA | ↔ | ↔ | NA | NA | ↔ | ↔ | PGB↓ | NA | NA | NA | NA | NA | ↔ | ↔ | NA | NA |
| LCM | ↔ | NA | ↔ | NA | NA | NA | NA | – | – | LEV↓ | H-OXC↓ | ? | NA | ↔ | NA | ? | NA | NA | NA | NA | ↔ | ↑ | ↑ | ↑ |
| LTG | ↔ | ↔ | CZP↓ | ↔ | ↔ | NA | NA | ↔ | – | LEV↓ | ↔ | ↔ | ↔ | ↔ | ↔ | ↔ | RTG↑ | ↔ | NA | NA | ↔ | VPA↓ | NA | ↓ |
| LEV | ↔ | ↔ | ↔ | ↔ | ↔ | NA | ↑ | ↔ | ↔ | – | NA | ↔ | ↔ | ↔ | ↔ | ↔ | ↔ | NA | NA | NA | ↔ | ↔ | NA | NA |
| OXC | CBZ↓ | ? | ? | NCCP | ? | ? | NA | ↔ | LTG↓ | LEV↓ | – | PMP⇓ | PB↑ | PHT↑ | NA | ? | ? | RFN↓ | ? | ? | TPM↓ | ↔ | NA | ↔ |
| PMP | CBZ↓ | CLB↓ | ? | ? | ? | ? | NA | NA | LTG↓ | ↔ | OXC↓[a] | – | ↔ | ↔ | NA | ? | ? | ? | ? | ? | ↔ | VPA↓ | NA | ↔ |
| PB | CBZ⇓ | CLB⇓ DMCLB⇑ | CZP⇓ | ? | ESM⇓ | ↔ | ↔ | LCM↓ | LTG⇓ | LEV↓ | H-OXC↓ | ↔ | AI | PHT↑↓ | ↔ | NCCP | RTG↑ RFN↓ | STP↓ | TGB⇓ | TPM⇓ | VPA⇓ | ↔ | | ZNS⇓ |
| PHT | CBZ⇓ | CLB⇓ DMCLB⇑ | CZP⇓ | ESL↓ | ESM⇓ | FBM⇓ | ↔ | LCM↓ | LTG⇓ | LEV↓ | H-OXC↓ | PMP⇓ | PB↑ | AI | PGB↓ | PRM↓ | RTG↓ | RFN↓ | STP⇓ | TGB⇓ | TPM⇓ | VPA⇓ | ↔ | ZNS⇓ |
| PGB | ↔ | NA | NA | NA | NA | NA | ↔ | NA | ↔ | ↔ | NA | NA | ↔ | ↔ | – | NA | NA | NA | NA | TGB↓ | ↔ | ↔ | NA | NA |
| PRM | CBZ↑ | ? | CZP⇓ | ? | ESM⇓ | ? | NA | ? | LTG⇓ | ↔ | ? | ? | NCCP | ↔ | NA | – | ? | RFN↓ | STP↓ | TGB⇓ | TPM⇓ | VPA⇓ | ↔ | ZNS⇓ |
| RTG | ↔ | NA | NA | NA | NA | NA | NA | NA | LTG↓ | NA | ? | ? | PB↑ | PHT↑ | NA | NA | – | NA | NA | NA | ↔ | ↔ | NA | NA |
| RFN | CBZ↓ | ↔ | NA | NA | NA | NA | NA | NA | LTG↓ | NA | ? | ? | PB↑ | PHT↑ | NA | NA | – | – | NA | NA | ↔ | ↔ | NA | NA |
| STP | CBZ⇑ | CLB⇑ | ? | ? | ESM↑ | ? | NA | NA | LTG↓ | NA | ? | ? | PB⇑ | PHT↑ | NA | PRM⇑ | ? | ? | – | ? | ? | VPA↑ | NA | ? |

| | DMCLB⇑ | | | | | | | | | | | | | | | | | | |
|---|---|---|---|---|---|---|---|---|---|---|---|---|---|---|---|---|---|---|---|
| TGB | ↔ | NA | NA | NA | NA | ↔ | NA | NA | ↔ | NA | NA | ↔ | NA | NA | NA | NA | ↔ | NA | NA |
| TPM | ↔ | ? | ? | ESL↓ | NA | ? | ↔ | ↔ | PMP⇓ | ↔ | PHT↑ | ↔ | PB⇑ | ↔ | RFN↑ | NA | ? | — | VPA↓ | NA |
| VPA | CBZ-E⇑ | ↔ | ? | ↔ | ESM↑↓ | FBM↑ | ↔ | LTG⇑ | ↔ | ↔ | PHT↓[b] | ↔ | PB⇑ | ↔ | RFN↑ | TPM↓ | — | ↔ | — | NA |
| VGB | CBZ↓ | NA | NA | ↔ | NA | ↔ | NA | ↔ | NA | NA | PHT↓ | NA | ↔ | NA | RFN↓ | NA | NA | ↔ | ↔ | NA |
| ZNS | CBZ-E↑ | ? | ? | NA | ? | ? | NA | ? | NA | NA | NA | ? | NA | ? | ? | NA | NA | NA | NA | NA |

CBZ, carbamazepine; CBZ-E, carbamazepine-10,11-epoxide (active metabolite of CBZ); CLB, clobazam; CZP, clonazepam; DMCLB, N-desmethylclobazam (active metabolite of CLB); ESL-a, eslicarbazepine (active metabolite of ESL-a); ESM, ethosuximide; FBM, felbamate; GBP, gabapentin; H-OXC, 10-hydroxycarbazepine (active metabolite of OXC); LCM, lacosamide; LEV, levetiracetam; LTG, lamotrigine; OXC, oxcarbazepine; PMP, perampanel; PB, phenobarbital; PHT, phenytoin; PGB, pregabalin; PRM, primidone; RFN, rufinamide; RTG, retigabine; STP, stiripentol; TGB, tiagabine; TPM, topiramate; VGB, vigabatrin; VPA, valproic acid; ZNS, zonisamide.

AI, autoinduction; NA, none anticipated; NCCP, not commonly co-prescribed; ↔, no change; ↓, a usually minor (or inconsistent) decrease in serum level; ⇓, a usually clinically significant decrease in serum level; ↑, a usually minor (or inconsistent) increase in serum level; ⇑, a usually clinically significant increase in serum level.

? unknown, an interaction could occur.

aThe effect on the active metabolite H-OXC is not known.

bFree (pharmacologically active) level may increase.

plasma proteins results in a fall in total drug concentration, but the free drug concentration and magnitude of the pharmacological effect remain practically unchanged. Nevertheless, awareness of these interactions is important for interpretation of plasma drug concentration measurements in clinical practice; in fact, in the presence of a plasma protein-binding interaction, therapeutic and toxic effects will occur at total drug concentrations lower than usual, and patient management may benefit from monitoring free unbound drug concentrations. The most commonly occurring plasma protein-binding interaction involving AEDs is the displacement of protein-bound phenytoin by valproic acid. Typically, this interaction results in a fall in total phenytoin concentration, while the concentration of free, pharmacologically active phenytoin is usually unaltered. In some patients, a modest rise in free phenytoin concentration may actually be seen due to a concomitant inhibition of phenytoin metabolism by valproic acid.

## Pharmacokinetic interactions between antiepileptic drugs and non-antiepileptic drugs

### Antimicrobials

#### Antibacterials

The macrolide antibiotics, erythromycin, troleandomycin, and clarithromycin, have potential to increase plasma carbamazepine concentrations up to twofold to fourfold. Oxcarbazepine, tiagabine, felbamate, and phenytoin are not affected by coadministration with erythromycin. Enzyme-inducing AEDs accelerate the elimination of doxycycline and metronidazole, reducing their effectiveness. Conversely, metronidazole can increase plasma carbamazepine levels by 60%. The carbapenem antibiotics (panipenem, meropenem, imipenem, ertapenem, and doripenem) can decrease plasma valproic acid concentrations by >99%; therefore, this combination is considered contraindicated.

#### Antifungal agents

Antifungals (miconazole, ketoconazole, and fluconazole) can increase plasma carbamazepine concentrations, resulting in carbamazepine intoxication. In contrast, ketoconazole has no significant effect on plasma phenytoin concentrations, while itraconazole and posaconazole can increase plasma concentrations

by a small amount (10% and 25%, respectively), and voriconazole, fluconazole, and miconazole are associated with substantial increases (70%, 128%, and 180%, respectively). Lacosamide is unaffected by omeprazole, while lamotrigine is unaffected by fluconazole. The possibility of AEDs interfering with response to antifungal agents also needs to be considered. For example, enzyme-inducing AEDs decrease plasma itraconazole concentrations, sometimes to undetectable levels, suggesting that this agent should probably be avoided.

#### Antituberculosis agents

Metabolism of various AEDs (carbamazepine, ethosuximide, phenytoin, lamotrigine, and valproic acid) can be inhibited by isoniazid, resulting in toxicity. In contrast, rifampicin enhances the metabolism of phenytoin, carbamazepine, valproic acid, ethosuximide, and lamotrigine and decreases their plasma concentrations. Interestingly, in combination, rifampicin counteracts the inhibiting effect of isoniazid on phenytoin metabolism.

#### Antiviral agents

Metabolism of many antiviral agents (nevirapine, efavirenz, delavirdine, indinavir, lopinavir, and ritonavir) is increased by enzyme-inducing AEDs, and this can lead to insufficient antiviral plasma concentrations. In contrast, valproic acid can inhibit the metabolism of antiviral agents (lersivirine, lopinavir, and zidovudine). Bidirectional interactions also occur whereby ritonavir increases phenytoin and carbamazepine plasma concentrations.

### Antineoplastic agents

Antineoplastic agents have a narrow therapeutic index, and any interaction affecting their activity may have serious consequences in terms of toxicity or loss of efficacy. Enzyme-inducing AEDs increase metabolism of many antineoplastic agents (9-aminocamptothecin, cyclophosphamide, busulfan, gefitinib, glufosfamide, ifosfamide, imatinib, irinotecan, lapatinib, procarbazine, temozolomide, temsirolimus, teniposide, topotecan, thiotepa, vincristine, etoposide, paclitaxel, and methotrexate) and decrease their plasma concentrations. Also, some antineoplastic agents (e.g., 5-fluorouracil, doxifluridine, and tamoxifen) inhibit phenytoin metabolism and cause toxicity. AEDs devoid of enzyme-inducing activity (lacosamide, levetiracetam, gabapentin, pregabalin) would be preferred when treating seizure disorders in cancer patients.

## Cardiovascular drugs

The metabolism of amiodarone, disopyramide, mexiletine, and quinidine is enhanced by phenytoin, which decreases their plasma concentrations. In contrast, while amiodarone is without effect on carbamazepine, it increases plasma phenytoin concentrations threefold and may precipitate signs of toxicity. Enzyme-inducing AEDs increase metabolism of atenolol, propranolol, metoprolol, diazoxide, losartan, nifedipine, felodipine, nilvadipine, nimodipine, nisoldipine, and verapamil. In contrast, valproic acid can inhibit metabolism of nimodipine and increase plasma nimodipine concentrations by 54%. Oxcarbazepine increases plasma felodipine concentrations by 35%. While topiramate is without effect on nisoldipine, it increases plasma diltiazem concentrations by 25%.

---

### ★ TIPS AND TRICKS

Narrow therapeutic index drugs:

*For digoxin* it is advisable to check plasma digoxin concentrations regularly and to adjust dosage accordingly. Phenytoin, topiramate, and eslicarbazepine acetate can decrease plasma digoxin concentrations. In contrast, lacosamide, levetiracetam, and tiagabine do not interact with digoxin.

*For warfarin* (and other anticoagulants), it is advisable to monitor the international normalized ratio (INR) whenever concomitant AED therapy is changed. Metabolism of warfarin is enhanced by carbamazepine, phenobarbital, phenytoin, and eslicarbazepine acetate. In contrast, levetiracetam, oxcarbazepine, and tiagabine do not interact with warfarin. Interaction between phenytoin and warfarin is complex in that after an initial enhancement in anticoagulant action, the latter can be subsequently decreased.

---

## Immunosuppressants

While cyclosporin A plasma concentrations are decreased by carbamazepine, phenobarbital, phenytoin, primidone, and oxcarbazepine, levetiracetam and valproic acid are without effect. However, valproic is associated with a risk of hepatotoxicity. Similarly, tacrolimus metabolism is enhanced by carbamazepine, phenytoin, and phenobarbital so that plasma tacrolimus concentrations are decreased, whereas levetiracetam is without effect. The interaction with phenytoin is bidirectional in that tacrolimus can also inhibit metabolism of phenytoin and increase plasma phenytoin concentrations by 97%. With sirolimus, only phenytoin has been reported to enhance its metabolism, resulting in a 74% decrease in plasma sirolimus concentrations.

## Psychotropic drugs

### Antidepressants

Enzyme-inducing AEDs can decrease plasma concentrations of various antidepressants including amitriptyline, nortriptyline, imipramine, desipramine, clomipramine, mianserin, mirtazapine, nefazodone, paroxetine, sertraline, doxepin, and viloxazine. Higher dosages of these antidepressants may be required for clinical efficacy. Valproic acid can inhibit metabolism of amitriptyline, nortriptyline, clomipramine, and paroxetine. With regard to amitriptyline and nortriptyline, their plasma concentrations can increase by 50–60%, which could lead to symptoms of overdosage, including worsening or precipitation of seizures. Topiramate can also inhibit amitriptyline metabolism, but the effect is not substantial, with amitriptyline and nortriptyline plasma concentrations increasing by 8% and 19%, respectively.

### Antipsychotics

Interactions between antipsychotics and AEDs are similar to those between antidepressants and AEDs. Thus, enzyme-inducing AEDs can decrease the plasma concentration of aripiprazole, bromperidol, clozapine, chlorpromazine, fluphenazine, haloperidol, olanzapine, quetiapine, risperidone, trazodone, and ziprasidone. The consequent decrease in concentration of the antipsychotic can lead to reemergence of psychopathology whereby following discontinuation of the enzyme-inducing AED, signs of antipsychotic overdosage may develop when the plasma concentration of the antipsychotic increases again.

Valproic acid can decrease aripiprazole and increases quetiapine plasma concentrations but does not affect asenapine, haloperidol, risperidone, and olanzapine plasma concentrations. Topiramate can increase plasma haloperidol concentration by 28% and its pharmacologically active metabolite by 50% but has no effect on clozapine, olanzapine or quetiapine.

**Table 13.3.** Interaction between AEDs and oral contraceptive steroids.

| AEDs that do not affect the efficacy of oral contraceptive steroids | AEDs that decrease the efficacy of oral contraceptive steroids |
| --- | --- |
| Clonazepam | Carbamazepine |
| Ethosuximide | Eslicarbazepine acetate |
| Gabapentin | Felbamate |
| Lacosamide | Oxcarbazepine |
| Lamotrigine | Phenobarbital |
| Levetiracetam | Phenytoin |
| Methsuximide | Primidone |
| Pregabalin | Rufinamide |
| Retigabine | |
| Tiagabine | |
| Valproic acid | |
| Vigabatrin | |
| Zonisamide | |

While lamotrigine has no effect on the estrogen component of the contraceptive pill and in most patients will not compromise contraception, lamotrigine does enhance metabolism of the progesterone component so that progesterone blood concentrations decrease by approximately 10%. This effect may be clinically significant in patients prescribed the progesterone-only contraceptive pill. Perampanel similarly does not affect the estrogen component but does enhance the metabolism of the progesterone component so that progesterone AUC values decrease by ~40% (>8 mg/day).

*Lithium*

Only acetazolamide has a substantial effect on lithium, with plasma lithium concentrations increasing five-fold. Other interactions include effects by clonazepam, which increases lithium plasma concentrations by 33–60%; lamotrigine, which increases them by 8%; and topiramate, which increases them by 12–140%. All interactions can result in clinically significant effects necessitating reduction in lithium dosage. AEDs with no known interaction with lithium include gabapentin and valproic acid.

**Oral contraceptives**

Table 13.3 summarizes the effects of AEDs on the metabolism of steroid oral contraceptives and the efficacy of the contraceptive pill. Women taking AEDs that enhance the metabolism of oral contraceptives should be prescribed an oral contraceptive containing 50 μg of ethinyl estradiol; if breakthrough bleeding occurs, ethinyl estradiol doses may need to be increased to 75 or 100 μg. For women taking enzyme-inducing AEDs, subdermal levonorgestrel implants are not recommended, whereas the efficacy of intrauterine progestogen-only contraceptives is not considered to be compromised by enzyme induction.

With regard to lamotrigine, a reverse interaction occurs whereby oral contraceptives enhance lamotrigine metabolism, decreasing plasma lamotrigine concentrations by 40–65%. This can result in reduced seizure control.

**Summary**

As a rule of thumb, only use AED polytherapy when absolutely essential, and choose those drugs that are least interacting (e.g., gabapentin, lacosamide, levetiracetam, pregabalin, and vigabatrin). However, whenever polytherapy with known interacting drugs is contemplated, it is best practice to monitor blood concentrations of the affected drug before and after the introduction of the interacting drug. Thus, a dosage adjustment can be undertaken to prevent unnecessary toxicity or seizure breakthrough consequent to the interaction.

**Acknowledgement**

The work by Professor Philip N. Patsalos was undertaken at UCLH/UCL and supported in part by funding from the Department of Health's NIHR Biomedical Research Centres funding scheme.

# Bibliography

Anderson GD. A mechanistic approach to antiepileptic drug interactions. *Ann Pharmacother* 1998; **32**:554–563.

Johannessen Landmark C, Patsalos PN. Drug interactions involving the new second and third generation antiepileptic drugs. *Exp Rev Neurother* 2010; **10**:119–140.

Johannessen Landmark C, Patsalos PN. Methodologies used to identify and characterise interactions among antiepileptic drugs. *Exp Rev Clin Pharmacol* 2012; **5**:281–292.

Patsalos PN. Drug interactions with the newer Antiepileptic Drugs (AEDs) – 1: Pharmacokinetic and pharmacodynamic interactions between AEDs. *Clin Pharmacokinet* 2013 [Epub ahead of print].

Patsalos PN. *Antiepileptic Drug Interactions: A Clinical Guide*, 2nd ed. London: Springer-Verlag, 2013.

Patsalos PN, Bourgeois BFD. *The Epilepsy Prescriber's Guide to Antiepileptic Drugs*. Cambridge, UK: Cambridge University Press, 2010.

Patsalos PN, Perucca E. Clinically important drug interactions in epilepsy: Interactions between antiepileptic drugs and other drugs. *Lancet Neurol* 2003; **2**:473–481.

Patsalos PN, Perucca E. Clinically important drug interactions in epilepsy: General features and interactions between antiepileptic drugs. *Lancet Neurol* 2003; **2**:347–356.

Patsalos PN, Froscher W, Pisani F, van Rijn CM. The importance of drug interactions in epilepsy therapy. *Epilepsia* 2002; **43**:365–385.

Patsalos PN, Berry DJ, Bourgeois BFD, et al. Antiepileptic drugs – Best practice guidelines for therapeutic drug monitoring: A position paper by the Subcommission on Therapeutic Drug Monitoring, ILAE Commission on Therapeutic Strategies. *Epilepsia* 2008; **49**:1239–1276.

Perucca E, Hebdige S, Frigo GM, Gatti G, Lecchini S, Crema A. Interaction between phenytoin and valproic acid: Plasma protein binding and metabolic effects. *Clin Pharmacol Ther* 1980; **28**:779–789.

Romanelli F, Jennings HR, Nath A, Ryan M, Berger J. Therapeutic dilemma: The use of anticonvulsants in HIV-positive individuals. *Neurology* 2000; **54**:1404–1407.

Sabers A. Pharmacokinetic interactions between contraceptives and antiepileptic drugs. *Seizure* 2008; **17**:141–144.

Spina E, Perucca E. Clinically significant pharmacokinetic interactions between antiepileptic and psychotropic drugs. *Epilepsia* 2002; **43** (Suppl. 2):37–44.

Yap KY, Chui WK, Chan A. Drug interactions between chemotherapeutic regimens and antiepileptics. *Clin Therapeut* 2008; **8**:1385–1407.

# Recognizing Intractability to Antiepileptic Medication

**Bassel W. Abou-Khalil**

Epilepsy Center, Vanderbilt University School of Medicine, Nashville, TN, USA

## Introduction

The treatment of epilepsy usually starts with antiepileptic drug (AED) therapy. However, a proportion of patients will prove drug resistant. This chapter addresses when to recognize intractability to medical therapy so that alternative treatments can be considered.

## Natural history of epilepsy and expected response to antiepileptic drug (AED) therapy

The recognition of intractability to AEDs is facilitated by understanding the natural history of epilepsy, best characterized with prospective studies of childhood-onset epilepsy. The longest study, which followed patients for several decades, found that two-thirds were in remission for at least 5 years, with about half achieving remission not interrupted by relapse. A remitting–relapsing pattern with terminal remission occurred in about a fifth of patients. Drug resistance was present from the outset in another one-fifth of patients, with emergence of drug resistance after remission in about one-seventh.

Drug resistance can be predicted with certain epileptic syndromes. Some idiopathic epileptic syndromes, such as benign epilepsy of childhood with centrotemporal spikes and childhood absence epilepsy, are expected to remit after puberty. Drug resistance is least common in idiopathic focal and generalized epilepsy and most common in symptomatic generalized epilepsy and symptomatic focal epilepsy, particularly temporal lobe epilepsy. In children, a high initial seizure frequency and seizure clustering during treatment predict drug resistance. Age at onset is also a predictor of seizure freedom. In children, age at onset between 5 and 9 years is the most favorable. In adults, the odds of remission are best in seniors.

### EVIDENCE AT A GLANCE

A large study of adults who had never received an AED, followed for a median of 5 years, revealed that 64% achieved remission. Drug resistance was predicted by the response to the first two AEDs. The first AED tried resulted in seizure freedom in 47% of individuals. If the first drug failed from adverse effects, the efficacy of the second drug was similar to the first one, but if the first AED failed from lack of efficacy, only 11% became seizure-free with the second. Only 10% of patients who failed two AEDs became seizure-free with subsequent trials. In an expanded follow-up study, 35% of patients were drug resistant throughout, and an additional 5% relapsed.

While children also have decreased likelihood of seizure control after failure of two AEDs, remissions are common in those who failed two AEDs, although these remissions are followed by relapse in the majority. However, one study with several decades of followup showed that half of the children who failed two AEDs eventually achieved sustained remission. Failure to enter remission and symptomatic etiology predicted long-term drug-resistant epilepsy. On the other hand, in adults, one study showed that after failing initial AED trials, additional trials achieved remission in 14% of patients, but this remission was not stable, and relapses eventually occurred in most.

### EVIDENCE AT A GLANCE

An adult study quantified response to AEDs based on past treatment failures. The odds of seizure freedom were 62% with the first AED, 42% after failing one AED, 17% after failure of two to five AEDs, and 0% after failure of six or seven AEDs. For every 1.5 AEDs that proved ineffective, the seizure-free rates decreased by 50%. Despite the 0% odds of seizure freedom after failure of six to seven past AEDs, there could still be benefit from additional AED trials, as greater than 50% reduction in seizure frequency occurred in almost a third of these patients.

## Definition of drug resistance in epilepsy

Based largely on the above evidence, the International League Against Epilepsy (ILAE) proposed a consensus definition of drug resistance in epilepsy as "failure of adequate trials of two tolerated and appropriately chosen AED schedules (whether as monotherapies or in combination) to achieve sustained seizure freedom." The definition may appear simple but does require elaboration. It excludes trials in which the AED was not tolerated. In addition, an appropriately chosen AED must have been proven effective for the specific seizure type. For example, the choice of carbamazepine would be appropriate for a patient with focal onset seizures, but its choice for a patient with myoclonic or absence seizures would not be appropriate, and its failure in that setting could not be counted towards the definition of drug resistance. Other examples in which drug failure cannot be considered are use of a low dose, failure to titrate an AED to maximum tolerated dose, or failure to appropriately prescribe the AED in the correctly divided daily dosing regimen. It should also be noted that success of an AED requires freedom from all seizures for at least 1 year or three times the longest interval between pretreatment seizures, whichever is longer.

Historically there has been considerable controversy regarding the definition of refractory epilepsy, and it has been recognized that the definition must vary depending on its intended purpose. The definition proposed by the ILAE was intended to identify a time point for reevaluation of the diagnosis and management of epilepsy, preferably in the setting of an epilepsy center. The reevaluation of the diagnosis after identification of drug resistance usually involves video–EEG monitoring. This testing can also help determine whether the patient has a surgically remediable focal epilepsy syndrome. The therapeutic implications are highly dependent on the specific epilepsy syndrome, etiology, and localization.

### ⚠ CAUTION!

Before determining epilepsy to be drug resistant, it is important to consider the possibility of wrong epilepsy diagnosis (psychogenic or physiological nonepileptic events), wrong epilepsy classification, seizure exacerbation by inappropriate AED treatment, and patient factors such as noncompliance, sleep deprivation, drug abuse, and comedication with a drug that reduces the seizure threshold.

## Intractability: Etiology and epilepsy syndrome

The underlying pathology and epileptic syndrome are important predictors of drug resistance. The highest chance of seizure control is in patients with idiopathic generalized epilepsy (up to 82%), but it is much lower (about 20%) with temporal lobe epilepsy and lowest (11%) for patients with focal epilepsy with hippocampal sclerosis. Patients with dual pathology (hippocampal sclerosis and another lesion) have only a 3% rate of seizure control. Similarly, in a study of children with temporal lobe epilepsy, one-third became seizure-free, but none with MRI lesions including hippocampal sclerosis were seizure-free. Once a specific syndrome has been diagnosed, there may be specific predictors for drug resistance. For example, in juvenile myoclonic epilepsy, the presence of all three seizure types (myoclonic, tonic–clonic, and absence) and psychiatric disorders predict drug resistance.

---

### ♗ SCIENCE REVISITED

The two key hypotheses regarding the pathophysiology of drug resistance in epilepsy are as follows:

1. Drug resistance proteins that transport AEDs out of neurons/glia/endothelium prevent them from reaching their targets.
2. Change in AED targets (such as channels or receptors) results in the target no longer being sensitive to the AED.

---

## Optimal strategy for trying medication that will make it possible to recognize intractability earlier

To minimize the misdiagnosis of drug resistance, it is essential to initiate AED therapy with the most appropriate AED for the specific seizure types and epilepsy syndrome, preferably using a drug that has demonstrated the optimal balance of efficacy and tolerability for the type of epilepsy in question (Chapter 11). For example, valproate appears to have an advantage over lamotrigine and topiramate for idiopathic generalized epilepsy and, in the absence of contraindication, should probably be considered first in a male patient with juvenile myoclonic epilepsy. AEDs that may exacerbate seizures should be avoided. For example, carbamazepine, phenytoin, oxcarbazepine, and gabapentin are usually not appropriate for an individual with idiopathic generalized epilepsy, as they may exacerbate generalized myoclonic and absence seizures. The appropriate AED should be titrated until seizure control is achieved or until the limit of tolerability is reached.

Despite optimal management, drug resistance may not become apparent before a long delay, with the time from latency to failure of a second drug ranging from 0 to 48 years, with an average of 9 years, and about a quarter of individuals having at least 1 year of seizure freedom. Seizure remissions are particularly common in patients with mesial temporal lobe epilepsy and hippocampal sclerosis.

---

### ☆ TIPS AND TRICKS

The identification of a patient as drug resistant does not preclude continued trials of AEDs and AED combinations not previously used. Chapter 15 further outlines strategies for optimizing AED use in patients who have been proven to be drug resistant but are not candidates for neurosurgical treatment.

---

## Conclusion and treatment implications of drug resistance in epilepsy

Defining an individual's epilepsy as drug resistant in a timely fashion should lead to alternate, potentially more effective treatments. These options depend on the specific epilepsy syndrome. Chapter 27 reviews surgical treatments for patients with focal epilepsy and a surgically remediable syndrome, such as hippocampal sclerosis; surgery is usually considered after two AEDs have failed. However, patients with nonlesional epilepsy who are not ideal candidates for surgery should not be considered for invasive EEG evaluation and epilepsy surgery until failure of five to six AEDs (Figure 14.1). Chapter 27 also reviews corpus callosotomy, a palliative treatment option for some patients with generalized tonic or atonic seizures, which should be considered only in highly refractory cases after failure of multiple AEDs and less invasive therapies. Chapter 28 reviews vagus nerve stimulation, a treatment that is also palliative, with low chance of seizure freedom. This is an option for patients who are not candidates for epilepsy surgery, including idiopathic and symptomatic generalized epilepsy (although it is not FDA approved for these syndromes). The five to six AED failure rule also seems appropriate for this device. Chapter 29 reviews dietary therapy, which can be considered after failure of two or more AEDs, in focal epilepsy as well as idiopathic and symptomatic generalized epilepsy. Finally, Chapter 15 outlines how AED therapies can be optimized in those patients that are not candidates for, or fail, these nonmedical treatments.

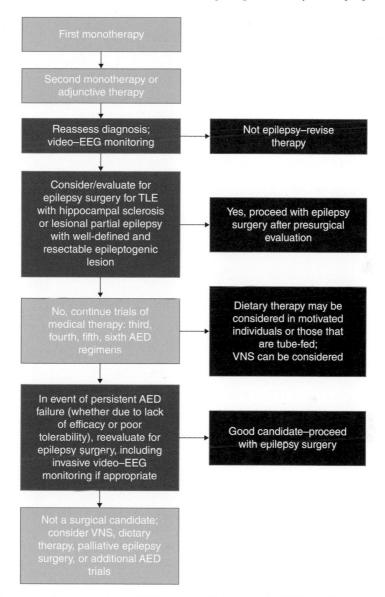

**Figure 14.1.** Spectrum of drug resistance. TLE, temporal lobe epilepsy; VNS, vagal nerve stimulation.

## Bibliography

Berg AT, Langfitt J, Shinnar S, et al. How long does it take for partial epilepsy to become intractable? *Neurology* 2003; **60**:186–190.

Berg AT, Levy SR, Testa FM, D'Souza R. Remission of epilepsy after two drug failures in children: A prospective study. *Ann Neurol* 2009; **65**:510–519.

Callaghan B, Schlesinger M, Rodemer W, et al. Remission and relapse in a drug-resistant epilepsy population followed prospectively. *Epilepsia* 2011; **52**:619–626.

Gelisse P, Genton P, Thomas P, Rey M, Samuelian JC, Dravet C. Clinical factors of drug resistance in juvenile myoclonic epilepsy. *J Neurol Neurosurg Psychiatry* 2001; **70**:240–243.

Kwan P, Brodie MJ. Early identification of refractory epilepsy. *N Engl J Med* 2000; **342**:314–319.

Kwan P, Arzimanoglou A, Berg AT, et al. Definition of drug resistant epilepsy: Consensus proposal by the ad hoc Task Force of the ILAE Commission on Therapeutic Strategies. *Epilepsia* 2010; **51**: 1069–1077.

Marson AG, Al-Kharusi AM, Alwaidh M, et al. The SANAD study of effectiveness of valproate, lamotrigine, or topiramate for generalised and unclassifiable epilepsy: An unblinded randomised controlled trial. *Lancet* 2007; **369**:1016–1026.

Schiller Y, Najjar Y. Quantifying the response to antiepileptic drugs: Effect of past treatment history. *Neurology* 2008; **70**:54–65.

Schmidt D, Löscher W. Drug resistance in epilepsy: Putative neurobiologic and clinical mechanisms. *Epilepsia* 2005; **46**:858–877.

Semah F, Picot MC, Adam C, et al. Is the underlying cause of epilepsy a major prognostic factor for recurrence? *Neurology* 1998; **51**:1256–1262.

Sillanpää M, Schmidt D. Natural history of treated childhood-onset epilepsy: Prospective, long-term population-based study. *Brain* 2006; **129**:617–624.

Sillanpää M, Schmidt D. Seizure clustering during drug treatment affects seizure outcome and mortality of childhood-onset epilepsy. *Brain* 2008; **131**:938–944.

Sillanpää M, Schmidt D. Is incident drug-resistance of childhood-onset epilepsy reversible? A long-term follow-up study. *Brain* 2012; **135**:2256–2262.

Spooner CG, Berkovic SF, Mitchell LA, Wrennall JA, Harvey AS. New-onset temporal lobe epilepsy in children: Lesion on MRI predicts poor seizure outcome. *Neurology* 2006; **67**:2147–2153.

# Optimizing Antiepileptic Drug Therapy in Refractory Epilepsy

**Nicholas P. Poolos**

Department of Neurology and UW Regional Epilepsy Center, University of Washington, Seattle, WA, USA

## Introduction: When are patients "refractory"?

Establishing whether your patient has refractory epilepsy is a topic well covered in Chapter 14. In general, epilepsy patients fall into two categories in terms of the ease of treatment: those for whom nearly anything will work and those for whom seemingly nothing will work. This bimodal distribution of patient characteristics was established clearly by a retrospective study by Kwan and Brodie of all patients presenting with a first seizure; about two-thirds of patients were rendered seizure-free with trials of the first one or two medications. Notably, the likelihood of successful treatment did not differ between newer-generation antiepileptic drugs (AEDs) and older drugs. Also, patients who achieve seizure freedom with initial monotherapy often do so at AED dosage below "standard" levels, such as carbamazepine at 600 mg/day. Thus, the majority of new-onset patients can be successfully treated with moderate doses of whichever AED presents the most favorable tolerability profile, assuming it is indicated for their seizure type. Although there is no sharp boundary between patients whose seizures will remit with treatment and those who will be refractory, it is clear that the odds of achieving seizure freedom drop off with each successive drug failure. Thus, many epileptologists consider the criteria for refractoriness to be the failure of two or three appropriate drug trials in either monotherapy or polytherapy.

Before declaring a treatment regimen a failure, it is important to avoid some dangerous pitfalls. The most notable of these is the possibility that the patient does not in fact have epilepsy. Patients with psychogenic nonepileptic episodes constitute a sizeable fraction of individuals admitted to the inpatient video–EEG monitoring service of any tertiary care epilepsy center, and these patients have often undergone several – sometimes many – fruitless AED trials. Identifying these patients after just one or two failed AED trials can spare years of needless AED exposure and open the possibility of successful psychiatric treatment. A more difficult problem is that of noncompliance. Missing even one dose of AEDs may be sufficient to provoke a seizure in some patients. It is hard for the epilepsy practitioner to know just how often this happens and how much it is a factor in apparent refractoriness to treatment. Subtherapeutic AED levels obtained at the time of emergency department visits are sometimes the only clear evidence of noncompliance, so I always ask ED providers to obtain these if they call about one of my patients, even for "sendout" levels of newer AEDs. Diabetes doctors have the benefit of tracking hemoglobin A1C levels and daily finger-stick glucose levels

*Epilepsy*, First Edition. Edited by John W. Miller and Howard P. Goodkin.

in their most difficult patients in order to assess compliance. Epilepsy doctors have no such luxury. Thus, I continually preach the importance of the low-tech pill container (subdivided into day-of-the-week compartments) as the best way to assure compliance. Another provoker of refractory seizures, especially in some forms of generalized epilepsy, is alcohol abuse. I've stumbled on the source of a few patients' refractoriness when a loved one tipped me off to their alcoholism – and witnessed a remarkable improvement when they cut down on their drinking.

☆ TIPS AND TRICKS

The low-tech pill box is the clinician's best friend in improving treatment compliance.

## More antiepileptic drug trials versus surgery

For some refractory localization-related epilepsy patients, epilepsy surgery is a viable option. Knowing when to quit further AED trials and when to offer surgical referral is a judgment call that has to be considered carefully because the surgical evaluation process is time-consuming and expensive and sometimes takes on a life of its own. I find it helpful to present the possible outcomes in rough probability terms that even unsophisticated patients can understand. For those who have gone through at least three AED trials and for whom the epilepsy diagnosis is secure, I suggest that the likelihood of seizure freedom with further AED trials is about 1 in 10, with temporal lobe resection about 6 in 10, and with extratemporal resection less than half. Many patients prioritize the possibility of discontinuing all AEDs as a reason for surgery. It's important to emphasize from the beginning that AEDs might only be reduced, not discontinued altogether, post-surgery, because only about half of patients successfully discontinue all AEDs after temporal lobectomy. Conversely, although some studies have shown that overall quality of life is most meaningfully increased if surgery results in seizure freedom, it is important to consider that a significant decrease in seizure frequency from "unsuccessful" surgery does mean a decreased risk of injury or sudden death from seizures. Presenting all of these contingencies to the patient contemplating surgery versus further medication trials may require multiple clinic visits so that the patient can fully digest the risks and benefits.

## General approach to the refractory patient

For those patients for whom further AED trials are warranted, there are some general principles to consider. First off, the statistical likelihood of success with further medical treatment applies to a population, but every individual is different. Thus, it is important not to deprive the patient of hope or of motivation to go forward. *Refractory* does not equate to impossible. (For this reason I avoid the word *intractable*, which I think has a more negative connotation.) Even in refractory patients exposed to multiple prior medications, success can be achieved if one tries enough different combinations of medications.

Establishing the epilepsy diagnosis is vital, and for most refractory epilepsy patients should involve long-term video–EEG monitoring to capture typical seizures. The utility of this test stems from multiple considerations: weeding out patients with non-epileptic spells (even patients with interictal abnormalities on routine EEG can have superimposed nonepileptic spells), establishing which localization-related epilepsy patients may be surgical candidates, and discriminating generalized from localization-related epilepsies so as to better refine AED choice (more on this in the succeeding text).

Once the epilepsy diagnosis is secure and the question of surgery settled, it is important to guide AED therapy on the basis of data. This means asking patients or their caregivers to keep a seizure diary. Most people know without a diary whether or not they are seizure-free but otherwise can lose track of how frequently seizures are occurring. Without this information, it is difficult to tell whether progress is being made as medication regimens are altered. Likewise, obtaining occasional AED serum levels will confirm compliance and provide some guidance as to whether reasonably therapeutic drug levels are being reached. While obtaining drug levels is not recommended as a substitute for decision making based on asking patients how they are doing, drug levels sometimes reveal pharmacokinetic surprises (e.g., low levels of lamotrigine while on oral contraceptives or when pregnant, low levels of P450-metabolized drugs in combination with hepatic inducers like carbamazepine).

On the topic of pharmacokinetics, it would seem that drugs with relatively long serum elimination half-lives might be more effective than those with greater diurnal variations in their serum concentrations. Unfortunately, there is little empirical evidence for this idea, but given the choice it is reasonable to opt for extended-release versions of drugs or drugs with intrinsically long half-lives (zonisamide, perampanel, lamotrigine in combination with valproate). In the USA extended-release versions of second-generation AEDs (lamotrigine, levetiracetam) are now available in generic versions. Conversely, drugs with shorter half-lives may need to be dosed three times daily (pregabalin, levetiracetam).

Most patients will have arrived at the refractory treatment pathway by virtue of having failed at least two drugs in monotherapy. The practice especially in the USA has been to titrate each drug in monotherapy to its limit of tolerability before declaring it a failure. It is typical at that point to begin treating with combinations of drugs, and it is safe to say that the majority of refractory patients will be treated with combinations of AEDs. It is reasonable to wonder what to expect from adding a second or third drug to a patient's regimen: Is there an added benefit in reduction in seizure frequency that is the sum of each drug's effect when used in monotherapy? Does adding three drugs produce more benefits than two? What about four or more AEDs at a time?

### EVIDENCE AT A GLANCE

A retrospective study (Poolos et al., 2012) examined the benefits of combination therapy in a developmentally disabled population and found that adding a second agent to monotherapy in a highly refractory population produced a 19% decrease in seizure frequency; surprisingly, adding a third agent to a two-drug regimen produced no added benefit. These results suggest that there may be diminishing returns from adding successive numbers of concurrent AEDs. Possible reasons for this may be increased pharmacokinetic interactions as drug number increases, poorer overall tolerability due to increased side effects, or even adverse pharmacodynamic (drug effects based on mechanisms of action) interactions. This study also demonstrated superior efficacy of the combination of lamotrigine and valproate against convulsive seizures. This was the only statistically superior AED combination out of 32 tested.

### ⚠ CAUTION!

More concurrent AEDs may not equal better efficacy, just increased adverse effects.

There is only a small amount of data addressing answers to these basic questions. Clinical trials of new AEDs typically occur in refractory patient populations for whom the new agent is added to existing regimens of one or two other drugs. These studies have typically shown a 15–30% (corrected for placebo) maximum improvement in seizure frequency from adding what is in essence a second or third agent. In practice, I would suggest that two-drug combinations in refractory epilepsy provide an efficacy benefit over a single agent; three-drug regimens should be attempted with caution; and four or more concurrent AEDs probably should not be used at all.

While it would appear that adding successive numbers of concurrent AEDs produces a benefit that it is less than the sum of their individual actions in monotherapy, much has been said over the years about the opposite idea: that some combinations of AEDs may exhibit "synergy" or actions together that exceed the sum of their parts. As can be imagined, this is an exceedingly difficult question to study considering the myriad possible combinations of the 20 or so AEDs in clinical use today. A study of the older agents phenytoin and carbamazepine suggested that either of these drugs worked better in combination with phenobarbital than paired with each other, supporting the idea that combining drugs with differing theoretical mechanisms of action was beneficial. Several prospective studies have suggested that combination therapy with lamotrigine and valproate produces benefits over either agent alone or lamotrigine in combination with phenytoin or carbamazepine. Whether the actions of lamotrigine and valproate together represent a pharmacokinetic or pharmacodynamic interaction is unclear; thus, the search for the holy grail of AED synergy goes on. One practical consideration of combining AEDs is the difficulty of ascertaining which drug is producing adverse effects if both have similar side effect profiles. This would suggest it is wise to avoid combinations of drugs with similar mechanisms: phenytoin with carbamazepine or lacosamide; topiramate with zonisamide; or two benzodiazepines together.

## Antiepileptic drugs in refractory generalized versus localization-related epilepsy

The most rationally based guidance for treating refractory epilepsy derives from observations of seizure exacerbation in generalized epilepsy. The utility of knowing whether the refractory patient has a generalized syndrome (often requiring long-term video–EEG monitoring) comes from avoiding those AEDs known to exacerbate generalized seizures. In mechanistic terms, the AEDs with theoretical mechanisms of action against voltage-gated sodium channels (principally phenytoin and carbamazepine) can worsen absence, myoclonic, and tonic–clonic seizures that are generalized from onset. Although lamotrigine is effective in absence epilepsy, it can occasionally provoke myoclonic seizures. Lacosamide and rufinamide have theoretical actions on sodium channels, and although lacosamide appears to have some efficacy in convulsions in primary generalized epilepsy and rufinamide is approved for Lennox–Gastaut syndrome, these drugs should be used with caution in generalized epilepsy. Drugs that indiscriminately act on GABA receptors (vigabatrin, tiagabine, pregabalin, and gabapentin) can have similar effects. However, $GABA_A$ receptor-selective drugs, such as benzodiazepines or phenobarbital, are effective in generalized epilepsy.

Sometimes the effect of drugs contraindicated in generalized epilepsy is observed not as provoking seizures outright but as rendering a patient refractory to drug regimens that include other, more appropriate, agents. Patients admitted for video–EEG monitoring and diagnosed with refractory epilepsy of unknown type are often ultimately found to have generalized epilepsy, often treated with contraindicated AEDs; once their regimens are rationalized to appropriate medications, a large proportion become seizure-free. A not uncommon scenario is the refractory patient whose only seizure type is a generalized convulsion, who has been on phenytoin all of his or her life, sometimes in conjunction with other AEDs, and whose routine EEGs are nonepileptiform. When video–EEG monitoring discloses the generalized onset of convulsions, phenytoin can be replaced with a more appropriate AED (see Table 11.1), and the patient's seizures often come under much better control.

Aside from the avoidance of seizure-exacerbating AEDs, there is little evidence-based guidance on the choice of drugs in generalized epilepsy. Several large prospective studies in nonrefractory, new-onset epilepsy have demonstrated valproate as the gold standard of efficacy in generalized epilepsy. This drug has serious dose-dependent and idiosyncratic toxicities, especially on the fetus in pregnant women with epilepsy, and so must be used with caution. Clonazepam is often helpful where myoclonus is predominant, such as in juvenile myoclonic epilepsy, whereas lamotrigine sometimes worsens seizures in this condition. This is also true in the relatively rare syndrome of severe myoclonic epilepsy of infancy (SMEI or Dravet syndrome), where drugs with sodium channel antagonism markedly worsen seizures, whereas benzodiazepines are helpful.

In focal-onset, localization-related refractory epilepsy, there is even less rational guidance for AED choice. Analogous to valproate in generalized epilepsy, carbamazepine has been the gold standard for efficacy (if not necessarily tolerability) in focal epilepsy, stemming from its modest superiority in new-onset epilepsy, as demonstrated in the VA Cooperative trials. However, a later prospective trial failed to show much efficacy difference between carbamazepine, oxcarbazepine, lamotrigine, and topiramate. Nonetheless, refractory patients should probably be exposed to carbamazepine at some point in their treatment course. Many clinicians feel that topiramate has comparable efficacy to carbamazepine, albeit with a number of dose-dependent cognitive adverse effects.

Two drugs are occasionally employed as "last-ditch" agents in refractory epilepsy: felbamate and vigabatrin. The experience with both of these drugs is that they are relatively effective, but their use comes with either a tiny but finite risk of death (felbamate) or a frequent, irreversible risk of vision loss (vigabatrin). My feeling is that neither of these drugs provides a sufficiently high chance of seizure freedom in refractory epilepsy to justify starting them in patients not already exposed, except in the most severely affected, for whom there are no other options. The chance of seizure freedom with less dangerous AEDs remains comparable given enough medication trials.

## Summary

Refractory epilepsy affects about one-third of all epilepsy patients, yet significant advances in treatment remain elusive. The likelihood of treatment success is increased by definitively establishing the epilepsy diagnosis through video–EEG monitoring, emphasizing compliance with treatment, avoiding AEDs that exacerbate seizures, and persistently varying the drug regimen in the hopes of arriving at the correct concoction of medications for the individual patient.

## Bibliography

Benbadis SR, Tatum WO, Gieron M. Idiopathic generalized epilepsy and choice of antiepileptic drugs. *Neurology* 2003; **61**:1793–1795.

Brodie MJ, Yuen AW. Lamotrigine substitution study: Evidence for synergism with sodium valproate? 105 Study Group. *Epilepsy Res* 1997; **26**:423–432.

Glauser TA, Cnaan A, Shinnar S, et al. Ethosuximide, valproic acid, and lamotrigine in childhood absence epilepsy. *N Engl J Med* 2010; **362**:790–799.

Kwan P, Brodie MJ. Early identification of refractory epilepsy. *N Engl J Med* 2000; **342**:314–319.

Luciano AL, Shorvon SD. Results of treatment changes in patients with apparently drug-resistant chronic epilepsy. *Ann Neurol* 2007; **62**:375–381.

Marson AG, Al-Kharusi AM, Alwaidh M, et al. The SANAD study of effectiveness of carbamazepine, gabapentin, lamotrigine, oxcarbazepine, or topiramate for treatment of partial epilepsy: An unblinded randomised controlled trial. *Lancet* 2007; **369**:1000–1015.

Marson AG, Al-Kharusi AM, Alwaidh M, et al. The SANAD study of effectiveness of valproate, lamotrigine, or topiramate for generalised and unclassifiable epilepsy: An unblinded randomised controlled trial. *Lancet* 2007; **369**:1016–1026.

Mattson RH, Cramer JA, Collins JF. A comparison of valproate with carbamazepine for the treatment of complex partial seizures and secondarily generalized tonic-clonic seizures in adults. The Department of Veterans Affairs Epilepsy Cooperative Study No. 264 Group. *N Engl J Med* 1992; **327**:765–771.

Poolos NP, Warner LN, Humphreys SZ, Williams S. Comparative efficacy of combination drug therapy in refractory epilepsy. *Neurology* 2012; **78**:62–68.

Schiller Y, Najjar Y. Quantifying the response to antiepileptic drugs: Effect of past treatment history. *Neurology* 2008; **70**:54–65.

# Rescue Medications for Home Treatment of Acute Seizures

**Peter Wolf[1] and Rūta Mameniškienė[2,3]**

[1]Danish Epilepsy Centre, Dianalund, Denmark
[2]Clinic of Neurology and Neurosurgery, Faculty of Medicine, Vilnius University, Vilnius, Lithuania
[3]Epilepsy Centre, Department of Neurology, Vilnius University Hospital Santariškių Klinikos, Vilnius, Lithuania

Epilepsy is a chronic disease and is treated with continuous medications aiming at sustained complete seizure control. However, in its course, emergency situations may sometimes arise that require acute interventions. In some epileptic conditions, seizures occur only occasionally but in series or prolonged states. These require rapid action, whereas continuous treatment may not be indicated. Rescue medication (RM) can also be used to prevent seizures when risk is perceived.

> ☆ **TIPS AND TRICKS**
>
> The home use of RMs can often help patients avoid emergency hospital admissions.

## Conditions requiring acute drug administration

### Febrile and nonfebrile serial seizures of childhood

Febrile seizures (FS) are the most frequent type of acute epileptic seizures and occur at the ages of 6 months to 5 years. There is a strong genetic predisposition. Although simple, uncomplicated FS have no sequelae, febrile status epilepticus has been correlated with the development of hippocampal sclerosis with the consequence of chronic temporal lobe epilepsy. It is therefore highly important that FS be treated as early and effectively as possible to prevent prolonged seizures. FS are often a once-in-a-lifetime event and not considered an indication for continuous antiepileptic drug (AED) treatment. However, recurrence occurs in up to one-third of children.

> ☆ **TIPS AND TRICKS**
>
> The risk of recurrence of FS is high enough that parents of a child who has had one should be provided with an RM and instructed how to administer it.

Recurrent prolonged and serial seizures unconnected with febrile illness are much more common in children than in adults and, in some patients, have a high risk of status epilepticus. RM should be made available.

### Epilepsies with habitual clusters of seizures

In some patients with epilepsy, seizures habitually occur in clusters of several seizures on one or subsequent days. These clusters may affect ability to work, independence, and life quality much more

*Epilepsy*, First Edition. Edited by John W. Miller and Howard P. Goodkin.
© 2014 John Wiley & Sons, Ltd. Published 2014 by John Wiley & Sons, Ltd.

than single seizures. In many cases, clusters can be effectively prevented by self-application of an RM after the first seizure.

### Prodromes and auras

Some patients have "warnings" before their seizures. These can be auras—that is, subjective symptoms that seem to precede the seizure but actually are the first seizure symptoms. These are quite common but usually last only seconds or fractions of seconds, too short for any drug intervention. In some patients, however, the auras last on the order of minutes, and a rapidly acting drug can possibly interrupt these.

A more rare kind of warning is the prodrome, which precedes a seizure for periods from 30 min upwards. Sometimes prodromes represent increased subclinical seizure activity or very mild forms of nonconvulsive status epilepticus, and sometimes their background cannot be clarified. They may be registered by the patients themselves or observed as behavioral changes by others. They are an indication for RM only if they stand out clearly from the habitual interictal state. In these cases, an oral benzodiazepine (BZD) can prevent an imminent seizure.

### ⚜ CAUTION!

Prodromes may impair a patient's ability to use RM as prescribed. It may therefore be necessary to have a family member or caregiver to administer it.

### Stress convulsions, provoked and lifestyle seizures, and social indications

Sleep disturbances increase the risk of seizures in many patients, especially when combined with excessive alcohol intake. Some patients with infrequent seizures even have exclusively provoked seizures that may also result from excessive psychophysical stress. They may be aware of the relationship but not necessarily willing to change their lifestyles. Prophylactic intake of an oral BZD at perceived risk can protect them against seizures. Prophylactic BZDs may also be recommended in cases of predictable sleep disturbances caused by overnight or transcontinental travel. People who travel a lot or have experienced a provoked seizure should have a small supply of a suitable BZD available.

Likewise, seizures can be prevented in socially important or potentially stigmatizing situations such

as church services, the theater, concerts, and sports events, or when the patient is in the spotlight, as when performing at cultural, political, or scientific events, applying for a job, or presenting a project to a committee.

### Reflex epileptic seizures (e.g., hot water epilepsy)

Reflex epilepsies are conditions where epileptic seizures habitually are precipitated by qualitatively, often even quantitatively, well-defined sensory or cognitive stimuli. Most patients also have spontaneous seizures that require continuous AED treatment. Others have only provoked seizures, or treatment controls the spontaneous but not the reflex seizures. If the seizure trigger cannot be avoided or attenuated (such as by the use of dark glasses to avoid photosensitive seizures), RM can be applied before the patient is exposed to the trigger. The best-known example is hot water epilepsy, a condition particularly common in South India, in which complex partial seizures habitually are provoked by pouring hot water over the head. In most cases, the application of 5–10 mg clobazam (CLB) 60–90 min before taking the head bath fully controls the seizures even without continuous AED treatment.

## Drugs for acute anticonvulsive intervention

### Benzodiazepines (BZDs)

Whereas BZDs are rarely used for sustained epilepsy treatment because of frequent development of secondary tolerance, they are clearly the first-line rescue medicines due to their rapid action and high anticonvulsant effect. The principal adverse effects are sedation and respiratory suppression, but these effects have not been reported to cause serious problems in studies of home RM. BZDs are differentiated from each other mainly by their pharmacokinetic properties.

### ⚜ CAUTION!

Persistent administration of BZDs often leads to tachyphylaxis that will limit their effectiveness.

#### Diazepam (DZP)

Diazepam (DZP) was the first BZD for which a solution for rectal use was introduced for home treatment as an alternative to IV administration. It has been extensively studied in both children and adults in double-blind, placebo-controlled studies. Absorption is rapid and complete, with peak concentrations attained within 5–15 min and a half-life of 20–40 h.

### Clonazepam (CLZ)

Oral clonazepam (CLZ) (tablets of 0.5 and 2 mg, orally disintegrating tablets of 5 strengths between 0.125 and 2 mg, or oral liquid of 2.5 mg/mL) is absorbed rapidly, with an absorption half-life of 24 min and without substantial differences between the formulations. Elimination half-life is 35–40 h. Rectal administration of CLZ has been investigated, and peak values were reached after 10–30 min, but no commercially available formulation for rectal use has been developed.

### Clobazam (CLB)

Clobazam is used almost exclusively for oral administration in tablets of 5, 10, and 20 mg, although rectal administration has been investigated and a liquid preparation is available in some countries. It is rapidly and completely absorbed, reaching peak levels after 1–3 h, and is metabolized with a half-life of 20–25 h. It has an active metabolite, desmethylclobazam, with a half-life of 36–46 h, so repetitive administration even at intervals of 2–3 days can be expected to produce accumulation to a steady state especially of the metabolite.

### Midazolam (MDZ)

Midazolam (MDZ) is a short-acting BZD developed in the 1970s, with rapid absorption and an elimination half-life of 1–4 h. It is available in tablets of 7.5 and 15 mg and in injectable form as ampoules of various sizes. Administration by the intranasal or the buccal route (absorption via the gums and cheek) as an alternative to rectally administered DZP is becoming increasingly popular for the emergency treatment of seizures because of high effectiveness for suppression of seizure activity and good tolerability. However, the main difficulty with the use of MDZ is tachyphylaxis, which becomes a problem within 48 h of initiation. A variety of liquid preparations for buccal and nasal administration are available. MDZ is absorbed directly via the mucosa into the bloodstream within 5–10 min.

### Lorazepam (LZP)

Oral, sublingual, and buccal administration of lorazepam (LZP) tablets (0.5, 1, or 2 mg) has been studied in several investigations. The absorption is rapid but too slow when immediate intervention is required. Absorption from a nasal spray is faster, and this formulation was not inferior to IV LZP in terminating acute seizures. LZP has a half-life of about 12 h, significantly longer than MDZ.

## Other

### Acetazolamide (AZM)

Acetazolamide (AZM) is a carbonic anhydrase inhibitor with antiepileptic properties that is not well established as an AED for sustained treatment, probably because of secondary tolerance. It has been used as interval therapy for catamenial epilepsy, with unconvincing results. There are no studies of AZM as RM for epilepsy, but it may be a possible alternative to BZDs if these are contraindicated, as in patients with a history of paradoxical reactions to BZDs, BZD addiction, or muscular weakness with increased risk of respiratory deficiency.

## Procedures

Home treatment normally excludes parenteral applications. RMs are available for oral, rectal, buccal, and nasal administration. The choice of route depends upon required speed of action, practicability, and availability, the latter differing much from country to country.

### Rectal

Diazepam is available in some countries as suppositories (5 or 10 mg) and in others as microclysmic gels (5 or 10 mg). DZP rectal gel is provided as unit doses of 2.5, 5, 7.5, 10, 12.5, 15, 17.5, and 20 mg, and the rectal delivery system includes a plastic applicator with a flexible, molded tip available in two lengths.

Leaking and defecation are potential obstacles to reliable rectal administration, especially as the application may provoke defecation. This is one of the reasons why other routes are now usually preferred when available.

### Buccal and nasal

The liquid formulation of MDZ for buccal administration can also be applied intranasally. The dose is given in two halves, one to each side. Traditionally, the liquid is provided in bottles from which the required dose is taken with a syringe and then delivered to the patient. For easier use and to improve speed of delivery, new ready-packed formulations are increasingly becoming available in some countries. LZP for nasal use comes with an atomizer or spray pump.

With buccal administration the patient must abstain from swallowing for 2 min. Nasal administration requires detailed instructions, and supporting materials are available, for example, at www.intranasal.net.

### Intramuscular

In some countries home treatment potentially includes intramuscular (IM) administration, which usually delivers the exact quantity of drug desired. For most AEDs, IM injection results in greater than 90% absorption, but the rate of absorption is highly variable. Formulations for IM administration are available for DZM, CLZ, MDZ, and LZP. Some patients and relatives prefer this rather than the rectal route. However, IM medications are absorbed more slowly than rectal formulations. Therefore, IM RM is used rarely, the alternative in most cases being oral administration. This may change in the future when autoinjectors that are under development for DZM, MDZ, and LZP become available.

### Strategies

> ★ **TIPS AND TRICKS**
>
> The rapidly absorbed buccal MDZ, nasal LZP, and rectal DZP will be used as interventions:
>
> For FS and habitually prolonged nonfebrile seizures in childhood
> To interrupt incipient recurrent status epilepticus (convulsive or nonconvulsive)
> In patients with habitual series of seizures occurring at short intervals; intervation is made at onset of a series, after the second or even the first seizure
> In patients at perceived risk of an imminent seizure (e.g., at aura onset)

In most instances, the buccal or nasal routes of administration will be preferred, especially if RM may be required out of the house. LZP acts longer than MDZ, which may determine individual choice depending on whether shorter action is desired to minimize side effects or longer action for more sustained therapeutic effect. In a semiconscious patient who could fight against buccal application

> ⚡ **CAUTION!**
>
> Rapidly acting BZD can produce a fall in blood pressure. Therefore, to prevent syncope, patients should rest in a recumbent position for some time after administration.

or when hypersalivation is present, the nasal route may be more reliable. Patients with a tendency toward resumption of seizure series or status after temporary interruption may benefit most from rectal DZP, which has the longest action of the three. This drug may also be easier to apply in bedridden and unconscious patients.

For recommended doses see Table 16.1.

> ★ **TIPS AND TRICKS**
>
> Oral CLB, DZP, and CLZ are indicated when onset of effective protection after 20–30 min is acceptable and sustained action is desired. This is the case when the RM is given to prevent seizures when risk is perceived, as with the following:
>
> - Prodromes
> - Seizures occurring in clusters
> - Lifestyle-provoked seizures
> - Overnight and transcontinental travel
> - Social situations
> - Reflex seizures

The time at which the preventive RM is taken depends on the time indicated by the individual's history. The therapeutic effect with all three drugs given orally starts approximately 20–30 min after intake, rapidly reaching its maximum. All three have sedation and drowsiness as unwanted effects, most pronounced with CLZ. CLB is the RM with which the most experience is available.

Most events that require RM end on the same day, but seizure clusters such as those in temporal lobe epilepsy may extend over two or more days. In these cases, doubling of the usual dose (such as 20 mg instead of 10 mg CLB) should be considered, and it may be necessary to repeat RM on the morning of the second day. These schemes may require adaptation in individual cases.

Some patients at perceived seizure risk may spontaneously take an extra dose of their regular AED,

**Table 16.1.** Recommended doses.

| Drug | Children | Adults | Remarks |
|---|---|---|---|
| DZP rectal gel | 0.5 mg/kg | 10–20 mg | 20 mg for cluster |
| Oral | | 10 mg | prevention |
| CLB oral | 5 mg for <30 kg; 10 mg for >30 kg body weight (for children more than 2 years old) | 10 mg | 20 mg for cluster prevention |
| CLZ oral | 0.02 mg/kg (from 0.01 to 0.03 mg/kg) | 1 mg | |
| MDZ buccal | 0.2 mg/kg | 10 mg | Rest recumbent after |
| Oral | 0.2 mg/kg | 10 mg | application |
| LZP nasal | 0.1 mg/kg | 2 mg | Rest recumbent after application |
| AZM oral | 8–30 mg/kg | 500 mg | |

AZM, acetazolamide; CLB, clobazam; CLZ, clonazepam; DZP, diazepam; LZP, lorazepam; MDZ, midazolam.

but the effect of this is doubtful and has not been established by any study.

Interventive, as well as preventive, RM is used only when a seizure is highly likely to occur. In some patients, however, the need for RM recurs rather frequently. The typical risks with repetitive administration of BZD, which accumulate because of a long half-life, are the development of tolerance and of drug dependence, so the question arises as to how often RM can be applied. This has been little discussed, but no such problems have been encountered with CLB used one to two times per week or even more frequently in the case of hot water epilepsy. No reports are available on DZM or on CLZ, which both may have a higher potential of dependence. In the case of reflex epilepsies, when frequent intake of RM may be required to provide protection only for brief periods, oral short-acting MDZ is probably the best option.

With some indications, the patients themselves can apply the acute medication. In most cases, however, the assistance of others is needed, and all should receive detailed instructions, which may need to be given repeatedly to ensure they are well understood and applied. The decision of whether or not to apply RM may be difficult and require a learning process before full success can be achieved. Camfield and colleagues recommend RM as the standard home treatment for FS "for a well-organized family."

Instructions to patients need to address the possibility that the RM might not have the desired effect and the seizures could thus continue or resume. In such instances, the most typical approach will be to repeat the RM one time along with calling an emergency doctor or an ambulance. Therefore, instructions should specify when the first RM should be considered unsuccessful, if and how often it can be repeated, and with what dose. Also, "home" treatment may include related situations such as school or kindergarten, where the immediate caretakers may be teachers or other nonmedical staff, unless a school nurse is available. These caregivers may have legal concerns about this responsibility and will usually feel more comfortable with buccal or nasal rather than rectal administration, which, in uninstructed observers, has raised suspicion of sexual assault. Questions such as how the RM may be stored where it is safe but rapidly accessible need to be discussed. Some issues may arise that cannot be resolved between the parents and caretakers and therefore need advice from the doctor. These matters have been discussed from a European perspective by Wait and colleagues.

## Conclusions

Several rapidly acting AEDs, especially BZD, are now available for rectal, buccal, nasal, and oral administration. This makes them applicable as RMs for home treatment by patients and caregivers. The advantages of RM are that emergency situations such as seizure clusters and status epilepticus can be stopped more rapidly, that patients at perceived risk can prevent seizures, and that emergency hospital admissions can be avoided.

## Bibliography

Camfield PR, Camfield CS, Eriksson KJ. Treatment of febrile seizures. In: Engel J, Pedley TA, eds. *Epilepsy: A Comprehensive Textbook*, 2nd ed. Philadelphia: Lippincott Williams & Wilkins, 2008, 1345–1349.

Meghana A, Sinha S, Sathyaprabha TN, Subbakrishna DK, Satishchandra P. Hot water epilepsy clinical profile and treatment – A prospective study. *Epilepsy Res* 2012; **102**(3):160–166.

Wait S, Lagae L, Arzimanoglou A, et al. The administration of rescue medication to children with prolonged acute convulsive seizures in the community: What happens in practice? *Eur J Paediatr Neurol* 2013; **17**(1):14–23.

Wolf P. Acute administration of benzodiazepines as part of treatment strategies for epilepsy. *CNS Neurosci Therap* 2011; **17**:214–220.

Wolf P. Acute drug administration in epilepsy. A review. *CNS Neurosci Therap* 2011; **17**:442–448.

# When and How to Stop Antiepileptic Drugs

**John D. Hixson**

Department of Neurology, University of California San Francisco,
San Francisco, CA, USA

## Introduction

When a patient is first diagnosed with epilepsy, the primary aim is to determine the appropriate treatment and stop further seizures. However, once seizure freedom is achieved, the eventual question becomes: how long should a patient remain on antiepileptic therapy? For other medical conditions, this question is more straightforward; antihypertensive therapy is generally considered a long-term commitment, while antibiotics have an intrinsically finite treatment plan. For epilepsy, the time frame is less clear. Some patients on antiepileptic drugs (AEDs) certainly benefit from prevented seizure recurrence, but other epilepsy patients may have entered a period of remission, even without medication. From the perspective of the healthcare provider, assigning a particular patient to a given category is difficult.

This chapter provides a summary of the evidence and resultant recommendations on this subject. A number of studies have examined this topic in imperfect conditions, using population-based methodology in both adults and children. This chapter will not review these studies exhaustively, but will summarize the primary approach to the concept of an AED withdrawal trial.

In general, for all patients with epilepsy who have been successfully treated with an AED, the seizure recurrence risk following medication withdrawal is significant, primarily in the first year following discontinuation. The overall seizure risk does not return to the population norm. However, depending on the situation, a withdrawal trial may be reasonable in many cases. Individual risk factors should be considered and discussed with each patient.

## When to stop an AED

Most studies that have examined this question in children and adult populations have had methodological shortcomings. Heterogeneity of epilepsy classification, variance in followup lengths, and different study designs prevent a definitive set of guidelines. However, some very clear trends emerge from the studies. First, even after a patient achieves seizure freedom, the risk of seizure recurrence after stopping an AED does not return to the healthy population norm. Second, certain risk factors predict an even higher rate of seizure recurrence following AED withdrawal. Thus, the best clinical practice is to have a detailed conversation with each patient about his or her relative risk (RR), focusing on the individual's fear of seizure recurrence versus the effect of continued therapy on quality of life and overall health.

Much of the practice of AED withdrawal trials has been guided by an American Academy of Neurology (AAN) practice parameter issued in the mid-1990s. This analysis examined 17 studies available at that

*Epilepsy*, First Edition. Edited by John W. Miller and Howard P. Goodkin.

time that dealt with AED withdrawal; only one study was a randomized controlled trial. The practice parameter noted pooled recurrence rates of 31.2% in children and 39.4% in adults. Across the different studies, the time of seizure freedom prior to AED withdrawal ranged from 1–2 years in children to 2–5 years in adults.

Since the publication of this AAN practice parameter, other studies have examined AED withdrawal in adults with epilepsy, demonstrating recurrence rates of 41–52%, depending on the length of followup. These investigations used a range of seizure freedom periods of 2–4 years, likely based on the guidance of the AAN practice parameter. It should also be noted that these studies suggested that the highest risk of recurrence occurred relatively early, within 6 months of the withdrawal period.

## EVIDENCE AT A GLANCE

In 2008, Lossius and colleagues reported a prospective randomized trial to explore the risks and benefits of AED withdrawal in adults. Although the primary aim of the study was to examine the effect of AED withdrawal on cognitive function and quality of life, it also provides evidence on seizure recurrence risk. Patients were required to be seizure-free for more than 2 years and were on AED monotherapy. The randomized withdrawal group exhibited an RR of 2.46 compared with the nonwithdrawal group (15% vs. 7%) in the initial 12-month followup. With longer followup, the withdrawal group demonstrated an increased relapse rate of 27%. The withdrawal group did show cognitive improvements on neuropsychological testing, supporting the rationale for the withdrawal attempt. The findings of this unique and important randomized, controlled adult study are largely consistent with the growing body of evidence concerning AED withdrawal.

In contrast, a randomized controlled trial of AED withdrawal in children that had been seizure-free for only 6 or 12 months, by Peters and colleagues, demonstrated relatively high recurrence rates of 55% and 49%, generally consistent with other studies performed since that time. Based on this study and others in children, a Camfield review in 2008 suggested a seizure-free period of 1–2 years as a reasonable pediatric benchmark for a trial of AED withdrawal. Notably, this standard for duration of seizure freedom is lower than

that of the adult population, possibly because some pediatric epilepsy syndromes are known to naturally remit over time. Thus, it is imperative to consider age when making this important decision.

It is also worth mentioning a special set of individuals that hopefully achieve seizure freedom: postsurgical epilepsy patients. By definition, these patients have risk factors for seizure recurrence (history of medication resistance, longer epilepsy duration), and the evidence of good long-term postsurgical seizure freedom rates depends on maintenance of AED therapy. However, several studies do support attempting AED withdrawal after 1–2 years of postsurgical seizure freedom. Although recurrence risk increases with duration of postoperative followup in most studies, the evidence suggests that this is not directly caused by AED withdrawal. Thus, it is reasonable to discuss this option with postsurgical patients while providing appropriate education and guidance after 1–2 years of complete seizure freedom.

It is important to recognize that a predefined period of seizure freedom cannot be broadly applied to all epilepsy patients. Intuitively, the length of the observation period depends on the pretreatment seizure frequency, which may differ widely among patients. The "rule of three" approach can be applied to this relationship: to be reasonably confident that a given treatment has improved seizure control, a span of at least three times the preintervention seizure interval is required. For example, in someone with one seizure every 3 months, seizure freedom for 9 months would be needed for confidence that control had truly been achieved. For those with very infrequent seizures, this "rule" may be less meaningful; however, it serves as a reminder that the necessary period of seizure freedom prior to considering AED withdrawal depends on the individual situation.

## ★ TIPS AND TRICKS

The decision to attempt an AED withdrawal trial should be individualized. In almost all cases, the risk of seizure recurrence is significant. This should be discussed with each patient. Practical considerations such as driving and work restrictions often affect the decision, perhaps even more than the long-term health consequences. Patients attempting AED withdrawal should enter a voluntary period of driving restriction and safe work practices.

## Risks and benefits

The decision to attempt an AED withdrawal trial should always be made after a careful consideration of the RR and benefits for each patient. This conversation with the patient needs to incorporate their wishes or those of the surrogate decision makers, in addition to the objective medical data.

There are a number of risk factors that increase the likelihood of seizure recurrence and the need for caution following AED withdrawal. In adults, considerations are abnormal neurological examination, IQ less than 70, longer epilepsy, higher number of historic seizures, multiple seizure types, focal epileptiform patterns on EEG, and worsening EEG patterns following AED withdrawal. For children, adolescent age of onset, symptomatic etiology, an abnormal neurological examination, and focal epileptiform patterns on EEG before or after withdrawal are associated with a higher risk of seizure recurrence. Additionally, certain epilepsy syndromes, such as juvenile myoclonic epilepsy and generalized tonic–clonic seizures upon awakening (idiopathic generalized epilepsy with pure grand mal), have known higher risks of seizure recurrence throughout a patient's lifetime.

For postsurgical patients, additional risk factors include longer duration of epilepsy, early postoperative seizures, abnormal EEG findings after surgery, preoperative normal MR imaging, and extratemporal resections.

**Table 17.1.** When to withdraw AEDs.

| Type of patient | Reasonable time to attempt withdrawal |
| --- | --- |
| Children with no risk factors | 2 years of seizure freedom (range 1–2 years) |
| Adults with no risk factors | 2 years of seizure freedom (range 2–5 years) |
| Adults following epilepsy surgery | 2 years of seizure freedom (range 1–2 years) |

In addition to considering these individual risk factors, it is also important for healthcare providers to anticipate and address the possible consequences of seizure recurrence. Even under the best circumstances, the seizure recurrence risk is significant, and it is important to prepare the patient for this possibility. Most commonly, a seizure recurrence may have negative psychological and quality of life effects on a patient who has previously been seizure-free. This will often have dramatic implications on driving- and work-related restrictions, and this scenario should be addressed with the patient in advance of AED withdrawal.

A final risk consideration is the possibility that seizure recurrence will change the natural course of a patient's epilepsy. After a period of seizure freedom, there is often a concern that the reappearance of seizures will result in a medically refractory state. Although this is a possibility, the evidence suggests that this is actually quite rare in the absence of the risk factors listed earlier. In general, patients with no risk factors and a prior history of successful seizure freedom will maintain a positive response to AEDs even after a failed withdrawal trial.

All of these risk considerations must be weighed against the benefits for an individual patient. Taking daily medications for epilepsy is a burden for most patients, and their quality of life would often be improved without this requirement. Additionally, eliminating the medication removes side effects, idiosyncratic reactions, and long-term adverse effects (Chapter 12). Finally, as many patients age and develop medical comorbidities, drug–drug interactions become increasingly problematic, particularly with older AEDs that exhibit enzymatic effects on hepatic metabolism (Chapter 13).

## How to stop an AED

Once a patient has decided to attempt AED withdrawal, the next decision is the method by which to accomplish this goal. Unfortunately, there are very few studies to guide this process. It is clear that a patient should not stop medications abruptly. This is particularly true for benzodiazepines or barbiturates due to the risk of precipitating a withdrawal seizure. Beyond this recommendation, there is little evidence to support a prolonged tapering period.

Several literature reviews have formally examined the approach to stopping an AED. For children, there was no difference in the risk of seizure recurrence between a "rapid" taper (over weeks) and a "slow" taper (over months), with the maximum seizure recurrence risk within 6 months of final AED discontinuation in both. Thus, prolonged tapering is not recommended, because it merely lengthens this overall process without adding benefit. In adult studies, a "slow" taper was defined as over 3 months and a "rapid" taper was defined as less than 3 months. A 2006 Cochrane review found that no studies possessed sufficiently strict criteria to guide recommendations. Overall, tapering in adults should adopt the same style as in the pediatric population.

## Conclusions

Healthcare providers and patients must individually weigh the benefits and risks when deciding to attempt an AED withdrawal trial after a period of seizure freedom. Population-based data can never provide a definitive predictive answer for an individual, and this should be stressed to patients. Even after successful treatment with an AED, risk of seizure recurrence is significant for all patients, regardless of situation or epilepsy etiology. Certain risk factors should be considered carefully and discussed with all patients or surrogate decision makers. And finally, all patients should be counseled about appropriate safety measures and possible ramifications if a seizure recurrence should occur. If these topics are all addressed, healthcare providers should feel comfortable offering the option of AED withdrawal to their seizure-free epilepsy patients.

## Bibliography

Aktekin B, Dogan EA, Oguz Y, Senol Y Withdrawal of antiepileptic drugs in adult patients free of seizure for 4 years: A prospective study. *Epilepsy Behav* 2006; **8**:616–619.

American Academy of Neurology. Practice parameter: A guideline for discontinuing antiepileptic drugs in seizure-free patients. *Neurology* 1996; **47**:600–602.

Berg AT, Shinnar S. Relapse following discontinuation of antiepileptic drugs: A meta-analysis. *Neurology* 1994; **44**:601–608.

Camfield P, Camfield C. The frequency of intractable seizure after stopping AEDs in seizure-free children with epilepsy. *Neurology* 2005; **64**:973–975.

Camfield P, Camfield C. When is it safe to discontinue AED treatment? *Epilepsia* 2008; **49**(Suppl. 9):25–28.

Cole AJ, Wiebe S. Debate: Should antiepileptic drugs be stopped after successful epilepsy surgery? *Epilepsia* 2008; **49**(Suppl. 9):29–34.

Kwan P, Arzimanoglou A, Berg AT, et al. Definition of drug resistant epilepsy: Consensus proposal by the ad hoc Task Force of the ILAE Commission on Therapeutic Strategies. *Epilepsia* 2010; **51**:1069–1077.

Lossius MI, Hessen E, Mowinckel P, et al. Consequences of antiepileptic drug withdrawal: A randomized, double-blind study. *Epilepsia* 2008; **3**:455–463.

Medical Research Council Antiepileptic Drug Withdrawal Study Group. Randomised study of antiepileptic drug withdrawal in patients in remission. *Lancet* 1991; **337**:1175–1180.

Peters ACB, Brouwer OF, Geerts AT, Arts WF, Stroink H, van Donselaar CA. Randomized prospective study of early discontinuation of antiepileptic drugs in children with epilepsy. *Neurology* 1998; **50**:724–730.

Ranganathan LN, Ramaratnam S. Rapid versus slow withdrawal of antiepileptic drugs. *Cochrane Database Syst Rev* 2006; **2**:CD005003.

Sirven J, Sperling MR, Wingerchuk DM. Early versus late antiepileptic drug withdrawal for people with epilepsy in remission. *Cochrane Database Syst Rev* 2001; **3**: Art. No.: CD001902.

Specchio LM, Tramacere L, La Neve A, Beghi E. Discontinuing antiepileptic drugs in patient who are seizure-free on monotherapy. *J Neurol Neurosurg Psychiatry* 2002; **72**:22–25.

# Using Parenteral Antiepileptic Medications

**Jane G. Boggs**

Neurology, Wake Forest University School of Medicine, Comprehensive Epilepsy Center, Winston Salem, NC, USA

## Introduction

Parenteral antiepileptic drugs (AEDs) are used for treatment of status epilepticus (SE) and acute repetitive seizures (ARS), as well as when enteral administration is not possible. Complexities inherent to use of parenteral AEDs include choosing how and when to use a loading dose, what maintenance doses to give, and whether and for how long to administer a continuous infusion. This chapter reviews these issues for those AED preparations clinically available for parenteral use. Approaches to treating SE are reviewed in Chapters 31 and 32.

## Agents

### Benzodiazepines

Although tachyphylaxis limits the role of most benzodiazepines (BZDs) in the long-term treatment of chronic epilepsy, these agents are typically the first treatment for SE and ARS. Pharmacokinetics of diazepam (DZP) and lorazepam (LZP) are given in Chapter 19. Pharmacodynamic drug interactions of BZDs with barbiturates may result in synergistic effects on respiration. Respiratory status must be carefully monitored and intubation considered before combining sedatives. Use of BZDs as out-of-hospital rescue medications is discussed in Chapter 16.

> **SCIENCE REVISITED**
>
> While gastrointestinal absorption delays the action of oral medication, the effects of parenteral drugs depend on lipophilicity, which affects the efficiency with which they traverse the blood–brain barrier. The BZDs vary in lipid solubility as well as redistribution rates from the site of action (neurons) to the remainder of the compartments of the cranium and, subsequently, the body. Drugs with the fastest egress from the brain may control seizures only briefly, with seizure recurrence resulting from the rapid loss of the pharmacological effect on GABA-mediated inhibition.

### Diazepam

Intravenous (IV) DZP has the fastest onset of CNS effect (less than 1 min) of current BZDs. Its 1–2 h distribution half-life $(t_{1/2})$ results in rapidly resolving sedation but mandates prompt introduction of longer-lasting AEDs in patients with repeated seizures. Initial DZP (5 mg/mL) adult IV dosing is 5–10 mg repeated every 10–15 min to reach a maximum of 30 mg. Dosing for neonates is 0.1–0.3 mg/kg/dose to a maximum of 2 mg, and for children, 0.04–0.3 mg/kg/dose

*Epilepsy*, First Edition. Edited by John W. Miller and Howard P. Goodkin.

to a maximum of 0.6 mg/kg/8 h. Injection rate should not exceed 5 mg/min and should be slower with cardiac, hepatic, or renal disease. Intramuscular (IM) injection may have erratic absorption. Tachyphylaxis may develop in less than 48 h. Other BZDs are preferred to DZP in kidney dysfunction, as renally eliminated active metabolites (e.g., desmethyldiazepam) may prolong sedation. DZP has modest cytochrome P450 induction (2B) and can accelerate clearance of other medications.

### Lorazepam

Intravenous LZP has high lipophilicity and affects the EEG within 2 min, with peak effect at 30 min. The effect is more sustained than that of DZP, with a distribution half-life of 2–3 h. The recommended dose is a 4 mg bolus (0.1 mg/kg), given no faster than 2 mg/min, with a repeat 4 mg after 10–15 min. Maximum recommended total adult dose is 8 mg. LZP may cause hypotension, somnolence, or respiratory depression. Continuous infusions for SE are at doses of 0.5–10 mg/h. While an IV 4 mg bolus gives a peak level of 70 ng/mL, IM administration has unpredictable absorption, with an average peak level of 48 ng/mL.

### Midazolam

Unlike DZP and LZP, midazolam (MDZ) does not contain propylene glycol. It is water soluble, making it suitable for IM injection. Because of conversion to the lipophilic form at physiological pH, its CNS effect is delayed up to 2 min, but it has rapid distribution $t_{1/2}$ (3.3–8.1 min). The initial recommended dose is 0.2 mg/kg over 2–3 min with a continuous infusion beginning at 2–4 mg/h, titrated to burst–suppression on the EEG. Tachyphylaxis often limits utility to <48 h. It can cause respiratory suppression.

### Phenytoin

Phenytoin (PHT) has been shown to stop 80% of acute seizures, and it is commonly used after BZD to treat SE. The usual initial PHT loading dose in adults and pediatrics is 15–20 mg/kg. An additional 10 mg/kg can be given, to a maximum total load of 30 mg/kg. Maintenance therapy (Chapter 19) should be promptly started.

Phenytoin has striking local toxicity due to poor water solubility, alkaline pH, and suspension in propylene glycol. Administration should be in large veins and not faster than 50 mg/min. Infusion is often associated with pain, phlebitis, and loss of IV access. Rates in children should be less than 1–3 mg/kg/min. "Purple glove syndrome" is a rare, devastating complication of PHT infusions that may lead to amputation. Systemic side effects of PHT infusion include hypotension, cardiac conduction abnormalities, and arrhythmias. Cardiac telemetry and blood pressure monitoring are required during infusion. Slowing the infusion rate may reduce these side effects. Adults with significant renal, hepatic, or cardiac disease should not receive PHT faster than 25 mg/min. IM injection is caustic and not recommended due to risk of abscesses and crystallization within muscle.

> ### ☞ CAUTION!
> Precipitation of PHT in IV tubing occurs when it is administered with glucose-containing solutions.

Fosphenytoin (FOS) is the water-soluble phosphorylated prodrug of PHT. Systemic phosphorylases immediately cleave off the phosphate group, converting it to PHT. FOS is dosed as "PHT equivalents" (mg PE) based on molecular weight after conversion to PHT. Maximal infusion rate is up to 150 mg PE/min. FOS still possesses PHT-related cardiovascular risks and should be infused only with telemetry and blood pressure monitoring. All such phosphorylated compounds can produce annoying pruritus, especially in the groin, which can be minimized by slowing the infusion rate. FOS can be safely administered intramuscularly but requires a high volume and should be divided into multiple injection sites.

### Barbiturates

#### Phenobarbital

Intravenous phenobarbital (PB) has an EEG onset of action within 5 min. Despite a terminal $t_{1/2}$ of several days, peak IV effects last 6–10 h, warranting two to three times daily dosing. Its effective $t_{1/2}$ is shortest in neonates, at 63 h; somewhat longer in children; and 80–100 h in adults. It is profoundly sedating, with significant potential for drug interactions, especially with BZDs.

The recommended adult and pediatric PB dose is 15–20 mg/kg, usually to a maximum of 1000 mg/dose. PB contains propylene glycol, limiting infusion rate to no faster than 60 mg/min, with reduced rates in cases of renal, hepatic, or cardiac impairment. Usual recommended maintenance IV therapy for patients over 12 years is 4–6 mg/kg/day. For children, recommended maintenance is 2.5–5 mg/kg/day. As with all barbiturates, tolerance may develop with prolonged use.

### Pentobarbital

Pentobarbital (PTB) is primarily used as a continuous infusion for refractory SE. A loading dose of 3–5 mg/kg followed by initial infusion rates of 1–4 mg/kg/h is typical. The infusion rate must be titrated based on effect on the CV-EEG. Onset of action is within 1 min following IV administration and within 10–25 min with IM administration. The systemic $t_{1/2}$ of PTB is ~20 h largely due to sequestration in systemic fat. Mobilization of these stores can result in prolonged sedation after infusion ends. The rates of entry of barbiturates into the brain are determined by cerebral blood flow, so low mean arterial pressure can lessen therapeutic response. Hypotension with PTB may warrant pressors to optimize cerebral blood flow.

---

### ☝ CAUTION!

DZP, LZP, PHT, PB, and PTB all are dissolved in propylene glycol with dose- and infusion rate-dependent cardiovascular instability. Risk of intravascular precipitation requires in-line filtering. The administration rate should be even slower in cases of cardiac, renal, or hepatic dysfunction. Patients receiving multiple doses or combinations of these agents should be monitored for increasing anion gap, hyperosmolality, and metabolic acidosis disproportionate to their underlying illness. Consider MDZ or FOS as alternatives.

---

### Other parenteral agents for seizures

### Propofol

Propofol is increasingly used in ICU management of SE. It is highly lipophilic and emulsified in a mixture of soybean oil, egg lecithin, and glycerol. Onset of effect is <1 min, with short duration of action (4–10 min). Although beneficial for rapid awakening after conscious sedation, this characteristic can result in recurrent seizures after SE. Prolonged use can lead to persistent sedation, suggesting significant redistribution to systemic fat. Continuous infusions are initiated at 5 µg/kg/min and titrated slowly in 5–10 µg increments to achieve burst–suppression on the EEG. Administration should be by central venous catheter due to the potential for peripheral irritation, with a new infusion setup every 12 h to prevent bacterial contamination. Hypotension is dose and rate dependent. At rates greater than 50 µg/kg/min for more than 48 h, serum triglycerides rise. Propofol infusion syndrome is a rare complication with a mortality rate of 60% or more. It occurs with high infusion rates sustained for 2 days and consists of cardiovascular collapse with refractory bradycardia, severe metabolic acidosis, rhabdomyolysis, and acute renal failure.

### Ketamine

Ketamine is an NMDA-receptor antagonist and anesthetic agent that has recently been used to treat refractory SE. It is water soluble and does not contain propylene glycol. It has been administered to adults as a 50 mg bolus given over at least 1 min, which is followed by an initial infusion of 40 mg/h (0.6 mg/kg/h) titrated to effect on EEG. Acute complications include respiratory depression and enhanced pressor response. Safety of infusions over longer periods remains to be established.

### Valproate sodium

Parenteral valproate sodium (VPA) is approved for IV substitution when VPA cannot be taken orally. It is bioequivalent to the standard-release (but not the extended-release) oral formulation. It is water soluble and does not contain propylene glycol. Although it is not approved for SE, several studies report benefit in the treatment of acute seizures and SE in adults and children. The recommended rate of infusion is 500 mg/h, but faster rates are commonly used. In acute seizures, initial loading doses of 15–20 mg/kg have been used at rates up to 6 mg/kg/min. Distribution $t_{1/2}$ is 30–60 min. Cardiovascular safety is high, and telemetry is not required.

### Levetiracetam

Intravenous levetiracetam (LEV) is bioequivalent to its oral counterpart. It is currently approved for parenteral replacement therapy. Successful treatment with LEV of acute seizures and SE in adults and children has been reported. It is renally eliminated and water soluble. Recommended dosing is by dilution of dos

(500–1500 mg) to 100 mL, infused over 15 min. There are reports of success in treating SE with infusions of 20 mg/kg over 15 min, followed by IV maintenance therapy of 1–3 g/day in three divided doses. Doses should be lower in cases of renal dysfunction. Complications of infusion are infrequent, and telemetry is not indicated.

*Lacosamide*

Parenteral lacosamide (LCS) formulation has similar bioavailability to the oral agent. It is approved for short-term replacement of the oral formulation. There are, however, reports of use in refractory SE and critical care seizure patients. After dilution, recommended infusion is over 15–30 min. Time to effect on the EEG has not been systematically studied, but the efficacy of LCS has been noted to be slower than that of other parenteral agents.

## Future perspectives

Parenteral versions of orally available AEDs have obvious utility when temporary replacement is needed. Other AEDs have parenteral forms under development, such as IV carbamazepine and the IV form of the monohydroxy derivative (MHD) of oxcarbazepine. Experience regarding parenteral AEDs will continue to be driven by treatment of ARS and SE. There is an ongoing need for additional effective therapies, especially for refractory SE. Until comparative prospective, blinded trials are performed, off-label use of these agents is supported by an ever-expanding literature of case series and retrospective reviews of parenteral agents for treatment of seizures in critical care.

## Bibliography

Alvarez V, Januel JM, Burnand B, Rossetti AO. Second-line status epilepticus treatment: Comparison of phenytoin, valproate and levetiracetam. *Epilepsia* 2011 July; **52**(7):1292–1296.

Appleton R, Sweeney A, Choonara I, Robson J, Molyneux E. Lorazepam versus diazepam in the acute treatment of epileptic seizures and status epilepticus. *Dev Med Child Neurol* 1995; **37**:682–688.

Biton V, Rosenfeld WE, Whitesides J, Fountain NB, Vaiciene N, Rudd GD. Intravenous lacosamide as replacement for oral lacosamide in patients with partial-onset seizures. *Epilepsia* 2008; **49**:418–424.

Browne TR, Kugler AR, Eldon MA Pharmacology and pharmacokinetics of fosphenytoin. *Neurology* 1996; **46**:S3–S7.

Claassen J, Hirsch LJ, Emerson RG, Mayer SA. Treatment of refractory status epilepticus with pentobarbital, propofol, or midazolam: A systematic review. *Epilepsia* 2002; **43**:146–153.

Greenblatt DJ, Divoll M. Diazepam versus lorazepam: Relationship of drug distribution to duration of clinical action. *Adv Neurol* 1983; **34**:487–491.

Jamerson BD, Dukes GE, Brouwer KL, Donn KH, Messenheimer JA, Powell JR. Venous irritation related to intravenous administration of phenytoin versus fosphenytoin. *Pharmacotherapy* 1994; **14**:47–52.

Knake S, Gruener J, Hattemer K, et al. Intravenous levetiracetam in the treatment of benzodiazepine refractory status epilepticus. *J Neurol Neurosurg Psychiatry* 2008; **79**:588–589.

Kramer AH, Early ketamine to treat refractory status epilepticus. *Neurocrit Care* 2012; **16**:299–305.

Limdi NA, Shimpi AV, Faught E, Gomez CR, Burneo JG. Efficacy of rapid IV administration of valproic acid for status epilepticus. *Neurology* 2005; **64**:353–355.

Stecker MM, Kramer TH, Raps EC, O'Meeghan R, Dulaney E, Skaar DJ. Treatment of refractory status epilepticus with propofol: Clinical and pharmacokinetic findings. *Epilepsia* 1998; **39**:18–26.

Venkataraman V, Wheless JW. Safety of rapid intravenous infusion of valproate loading doses in epilepsy patients. *Epilepsy Res* 1999; **35**:147–153.

Wilson KC, Reardon C, Theodore AC, Farber HW. Propylene glycol toxicity: A severe iatrogenic illness in ICU patients receiving IV benzodiazepines: A case series and prospective, observational pilot study. *Chest* 2005 September; **128**(3):1674–1681.

# 19

# Pharmacopeia

**Gail D. Anderson**

Department of Pharmacy, UW Regional Epilepsy Center, University of Washington, Seattle, WA, USA

**Table 19.1.** Approved indications of the antiepileptic drugs.

| Drug | Indications | Approval for monotherapy | Approval in children |
|---|---|---|---|
| Acetazolamide | Epilepsy | Yes | No |
| Carbamazepine | Partial, generalized, and mixed types of epilepsy | Yes | All ages |
| Clobazam | Lennox–Gastaut syndrome | No | ≥2 years of age |
| Clonazepam | Lennox–Gastaut syndrome; absence, akinetic, myoclonic seizures | Yes | All ages |
| Diazepam | Status epilepticus, seizures (refractory) | Yes | ≥6 months of age |
| Eslicarbazepine acetate | Partial seizures with and without secondary generalization | No | ≥6 months of age |
| Ethosuximide | Absence seizures | Yes | ≥3 years of age |
| Ezogabine | Partial seizures | No | ≥18 years of age |
| Felbamate | Lennox–Gastaut syndrome | No | ≥2 years of age |
| | Partial seizures with and without secondary generalization | No | ≥14 years of age |
| Gabapentin | Partial seizures | No | ≥3 years of age |
| Lacosamide | Partial seizures | No | ≥18 years of age |
| Lamotrigine | Lennox–Gastaut syndrome, primary generalized tonic–clonic seizures | No | ≥2 years of age |
| | Partial seizures | Yes | ≥2 years of age |

*Epilepsy*, First Edition. Edited by John W. Miller and Howard P. Goodkin.

**Table 19.1.** (*Continued*)

| Drug | Indications | Approval for monotherapy | Approval in children |
|---|---|---|---|
| Levetiracetam | Partial seizures<br>Myoclonic seizures<br>Primary generalized tonic–clonic seizures | No<br>No<br>No | ≥1 month of age<br>≥12 years of age<br>≥6 years of age |
| Lorazepam | Status epilepticus | Yes | ≥18 years of age[a] |
| Oxcarbazepine | Partial seizures | Yes | ≥2 years of age |
| Perampanel | Partial seizures | No | ≥12 years of age |
| Phenobarbital | Epilepsy | Yes | All ages |
| Phenytoin | Generalized tonic–clonic seizures, partial seizures | Yes | All ages |
| Pregabalin | Partial seizures | No | ≥18 years of age |
| Primidone | Epilepsy | Yes | All ages |
| Rufinamide | Lennox–Gastaut syndrome | No | ≥4 years of age |
| Stiripentol | Intractable atypical absence, partial or generalized seizures | No | ≥6 years of age |
| Tiagabine | Partial seizures | No | ≥12 years of age |
| Topiramate | Lennox–Gastaut syndrome, partial or primary generalized tonic–clonic seizures | Yes | ≥2 years of age |
| Valproate | Absence, complex partial, multiple seizure types | Yes | ≥10 years of age |
| Vigabatrin | Complex partial seizures<br>West syndrome | No<br>Yes | ≥16 years of age<br>1 month to 2 years |
| Zonisamide | Partial seizures | No | ≥16 years of age |

[a]Not FDA approved for ages less than 18 years. Recommendations for treatment of status epilepticus in children include lorazepam as an accepted agent for initial treatment.

**Table 19.2.** Chemistry and pharmacology of the antiepileptic drugs.

| Drug | Chemical structure | Proposed mechanism of action |
|---|---|---|
| Acetazolamide | 5-Acetamido-1,3,4-thiadiazole-2-sulfonamide | Inhibits carbonic anhydrase |
| Carbamazepine | 5-Carbamoil-5H-dibenz[b,f]azepine | Inhibits voltage-gated sodium channels Stabilizes neuronal membranes and limits sustained repetitive firing |
| Clobazam | 7-chloro-1-methyl-5-phenyl-1H-1,5-benzodiazepine-2,4(3H,5H)dione | Enhances GABA$_A$ receptor-mediated chloride currents |
| Clonazepam | 5-(2-Chlorophenyl)-1,3-dihydro-7-nitro-2H-1,4 benzodiazepin-2-one | Enhances GABA$_A$ receptor-mediated chloride currents |
| Diazepam | 7-Chloro-1,3-dihydro-1-methyl-5-phenyl-1,4 benzodiazepin-2(3H)-one | Enhances GABA$_A$ receptor-mediated chloride currents |

(*Continued*)

**Table 19.2.** (*Continued*)

| Drug | Chemical structure | Proposed mechanism of action |
|---|---|---|
| Eslicarbazepine acetate | S-(−)-10-acetoxy-10,11-dihydro-5H-dibenzo[b,f]azepine-5-carboxamide | Voltage-gated sodium channel blocker |
| Ethosuximide | 2-Ethyl-2-methylsuccinimide | Attenuates voltage-sensitive calcium channels |
| Ezogabine | N-(2-amino-4-(4-fluorobenzyl-amino)-phenyl) carbamic acid ethyl ester | Opens/activates voltage-gated potassium channels (KCNQ2/3, KCNQ3/6) Potentiates GABA-evoked currents |
| Felbamate | 2-Phenyl-1,3-propanediol dicarbamate | Inhibits voltage-gated sodium channels Inhibits calcium currents through NMDA receptors Enhances GABA$_A$ receptor-mediated chloride channels |
| Gabapentin | 1-Aminomethyl-cyclohexane acetic acid | Binds to $\alpha_2\delta$ subunit of the L-type calcium channel Increases GABA levels by increasing GABA turnover Inhibits monoamine neurotransmitter release Decreases sustained repetitive firing |
| Lacosamide | (R)-2-acetamido-N-benzyl-3-methoxypropionamide | Enhances slow inactivation of sodium channels |
| Lamotrigine | 3,5-Diamino-6-(2,3-dichlorophenyl)-1,2,4-triazine | Inhibits sodium currents Inhibits high-threshold activated calcium channels |
| Levetiracetam | (S)-$\alpha$-ethyl-2-oxo-1-pyrrolidine acetamide | Limits calcium influx through an N-type voltage-sensitive calcium channel Binds to synaptic vesicle protein 2A |
| Lorazepam | 7-Chloro-5(2-chlorophenyl)-1,3-dihydro-3-dihydroxy-2H-1,4-benzoidazepin-2-one | Enhances GABA$_A$ receptor-mediated chloride currents |
| Oxcarbazepine | 10,11-Dihydro-10-oxo-carbamazepine | Active metabolite, 10-OH-carbazepine, inhibits sustained repetitive firing |
| Perampanel | | Reduces neuronal excitation via the noncompetitive antagonism of the ionotropic AMPA-glutamate receptor on postsynaptic neurons |
| Phenobarbital | 5-Ethyl-5-phenylbarbituric acid | Enhances GABA$_A$ receptor-mediated chloride currents |
| Phenytoin | 5,5-Diphenylhydantoin | Inhibits voltage-gated sodium channels Stabilizes neuronal membranes and limits sustained repetitive firing |
| Pregabalin | S-(+)-3-aminomethylhexanoic acid; Isobutyl-$\gamma$-aminobutyric acid | Selective inhibitor of L-type voltage-gated calcium channels containing the $\alpha_2\delta$ subunit |

**Table 19.2.** (*Continued*)

| Drug | Chemical structure | Proposed mechanism of action |
|------|--------------------|------------------------------|
| Primidone | 5-Ethyldihydro-5-phenyl-4,6 (1H,5H) pyrimidine-dione | Enhances GABA$_A$ receptor-mediated chloride currents |
| Rufinamide | 1-(2,6-Difluorophenyl) methyl-1H-1,2,3-triazole-4-carboxamide | Sodium channel blocker |
| Stiripentol | 4,4-Dimethyl-1-[(3,4 methylenedioxy) phenyl]-1-penten-3-ol | Enhances GABAergic neurotransmission by increasing the release of GABA and the duration of the activation of GABA$_A$ receptors |
| Tiagabine | (−)-*R*-1-[4,4-bis(3-methyl-2-thienyl)-3-butenyl]-3-piperidinecarboxylic acid | Selective blocker of neuronal and glial GABA transporters resulting in increased brain GABA levels |
| Topiramate | 2,3:4,5-bis-*O*-(1-methylethylidene)-β-D-fructopyranose sulfamate | Blocks sustained repetitive firing and inhibits sodium currents<br>Decreases glutamate-mediated excitation via the AMPA/kainate receptor<br>Enhances GABA$_A$ currents<br>Potentiates hyperpolarizing potassium currents<br>Inhibits high-threshold activated calcium channels<br>Inhibits carbonic anhydrase |
| Valproate | 2-Propylpentanoic acid | Attenuates voltage-sensitive calcium channels, inhibits sodium channels, and stabilizes neuronal membranes<br>Enhances GABAergic-mediated inhibition |
| Vigabatrin | 4-Amino-5-hexenoic acid; γ-vinyl GABA | Irreversibly inhibits GABA transaminase, resulting in increased brain GABA levels |
| Zonisamide | 1,2-Benzisoxazole-3-methane sulfonamide | Blocks sustained repetitive firing through an effect on voltage-sensitive sodium channels<br>Reduces T-type calcium currents<br>Alters ligand binding to GABA$_A$ receptor<br>Inhibits carbonic anhydrase |

**Table 19.3.** Average daily doses of the antiepileptic drugs (monotherapy).

| Drug | Neonates | Infants | Children | Adults | Serum reference range |
|---|---|---|---|---|---|
| Acetazolamide | NE | NE | 10–20 mg/kg/day | 375–1000 mg/day | 10–14 mg/L |
| Carbamazepine | NE | 10–16 mg/kg/day | <6 years: 10–20 mg/kg/day 6–12 years: 400–1000 mg/day | 800–2400 mg/day | 4–12 mg/L |
| Clobazam | NE | 2.5 mg | ≦30 kg: 5–20 mg/day >30 kg: 10–40 mg/day | 10–40 mg/day | 30–300 µg/L[a] |
| Clonazepam | 0.01 mg/kg/day | 0.01–0.05 mg/kg/day | ≦30 kg: 0.01–0.05 mg/kg/day >30 kg 0.03–0.2 mg/kg/day | 2–20 mg/day | 20–80 µg/L[a] |
| Diazepam | NE | 0.3 mg/kg | 0.3–0.5 mg/kg | 5–30 mg | 0.1–100 µg/L[a] |
| Eslicarbazepine | NE | NE | NE | 800–1200 mg/day | NE |
| Ethosuximide | NE | NE | 20–30 mg/kg/day | 500–1500 mg/day | 40–100 mg/L |
| Ezogabine | NE | NE | NE | 200–400 mg/day | NE |
| Felbamate | NE | NE | 15–45 mg/kg/day | 1200–3600 mg/day | 30–60 mg/L[a] |
| Gabapentin | NE | NE | 10–45 mg/kg/day | 1800–3600 mg/day | 2–20 mg/L[a] |
| Lacosamide | NE | NE | NE | 200–400 mg/day | NE |
| Lamotrigine | NE | NE | 2–8 mg/kg/day | 100–600 mg/day | 4–20 mg/L[a] |
| Levetiracetam | NE | 1–6 months: 28–42 mg/kg/day | 6–<4 years: 20–50 mg/kg/day 4–16 years: 20–60 mg/kg/day | 1000–3000 mg/day | 5–40 mg/L[a] |
| Lorazepam | NE | 0.1 mg/kg | 0.1 mg/kg, max: 5–8 mg | 2–10 mg | 10–30 µg/L[a] |
| Oxcarbazepine | NE | NE | 2–4 years: 20–60 mg/kg/day 4–16 years – if weight is: 20–29 kg: 900 mg/day 29.1–39 kg: 1200 mg/day >39 kg: 1800 mg/day | 600–2100 mg/day | MDH: 12–30 mg/L[a] |
| Perampanel | NE | NE | 4–12 mg/day | 4–12 mg/day | NE |

| | | | | | |
|---|---|---|---|---|---|
| Phenobarbital | 3–4 mg/kg/day | 5–6 mg/kg | 4–8 mg/kg/day | 60–300 mg/day | 10–40 mg/L |
| Phenytoin | 5–8 mg/kg | 4–8 mg/kg/day | 4–8 mg/kg/day | 200–500 mg/day | 10–20 mg/L |
| Pregabalin | NE | NE | NE | 200–600 mg/day | NE |
| Primidone | NE | NE | <8 years: 10–25 mg/kg/day ≥8 years: 750–1000 mg/day | 750–1000 mg/day | Primidone: 5–12 mg/L Phenobarbital: 10–40 mg/L |
| Rufinamide | NE | NE | 10–45 mg/kg/day | 1600–3200 mg/day | 10–40 mg/L |
| Stiripentol | NE | NE | If weight is: 12–14 kg: 1000 mg/day 15–19 kg: 1500 mg/day 20–29 kg: 2000 mg/day 30–39 kg: 2500 mg/day >39 kg: 3000 mg/day | 1000–3000 mg/day | NE |
| Tiagabine | NE | NE | 0.375–1.25 mg/kg/day | 16–56 mg/day | 100–300 mg/L [a] |
| Topiramate | NE | NE | 5–9 mg/kg/day | 100–400 mg/day | 2–25 mg/L [a] |
| Valproate | NE | 15–30 mg/kg | 15–30 mg/kg | 1000–5000 mg/day | 50–100 mg/L |
| Vigabatrin | NE | 50–150 mg/kg/day | NE | 500–1500 mg/day | NE |
| Zonisamide | NE | NE | 4–12 mg/kg/day | 100–600 mg/day | 10–40 mg/L [a] |

NE, not established.

[a] No established therapeutic range.

**Table 19.4.** Pharmacokinetic parameters of antiepileptic drugs.

| AED | Vd (L/kg) | Protein binding (%) | $t_{1/2}$ (h) | Renal (%) | Hepatic isozymes involved if known | Active metabolite |
|---|---|---|---|---|---|---|
| Acetazolamide | 0.2 | 70–90 | 4–8 | 90 | None | No |
| Carbamazepine | 0.8–2 | 75 | 12–17 | <1 | CYP3A4 (major), CYP1A2, CYP2C8 | Yes |
| Clobazam | 0.9–1.4 | 85–93 | 10–30 | 2 | CYP2C19, CYP3A4 | Yes |
| Clonazepam | 3.2 | 85 | 22–40 | <1 | CYP3A4 | Yes |
| Diazepam | 1–2 | 98 | 24–48 | <3 | CYP2C19, CYP3A4 | Yes |
| Eslicarbazepine acetate | | | | | | Yes |
| Eslicar-bazepine | nk | 30 | 20–24 | 66 | UGT1A4, UGT1A9,UGT2B4,UGT2B7, UGT2B7 | No |
| Ethosuximide | 0.6–0.7 | 0 | 13–20 | 20 | CYP3A4 (major), CYP2E1 | No |
| Ezogabine | 2–3 | 80 | 25–60 | 33 | UGT, NAT | No |
| Felbamate | 0.7–1.0 | 22–25 | 20–23 | 50 | UGT, CYP3A4 (20%),CYP 2E1 | No |
| Gabapentin | 0.85 | 0 | 5–9 | >90 | None | No |
| Lacosamide | 0.6 | <15 | 13 | 40 | Not identified | No |
| Lamotrigine | 0.9–1.3 | 55 | 12–60 | <1 | UGT1A4 | No |
| Levetiracetam | 0.5–0.7 | <10 | 6–8 | 66 | Amidase | No |
| Lorazepam | 0.8–1.5 | 93 | 17–56 | <1 | UGT2B15 | |
| Oxcarbazepine | nk | 40–60 | 1–2.5 | <1 | Cytosolic arylketone reductase | Yes |
| MHD | 0.7–0.8 | 33–40 | 8–11 | 20 | UGT | No |
| Perampanel | nk | 95 | 105 | 22 | CYP3A4, CYP3A5, other CYPs | No |
| Phenobarbital | 0.5–1.0 | 20–60 | 36–118 | 20 | Glucosides, CYP2C9, CYP2C19, CYP2E1 | No |
| Phenytoin | 0.5–1.0 | 88–93 | 7–42 | 2 | CYP2C9 (major), CYP2C19 (minor) | No |
| Pregabalin | 0.5 | 0 | 5–6.5 | >95 | None | No |
| Primidone | 0.85 | <10 | 10–15 | 40–60 | Not identified | Yes |
| Phenobarbital | 0.5–1.0 | 20–60 | 36–118 | 20 | Glucosides, CYP2C9, CYP2C19, CYP2E1 | |
| PEMA | 0.69 | <10 | 29–36 | nk | | |
| Rufinamide | 0.7 | 34 | 6–10 | <2 | Non-CYP dependent hydrolysis | No |
| Stiripentol | nk | 99 | 13 | <1 | UGT and CYPs, isozymes not identified | No |
| Tiagabine | nk | 96 | 3–8 | <2 | CYP3A4 (22%) | No |

**Table 19.4.** (*Continued*)

| AED | Vd (L/kg) | Protein binding (%) | $t_{1/2}$ (h) | Renal (%) | Hepatic isozymes involved if known | Active metabolite |
|---|---|---|---|---|---|---|
| Topiramate | 0.6–0.8 | 9–41 | 21 | 30 | Not identified | No |
| Valproate | 0.1–0.2 | 5–15 | 6–17 | <5 | β-oxidation, UGT1A6,1A9,2B7, CYP2C9, 2C19 | Yes |
| Vigabatrin | 0.8 | 0 | 5–8 | >90 | None | No |
| Zonisamide | 0.8–1.6 | 40–60 | 27–70 | 35 | NAT2 (15%), CYP3A4 (major), CYP2C19 | No |

CYP, cytochrome P450; NAT, *N*-acetyltransferase; nk, not known; UGT, UDP glucuronosyltransferase.

**Table 19.5.** Antiepileptic drug adverse effects.

| Drug | Acute adverse effect: concentration related | Acute adverse effect: idiosyncratic | Chronic adverse effects |
|---|---|---|---|
| Acetazolamide | Confusion<br>Diarrhea<br>Drowsiness<br>Loss of appetite<br>Nausea/vomiting<br>Paresthesia<br>Seizure<br>Somnolence<br>Taste sense alteration<br>Tinnitus | Agranulocytosis<br>Aplastic anemia<br>Bone marrow depression<br>Hepatotoxicity<br>Leukopenia<br>Multiorgan hypersensitivity<br>Photosensitivity<br>Rash<br>Stevens–Johnson syndrome<br>Thrombocytopenia<br>Toxic epidermal necrolysis<br>Urolithiasis | Angle-closure glaucoma<br>Hyperglycemia<br>Hyperuricemia<br>Hypokalemia<br>Metabolic acidosis<br>Nephrolithiasis<br>Nephrotoxicity<br>Polyuria<br>Reduced libido<br>Renal calculi<br>Teratogenicity |
| Carbamazepine | Ataxia<br>Blurred vision<br>Diplopia<br>Dizziness<br>Drowsiness<br>Impaired cognition<br>Lethargy<br>Nausea/vomiting | Agranulocytosis<br>Aplastic anemia<br>Bone marrow depression<br>Hepatotoxicity<br>Leukopenia<br>Multiorgan hypersensitivity<br>Rash<br>Stevens–Johnson syndrome<br>Thrombocytopenia<br>Toxic epidermal necrolysis | Hyponatremia<br>Lipid abnormalities<br>Osteomalacia<br>Paresthesia<br>Teratogenicity<br>Thyroid abnormalities |

(*Continued*)

**Table 19.5.** (*Continued*)

| Drug | Acute adverse effect: concentration related | Acute adverse effect: idiosyncratic | Chronic adverse effects |
|---|---|---|---|
| Clobazam | Ataxia<br>Constipation<br>Irritability<br>Nausea/vomiting<br>Sedation | | Behavioral effects<br>Tolerance |
| Clonazepam | Ataxia<br>Confusion<br>Diplopia<br>Dizziness<br>Fatigue<br>Impaired coordination<br>Memory impairment | Rash<br>Hypersalivation | Behavioral effects<br>Depression<br>Tolerance |
| Eslicarbazepine acetate | Abnormal<br>  coordination<br>Diplopia<br>Dizziness<br>Headache<br>Nausea/vomiting<br>Somnolence | | |
| Ethosuximide | Anorexia<br>Ataxia<br>Drowsiness<br>Epigastric pain<br>Headache<br>Lethargy<br>Hiccups<br>Nausea/vomiting<br>Unsteadiness | Agranulocytosis<br>Aplastic anemia<br>Bone marrow depression<br>Leukopenia<br>Multiorgan hypersensitivity<br>Pancytopenia<br>Rash<br>Stevens–Johnson<br>  syndrome<br>Systemic lupus<br>  erythematosus | Behavioral effects<br>Psychiatric symptoms |
| Ezogabine | Blurred vision<br>Confusion<br>Diplopia<br>Dizziness<br>Dysuria<br>Fatigue<br>Gait disturbance<br>Nausea<br>Somnolence<br>Tremor<br>Urinary retention | Prolonged QTc interval | Hallucinations<br>Psychiatric symptoms<br>Weight gain<br>Blue discoloration of skin,<br>  nail beds, and lips<br>Retinal pigmentary<br>  changes |
| Felbamate | Anorexia<br>Headache<br>Insomnia<br>Nausea/vomiting | Aplastic anemia<br>Acute hepatic failure | Weight loss |
| Gabapentin | Ataxia<br>Constipation<br>Diarrhea<br>Diplopia<br>Dizziness<br>Fatigue<br>Nausea/vomiting<br>Somnolence<br>Tremor | Peripheral edema | Weight gain<br>Psychiatric effects<br>  (children) |

**Table 19.5.** (*Continued*)

| Drug | Acute adverse effect: concentration related | Acute adverse effect: idiosyncratic | Chronic adverse effects |
|---|---|---|---|
| Lacosamide | Ataxia<br>Blurred vision<br>Diplopia<br>Dizziness<br>Drowsiness<br>Nausea/vomiting<br>Tremor<br>Unsteady gait | Prolonged PR interval | |
| Lamotrigine | Blurred vision<br>Diplopia<br>Dizziness<br>Headache<br>Insomnia<br>Nausea/vomiting<br>Tremor<br>Unsteadiness | AED hypersensitivity<br>  syndrome<br>Aseptic meningitis<br>Multiorgan<br>  hypersensitivity<br>Rash<br>Stevens–Johnson<br>  syndrome<br>Toxic epidermal<br>  necrolysis | |
| Levetiracetam | Coordination<br>  difficulties<br>Dizziness<br>Fatigue<br>Sedation<br>Somnolence | Rash<br>Stevens–Johnson<br>  syndrome<br>Toxic epidermal<br>  necrolysis | Behavioral<br>  abnormalities<br>Psychiatric effects |
| Oxcarbazepine | Abnormal gait<br>Ataxia<br>Dizziness<br>Fatigue<br>Nausea/vomiting<br>Sedation<br>Somnolence<br>Tremor | Rash<br>Stevens–Johnson<br>  syndrome<br>Toxic epidermal<br>  necrolysis | Hyponatremia<br>Thyroid abnormalities<br>Weight gain |
| Perampanel | Ataxia<br>Blurred vision<br>Diarrhea<br>Dizziness<br>Fatigue<br>Headache<br>Irritability<br>Somnolence | Contusion<br>  (bruising)<br>Convulsions<br>Fall<br>Peripheral edema<br>Rash | |
| Phenobarbital | Ataxia<br>Headache<br>Hyperactivity<br>Impaired cognition<br>Nausea<br>Sedation<br>Somnolence<br>Unsteadiness | AED hypersensitivity<br>  syndrome<br>Blood dyscrasia<br>Rash<br>Stevens–Johnson<br>  syndrome | Behavioral effects<br>Cerebellar syndrome<br>Folate deficiency<br>Gingival hyperplasia<br>Hirsutism<br>Lipid abnormalities<br>Osteomalacia/<br>  osteoporosis<br>Teratogenicity |

(*Continued*)

**Table 19.5.** (*Continued*)

| Drug | Acute adverse effect: concentration related | Acute adverse effect: idiosyncratic | Chronic adverse effects |
|---|---|---|---|
| Phenytoin | Ataxia<br>Cognitive impairment<br>Confusion<br>Coordination problems<br>Dizziness<br>Headache<br>Lethargy<br>Nystagmus<br>Sedation<br>Visual blurring | AED hypersensitivity syndrome<br>Multiorgan hypersensitivity<br>Hepatotoxicity<br>Rash<br>Stevens–Johnson syndrome<br>Toxic epidermal necrolysis | Behavioral effects<br>Folate deficiency<br>Gingival hyperplasia<br>Hirsutism<br>Lipid abnormalities<br>Lymphadenopathy<br>Osteomalacia/osteoporosis<br>Peripheral neuropathy<br>Teratogenicity |
| Pregabalin | Blurred vision<br>Dizziness<br><br>Somnolence<br>Tremor | Constipation<br>Creatine kinase elevation<br>Peripheral edema | Weight gain |
| Primidone | Ataxia<br>Headache<br>Hyperactivity<br>Impaired cognition<br>Nausea<br>Sedation<br>Somnolence<br>Unsteadiness | Agranulocytosis<br>Megaloblastic anemia<br>Rash<br>Systemic lupus erythematosus<br>Thrombocytopenia | Connective tissue disorders<br>Personality changes<br>Teratogenicity<br>Other adverse effects as listed for phenobarbital |
| Rufinamide | Abnormal gait<br>Ataxia<br>Blurred vision<br>Diplopia<br>Dizziness<br>Nausea/vomiting<br>Somnolence | Multiorgan hypersensitivity<br>Pruritus<br>Rash | |
| Stiripentol | Ataxia<br>Diplopia<br>Drowsiness<br>Nausea/abdominal pain<br>Slowing of mental function | Neutropenia | Weight loss |
| Tiagabine | Blurred vision<br>Dizziness<br>Difficulty concentrating<br>Fatigue<br>Nervousness<br>Tremor<br>Weakness | Spike–wave stupor | Depression |
| Topiramate | Concentration difficulties<br>Dizziness<br>Fatigue<br>Headache<br>Psychomotor slowing<br>Speech/language problems<br>Somnolence | Acute-angle glaucoma<br>Hepatotoxicity<br>Metabolic acidosis<br>Oligohydrosis | Depression/psychosis<br>Kidney stones<br>Weight loss |

**Table 19.5.** (*Continued*)

| Drug | Acute adverse effect: concentration related | Acute adverse effect: idiosyncratic | Chronic adverse effects |
|------|---------------------------------------------|-------------------------------------|-------------------------|
| Valproate | Ataxia<br>Blurred vision<br>Diplopia<br>Dizziness<br>Nausea/vomiting<br>Sedation<br>Tremor | Alopecia<br>Elevated liver function test<br>Hematological abnormalities<br>Hepatotoxicity<br>Pancreatitis<br>Thrombocytopenia | Hyperammonemia<br>Menstrual cycle irregularities<br>Polycystic ovary-like syndrome<br>Teratogenicity<br>Weight gain |
| Vigabatrin | Abnormal gait<br>Blurred vision<br>Diplopia<br>Concentration difficulties<br>Coordination problems<br>Dizziness<br>Nausea/vomiting<br>Somnolence | Hematological abnormalities<br>Rash | Behavioral abnormalities<br>Permanent vision loss<br>Visual field defects<br>Weight gain |
| Zonisamide | Cognitive impairment<br>Dizziness<br>Nausea/vomiting<br>Sedation | Metabolic acidosis<br>Oligohydrosis<br>Paresthesia<br>Rash<br>Stevens–Johnson syndrome<br>Toxic epidermal necrolysis | Depression<br>Kidney stones<br>Visual hallucinations<br>Weight loss |

## Bibliography

Bialer M, Johannessen SI, Levy RH, Perucca E, Tomson T, White HS. Progress report on new antiepileptic drugs: A summary of the Tenth Eilat Conference (EILAT X). *Epilepsy Res* 2010; **92**:89–124.

Levy RH, Mattson RH, Meldrum BS, Perruca P (eds). *Antiepileptic Drugs*, 5th ed. Philadelphia: Lippincott Williams & Wilkins, 2002.

Pellock JM, Dodson W, Bourgeois B (eds). *Pediatric Epilepsy: Diagnosis and Therapy*, 2nd ed. New York: Demos Medical Publishing, 2001.

Rho JM, Sankar R. The pharmacologic basis of antiepileptic drug action. *Epilepsia* 1999; **40**:1471–1483.

Stephen LJ, Brodie MJ. Pharmacotherapy of epilepsy: Newly approved and developmental agents. *CNS Drugs* 2011; **25**:89–107.

Thomson Micromedex™. Available at www.micromedex.com (accessed on September 2, 2013).

# Part IV

# Special Topics in Pediatric Epilepsy

# Seizures in the Neonate

**Adam L. Hartman[1] and Frances J. Northington[2]**

[1] Divisions of Epilepsy and Pediatric Neurology, Neurosciences Intensive Care Nursery, Johns Hopkins Medicine Baltimore, MD, USA
[2] Division of Neonatology, Neurosciences Intensive Care Nursery, Neonatal Research Laboratory, Johns Hopkins Medicine, Baltimore, MD, USA

## Introduction

Seizures are common during the neonatal period, occurring at a rate of approximately 2/1000 live births. Although the neonate with seizures may have an otherwise normal appearance, seizures reflect the presence of central nervous system pathology, such as hypoxic–ischemic injury. The presence of a seizure in a neonate should be considered an urgent condition requiring close monitoring and a thorough diagnostic evaluation for treatable and life-threatening conditions.

### SCIENCE REVISITED

In the developed nervous system, GABA is considered an inhibitory neurotransmitter. However, in immature neurons, GABA can lead to depolarization (rather than hyperpolarization) due to reversals of the chloride gradient. It has been posited that this depolarizing effect of GABA contributes to the propensity for seizures during the neonatal period and may complicate treatment with drugs that target the GABAergic system.

## Clinical features

### Electroclinical seizures

The clinical features of neonatal seizures may involve focal clonic activity (unifocal or multifocal), focal tonic activity (which may involve limbs, trunk, or sustained ocular deviation), myoclonic activity, or spasms (either flexor, extensor, or both). Myoclonus may be either epileptic or nonepileptic, making it one of the more challenging semiologies to evaluate.

### ★ TIPS AND TRICKS

At the bedside, the most straightforward way to differentiate a seizure from other adventitious movements is to determine whether the suspicious activity can be provoked or, conversely, can be easily suppressed (i.e., by gently restraining the affected limb). In both cases, the likelihood of a seizure is decreased.

Classically, the EEG during neonatal seizures is associated with rhythmic sharp or sharply contoured slow activity that evolves from higher to

*Epilepsy*, First Edition. Edited by John W. Miller and Howard P. Goodkin.
2014 John Wiley & Sons, Ltd. Published 2014 by John Wiley & Sons, Ltd.

lower frequencies, sometimes followed by postictal slowing (i.e., a typical ictal evolution). One variant that may be missed by automated EEG detection systems is low-amplitude, low-frequency activity with a typical ictal evolution. Most neonatal seizures last less than 5 min and originate in the central or temporal regions. According to one convention, in order to be labeled a seizure, ictal EEG changes must have a duration greater than 10 s. Some neonates have bursts of epileptiform activity that are brief in duration (i.e., >10 s), referred to as "brief rhythmic discharges" or BRDs. Although not typically treated as seizures, BRDs may be an indicator of other types of underlying pathology, including periventricular leukomalacia.

**Electrographic seizures**

It is not uncommon in the setting of a neonatal encephalopathy to observe on brain monitoring periods of abnormal activity that have a typical electrographic ictal evolution without clinical changes. These "electrographic-only" seizures typically portend a poor long-term outcome or death. There are a number of conditions associated with these "electrographic-only" seizures. The most obvious is that the neonate has been paralyzed (i.e., for ventilation) and is not capable of manifesting motor activity. The second reason is that the neonate has been sedated to the point that motor and/or autonomic changes have been masked (i.e., electroclinical dissociation). The third and most concerning reason is that the initial injury prevents the expected clinical manifestations from occurring. Occasionally, these circumstances may occur in combination.

*Neonatal epilepsy syndromes*

Although the distinction is rarely considered initially, there are both malignant and benign neonatal epilepsy syndromes. The malignant epilepsy syndromes include early infantile epileptic encephalopathy (EIEE, also known as Ohtahara syndrome) and early myoclonic encephalopathy (EME). The EEG in both syndromes shows a burst–suppression pattern. At the bedside, the distinction between these two syndromes is not always clear, and both share a poor prognosis in terms of seizures, development, and survival. Neonates with EIEE typically have frequent tonic spasms (i.e., hundreds per day) that may occur during the awake or asleep states. Myoclonic and partial seizures also can occur. The most common

associated pathology is structural brain lesions, including hemimegalencephaly, porencephaly, and malformations of cortical development. Some patients have mutations in *STXBP1*, *CDKL5*, *ARX*, and other genes. Neonates with EME typically have recurrent myoclonic seizures but also can have focal seizures or tonic spasms. The most common associated pathologies are inborn errors of metabolism, including glycine encephalopathy and organic acidurias. Because of some overlap in signs and symptoms, with either electroclinical presentation, extensive genetic and metabolic testing is typically performed. In both EIEE and EME, the mortality rate is high in early infancy and survivors have poor neurodevelopmental outcomes. Seizures are highly resistant to treatment.

Fortunately, not all neonatal epilepsy syndromes are malignant. Benign familial neonatal seizures (BFNS), also known as "third-day fits," are associated with mutations in *KCNQ2* and *KCNQ3*. In most patients, seizures are focal or generalized and there may be associated apnea. The interictal EEG usually is normal. The ictal EEG shows a voltage decrement followed by spikes or slowing (either focal or generalized). Focal epileptiform activity is seen rarely. Other types of seizures may occur later in life.

**⚠ CAUTION!**

Not all patients with mutations in *KCNQ2* have a benign course, although a malignant course is rare. Recently, mutations in *KCNQ2* were found in neonates with treatment-resistant seizures. Unlike in "typical BFNS," in this syndrome tonic seizures are prominent and the EEG has a burst–suppression pattern. Although the seizures may cease, many of the patients in the study were found later to have motor and intellectual disabilities.

The syndrome of benign idiopathic neonatal seizures (BINS) also is known as "fifth-day fits." The seizures associated with this rare syndrome can include multifocal clonic seizures that may occur in clusters or be associated with apnea. Tonic–clonic seizures have been reported as having episodes of eye deviation and oral-motor movements. The interictal EEG may be normal but occasionally shows a pattern known as *theta pointu alternant*, which consists of theta-range activity with intermixed sharp activity (this may b asynchronous between hemispheres). Importantly, this pattern is nonspecific and may be seen in BFNS and in patients with seizures of other etiologies. Another variant, benign familial neonatal–infantile seizures, is associated with a positive family history of similar seizures. Seizure onset usually is at 2–3 months of age but can occur as early as 2 days of life. The seizure semiology usually is focal onset with secondary generalization, but apnea and cyanosis have been reported. This syndrome is associated with mutations in *SCN2A*, *PRRT2*, and *ASC-1* genes (and possibly others), but seizures resolve after the first year of life.

## Diagnosis

The goal of finding an underlying cause for neonatal seizures is to make a diagnosis with therapeutic or prognostic implications (Figure 20.1). Underlying causes of neonatal seizures include hypoxic–ischemic injury, infection (congenital or perinatal), metabolic abnormalities (both acute and inborn errors of metabolism), genetic abnormalities, hemorrhage, infarction, cortical dysgenesis, drug withdrawal, and neonatal epilepsy syndromes.

At a minimum, all neonates with seizures should have a neonatal montage EEG. The American Clinical Neurophysiology Society has released a guideline on continuous electroencephalography monitoring in neonates, citing continuous video–EEG monitoring as the gold standard for characterization of abnormal paroxysmal events. Many institutions also use amplitude-integrated EEG (aEEG) for prolonged monitoring if video–EEG resources are limited.

### ★ TIPS AND TRICKS

Although aEEG still has limitations, its ease of use by non-neurophysiologists and ability to monitor for prolonged periods (days), along with increasing recognition of the possibility of electroclinical dissociation in infants in the ICU, have contributed to growth in its popularity. Evolution of the technology to include more than one channel and simultaneous display of both the "real time" and compressed trace has improved the diagnostic accuracy of the device, but in general, most studies find that it is still significantly less sensitive than an EEG with a standard neonatal montage. This difference is to be expected because of the relative paucity of the cortical surface surveyed with 2 channels compared to the 14–16 channels on a standard neonatal EEG and the availability of synchronized video with conventional EEG.

At the time of the first seizure, neonates also should have a bedside fingerstick glucose test; a complete blood count; tests of electrolytes, liver function, calcium, magnesium, and cholesterol; toxicology screens; and some form of imaging (i.e., bedside ultrasound) performed as soon as possible. A lumbar puncture should be considered, with tests including cell count, glucose, protein, Gram stain, bacterial culture, and polymerase chain reaction tests for herpes simplex virus, cytomegalovirus, varicella zoster virus, enterovirus, human parechovirus, and Epstein–Barr virus. Ideally, a tube of CSF can be held in the laboratory for additional studies if the initial screen is negative.

An inborn error of metabolism should be rapidly suspected if seizures are refractory to initial treatment, if other signs of encephalopathy are present, or if there are abnormal metabolic screening labs (i.e., hypoglycemia or persistent acidosis). In this setting, additional tests may include serum lactate, plasma amino acids, ammonia, acylcarnitine profile, urine organic acids, urine-reducing substances, and studies for sulfite oxidase/molybdenum cofactor deficiency. Cerebrospinal fluid studies should include amino acids and neurotransmitters. If seizures persist or refractory status epilepticus (defined as lack of response to the first two medicines tried) is present, pyridoxine dependency should be suspected. In this setting, a trial of vitamin B6 should be performed using pyridoxine 100 mg (intravenous) with continuous video–EEG running (this can be repeated two to three times in 24 h). If this trial is unsuccessful, a trial of pyridoxine 5–10 mg/kg/day by mouth can be performed for 2 weeks, as some patients respond to chronic dosing. Both false positives and negatives can be seen with this type of medication trial, so a definitive diagnosis is based on genetic testing (*ALDH7A1*). Genetic testing for other disorders is constantly evolving, so a local genetics expert should be consulted regarding the most efficient means of diagnosing these abnormalities.

144 · Special Topics in Pediatric Epilepsy

## Treatment

Step 1
  Phenobarbital 20 mg/kg IV x 1
  If seizures stop, then no further doses of
  phenobarbital. (Consider antibiotics and
  antivirals, per the clinical situation and
  findings from lab studies.)

Step 2
If seizures recur within 30 min,* then

Options

a.  Phenobarbital 10 mg/kg IV x 1
b.  Fosphenytoin 20 mg/kg IV x 1
c.  Levetiracetam 20–30 mg/kg IV x 1
d.  Midazolam (protocols vary; one published is a
    bolus dose of 60 mcg/kg followed by an infusion
    of 150 mcg/kg/h)
e.  Lorazepam 0.05–0.1 mg/kg IV x 1

If seizures stop, then continue on maintenance
medication of choice.

Step 3
If seizures recur, then repeat dosing of one of the
medicines used previously or, alternatively, one
that was not used previously.

Step 4
If the evaluation thus far is negative, consider
pyridoxine 100 mg IV x 1 with continuous video–
EEG running (can be repeated 2–3 times in 24 h).
Consider 5–10 mg/kg/day PO x 2 weeks (some
patients respond to chronic dosing). If response is
incomplete, can try folinic acid 2.5–5 mg PO BID.

If seizures stop, then continue on maintenance
medication of choice.

Other options for seizure control include lidocaine
(use caution if fosphenytoin was administered
previously), topiramate, zonisamide, lacosamide,
valproate, and the ketogenic diet, among others.
Additional treatment options may include pyridoxal
phosphate or folinic acid.

*If seizures recur after more than 30 min, then
options may include a repeat dose of
phenobarbital, lorazepam, or fosphenytoin.

## Diagnostic studies

Initial studies
Consider:

✓ STAT blood glucose (to detect hypoglycemia and
  to correlate with LP), CBC, CMP, phosphate,
  magnesium, blood cultures, ABG, ammonia,
  toxicology (incl. meconium)
✓ LP (culture, cell count, glucose, protein, HSV and
  other viral PCRs)
✓ Imaging (head ultrasound, MRI, or CT, depending
  on patient, history, etc.)
✓ Routine EEG

Additional studies
Consider:

✓ Blood for amino acids, lactate, acyl carnitines,
  urine for organic acids, cholesterol
✓ Urine-reducing substances, studies for sulfite
  oxidase/molybdenum cofactor deficiency
✓ Expedite state newborn screening results
✓ Other genetics/metabolism studies may include
  SNP array, CDG, VLCFA, pipecolic acid, *ALDH7A1*,
  CSF amino acids, CSF neurotransmitters, and
  others

**Figure 20.1.** Algorithm of initial diagnostic studies and treatments for neonatal seizures.

Abbreviations: CBC, complete blood count; CDG, congenital disorders of glycosylation; CMP, complete metabolic panel; CSF, cerebrospinal fluid; CT, computed tomography; EEG electroencephalography; HSV, herpes simplex virus; LP, lumbar puncture; MRI, magnetic resonance imaging; PCR, polymerase chain reaction; SNP, single-nucleotide polymorphism; VLCFA, very long-chain fatty acids.

## Differential diagnosis

The most common alternative diagnosis of seizures is jitteriness, which can be distinguished from seizures by the relative ease with which it can be suppressed (using gentle restraint). Seizures are not inducible by environmental stimuli, whereas jitteriness can be. Jitteriness also is not associated with changes in level of consciousness. Neonates frequently have sleep-associated myoclonus and shuddering, both of which are benign. One diagnosis that should not be overlooked is hyperekplexia (which clinically looks like an exaggerated startle response, sometimes in response to gently tapping the neonate's nose), which in some cases involves abnormalities in spinal cord inhibitory glycine receptors. This diagnosis may involve the diaphragm and, thus, can cause respiratory arrest. Benzodiazepines typically are used for treatment, and the symptoms usually resolve in the first 2 years of life.

### ☆ TIPS AND TRICKS

In neonates with hyperekplexia, forced flexion of the head and legs during an event of tonic stiffening with respiratory distress has proven to be lifesaving.

Neonates can have other types of movements that are very similar to reflex movements noted in animal models. These events, which some have labeled subtle seizures, do not have an EEG correlate and thus are not managed like the electroclinical events noted previously. In some cases, these abnormal movements may be associated with underlying brain pathology. As mentioned previously, myoclonus may be either epileptic or nonepileptic. Video–EEG may be required to determine the nature of myoclonus in a specific patient. Other examples include eye movements (e.g., dysconjugate gaze or roving eye movements), oral movements (e.g., sucking, chewing, or tongue protrusion), extremity movements (e.g., rowing, swimming, or pedaling), and generalized tonic posturing. Only rarely are changes in vital signs (e.g., apnea, tachycardia, bradycardia) the only sign of seizures, but their presence should increase awareness for other seizure-associated behaviors.

## Treatment

Neonatal seizure treatment includes antiepileptic drugs (AEDs) and therapy for specific underlying problems, if known. Diagnosis and treatment typically are pursued in tandem (Figure 20.1). The most commonly used first line of treatment is phenobarbital. Consideration has been given to other medicines as first-line treatment because of concerns about side effects after long-term use of phenobarbital. If only one seizure occurs, and it is limited in duration, then further treatment may not be necessary, as further benefit may not outweigh some of the risks of AEDs. If the initial seizure persists, options include additional doses of phenobarbital or the initiation of phenytoin/fosphenytoin, levetiracetam, midazolam, or lorazepam. In our institution, an intravenous dose of pyridoxine (typically administered with simultaneous continuous cardiorespiratory and EEG monitoring) is considered for refractory status epilepticus or recurrent seizures fairly early in the course. If seizures stop, then the medication that worked is continued as a maintenance medication. Lidocaine has been studied for neonatal seizures. Although effective, there is a concern about a synergistic adverse effect with medicines that act on voltage-gated sodium channels (e.g., fosphenytoin) because of their similar mechanisms of action. Lidocaine use requires monitoring of metabolite levels, as their accumulation can be toxic. Other options for seizure control include topiramate, zonisamide, lacosamide, valproate, and the ketogenic diet, among others. Additional treatment options may include pyridoxal phosphate or folinic acid.

### ✋ CAUTION!

If treatment with pyridoxine is incomplete, a trial of folinic acid (2.5–5 mg twice a day) may stop seizures (as both pyridoxine-dependent and folinic acid-responsive seizures are due to mutations in the *ALDH7A1* gene). Some also have described the initial use of pyridoxal-5'-phosphate, the biologically active form of pyridoxine, followed by maintenance dosing with pyridoxine.

Long-term developmental outcome is an important factor behind the decision of how aggressively neonatal seizures should be treated. In general, neonates with benign epilepsy syndromes or seizures that are readily diagnosed and treated, such as brief neonatal hypoglycemia, have a good prognosis. Neonates with seizures due to severe brain pathology may not fare as well. A practical (and fairly common) clinical conundrum is whether "electrographic-only" seizures should be treated like those with overt clinical manifestations (i.e., electroclinical seizures). There has been some controversy surrounding whether the prognosis is due primarily to underlying pathology (i.e., structural sequelae of neonatal encephalopathy) or whether the seizures themselves make a substantial contribution to the prognosis. As of this writing, this question has not been resolved. The neonatal brain appears to tolerate brief seizures better than the adult brain, but animal data and some human studies support the notion that repetitive electrographic seizures in the injured brain contribute to a poor prognosis, independent of underlying pathology.

Clinical factors associated with a poor prognosis following neonatal seizures include preterm delivery, severe encephalopathy, cerebral dysgenesis, complicated intraventricular hemorrhage, abnormal EEG, use of multiple AEDs, and, in preterm infants, infection or generalized myoclonic seizures. In many studies, both neonatal status epilepticus and abnormal MRI findings have been shown to predict future epilepsy. Other studies have shown that EEG findings associated with a poor long-term neurodevelopmental prognosis include the presence of BRDs, multifocal seizure onset, and contralateral spread of an initially unilateral seizure focus.

Another challenging decision is when to discontinue AEDs. As a general guide, we attempt to discontinue AEDs as soon as it appears to be safe (i.e., normal exam and EEG without paroxysmal abnormalities). Neonates with continuing seizures or EEGs with clear epileptiform abnormalities are discharged from the NICU on oral AEDs (typically phenobarbital but occasionally other agents), with close followup in neurology clinic. AEDs are discontinued at the earliest opportunity, but if this is not possible, we attempt to switch the infant to something other than phenobarbital.

## Future perspectives

There is much to be learned about the management of neonatal seizures. The timing of diagnostic studies (i.e., how to perform them in a cost-effective manner) remains to be defined. The value (in terms of long-term outcomes) of continuous monitoring remains to be defined. There is a question of whether aggressive treatment of electrographic seizures changes long-term outcomes. The use of phenobarbital as a first-line agent also is being actively debated, given the alternatives available now. The use of continuous monitoring and implementation of cooling in neonatal encephalopathies has revolutionized care in this age group. Neonatal seizure treatment benefits from some of these advances, but the results of ongoing clinical trials provide further reason to be optimistic that antiseizure care for this vulnerable population will continue to improve in the near future.

### ✋ CAUTION!

As neonatal seizures are typically unexpected, seizures in the neonate can lead to anxiety for caregivers and parents alike. Thus, communication with an expert is suggested in situations that are not straightforward.

## Bibliography

Abend NS, Wusthoff CJ. Neonatal seizures and status epilepticus. *J Clin Neurophysiol* 2012; **29**:441–448.

Mizrahi EM. Neonatal seizures. In: Swaiman KF, Ashwal S, Ferriero DM, eds. *Pediatric Neurology: Principles and Practice*, 4th ed. Philadelphia: Mosby, 2006, 257–277.

Mizrahi EM, Kellaway P. Characterization and classification of neonatal seizures. *Neurology* 1987; **37**:1837–1844.

Mizrahi EM, Hrachovy RA, Kellaway P. *Atlas of Neonatal Electroencephalography*, 3rd ed. Philadelphia: Lippincott Williams & Wilkins, 2003.

Pearl PL. New treatment paradigms in neonatal metabolic epilepsies. *J Inherit Metab Dis* 2009; **32**:204–213.

Ronen GM, Buckley D, Penney S, Streiner DL. Long-term prognosis in children with neonatal seizures: A population-based study. *Neurology* 2007; **69**: 1816–1822.

Shellhaas RA, Chang T, Tsuchida T, et al. The American clinical neurophysiology society's guideline on continuous electroencephalography monitoring in neonates. *J Clin Neurophysiol* 2011; **28**:611–617.

Volpe JJ. *Neurology of the Newborn*, 5th ed. Philadelphia: Saunders, 2008.

# Benign and Malignant Childhood Epilepsies

Katherine C. Nickels and Elaine C. Wirrell

Mayo Clinic, Rochester, MN, USA

Epilepsy is one of the most common chronic neurological disorders in children, with an incidence of 33–82 per 100,000 children. It is most likely to begin early, with the highest incidence rates in the first year of life. Fortunately, approximately 60% of children will outgrow their epilepsy, becoming seizure-free and discontinuing antiepileptic medication. Conversely, approximately 20% are medically intractable, continuing to have uncontrolled seizures despite trials of two or more antiepileptic drugs.

This chapter will provide an overview of the various types of epilepsy syndromes and constellations (see Chapter 2 on classification) that occur in the pediatric age range, outside the neonatal period (see Chapter 20 on neonatal epilepsy). Those epilepsies that are pharmacoresponsive and self-limited are "benign," whereas the epilepsies that respond poorly to antiepileptic medications (pharmacoresistant), are not self-limited, and are associated with encephalopathy that is present or worsens after seizure onset (i.e., epileptic encephalopathy) are designated "malignant."

> ★ **TIPS AND TRICKS**
>
> Approximately one-third to one-half of epilepsy cases in children can be classified into distinct electroclinical syndromes

or epilepsy constellations. Such classification provides important information on the best (and contraindicated) therapies and long-term prognosis.

## "Benign" childhood epilepsies

### Infantile onset

*Benign infantile epilepsy/benign familial infantile epilepsy*

The benign infantile epilepsies comprise several entities, all self-limited and associated with favorable neurological and intellectual outcome (Table 21.1). Benign (nonfamilial) infantile epilepsy presents in neurologically normal infants in the first year of life. Seizures can be focal dyscognitive, with motion arrest, decreased responsiveness, and mild clonic activity, or can evolve to generalized tonic–clonic activity. Seizures typically occur in a cluster over several days and are very pharmacoresponsive. The interictal EEG is normal. Ictal recordings show temporal foci with focal dyscognitive seizures and centroparietal foci in those that evolve to bilateral convulsive activity. Neuroimaging is normal.

*Epilepsy*, First Edition. Edited by John W. Miller and Howard P. Goodkin.
2014 John Wiley & Sons, Ltd. Published 2014 by John Wiley & Sons, Ltd.

**Table 21.1.** Pharmacoresponsive childhood epilepsies.

| Syndrome | Typical age at onset | Seizure types | Self-limited | Pharmaco-responsive | Associated epileptic encephalopathy | EEG | Etiology | Initial treatment |
|---|---|---|---|---|---|---|---|---|
| Benign epilepsy in infancy | First year | Focal seizures that may evolve to bilateral GTCS, often occur in rare clusters | Yes | Yes | No | Normal background, focal discharges (temporal, centroparietal) | Unknown | Carbamazepine, oxcarbazepine, levetiracetam |
| Benign familial infantile epilepsy | First year | Focal seizures that may evolve to bilateral GTCS, often occur in rare clusters | Yes | Yes | No | Normal background, focal discharges (temporal, centroparietal) | Genetic | Carbamazepine, oxcarbazepine, levetiracetam |
| Myoclonic epilepsy in infancy | 4 months to 3 years | Myoclonic jerks | Usually | Usually | Rarely | Generalized spike–wave with normal background | Genetic | Valproate most commonly used |
| GEFS+ | 4 months to 10 years | Febrile and afebrile, usually generalized but occasionally focal | Usually | Yes | Rarely | Usually generalized spike–wave but may see focal/multifocal discharges | Genetic | Depends on mode of onset |
| Panayiotopoulos syndrome | Preschool years | Focal, with prominent autonomic features | Yes | Yes | No | Normal background, benign focal sharp waves | Unknown | Carbamazepine, oxcarbazepine, levetiracetam |
| Benign epilepsy of childhood with centrotemporal spikes | Early school years | Focal, affecting lower face with dysarthria, drooling, may evolve to bilateral GTCS in sleep | Yes | Yes | No | Normal background, high-amplitude centrotemporal spikes | Unknown | Carbamazepine, oxcarbazepine, levetiracetam |

| Syndrome | Age of onset | Seizure types | | | | EEG | Etiology | Treatment |
|---|---|---|---|---|---|---|---|---|
| | 5–10 years | Typical absences | Usually | Usually | No | Normal background, 3-Hz generalized spike–wave, often triggered with hyperventilation | Genetic | Ethosuximide, lamotrigine, valproate |
| Autosomal dominant frontal lobe epilepsy | Childhood to adolescence | Focal nocturnal frontal lobe seizures | Unknown | Usually | No | Normal background, may see frontal spikes | Genetic – nicotinic ACh receptor mutation | Carbamazepine or any medication for focal seizures |
| JAE | 10–16 years | Typical absences, 80% also have GTCS | Rarely | Usually | No | Normal background, 3–4-Hz generalized spike and wave | Genetic | Valproate, lamotrigine, levetiracetam |
| JME | Teens to early adult years | Myoclonic jerks, GTCS, occasional absences | Rarely | Usually | No | Normal background, fast, generalized polyspike and wave, often photosensitivity present | Genetic | Valproate, lamotrigine, levetiracetam |
| Idiopathic generalized epilepsy with pure grand mal | Teens to early adult years | GTCS alone | Rarely | Usually | No | Normal background, 3–5-Hz generalized spike and wave | Genetic | Valproate, lamotrigine, levetiracetam |
| Familial mesial temporal lobe epilepsy | Teens to early adult years | Focal – déjà vu, nausea, altered awareness | Unknown | Usually | No | Normal background, temporal sharp waves/spikes | Presumed genetic | Any AED for focal seizures |
| Familial lateral temporal lobe epilepsy | 10–30 years | Focal seizures with prominent auditory aura | Unknown | Usually | No | Normal background, temporal sharp waves/spikes | Genetic – LGI1 gene mutation | Any AED for focal seizures |

ACh, acetylcholine; CAE, childhood absence epilepsy; GEFS+, generalized epilepsy with febrile seizures plus, GTCS, generalized tonic–clonic seizures, JAE, juvenile absence epilepsy; JME, juvenile myoclonic epilepsy.

Benign familial infantile epilepsy also affects otherwise healthy infants, with onset between 2 and 20 months of focal dyscognitive seizures, often clustering. Similarly affected family members are usually identified, as this entity is autosomal dominant. Three genetic loci have been identified: chromosomes 19 and 2, which lead to seizures alone, and chromosome 16, which leads to seizures with choreoathetosis. The EEG is normal interictally and shows occipitoparietal discharges with ictal recording.

Other "benign" infantile epilepsies have been described but have significant clinical overlap. These disorders may be best distinguished based on genotype.

### ☝ CAUTION!

Benign infantile epilepsy can be mimicked by focal cortical dysplasia. Detection of cortical dysplasia in infants is challenging as the ongoing myelination makes detection difficult particularly between 6 and 24 months of age. Children with presumed benign infantile epilepsy should be followed carefully, and if seizures do not resolve by 24 months, strong consideration should be given to repeating the MRI using an epilepsy-specific protocol.

### Myoclonic epilepsy in infancy

Myoclonic epilepsy in infancy is rare and presents with myoclonic seizures starting between 4 months and 3 years of age in otherwise healthy infants. Myoclonus is often subtle at presentation but increases in intensity and frequency. Nearly one-third have preceding febrile convulsions and a few progress to generalized tonic–clonic seizures (GTCS). A family history of generalized epilepsy is present in one-third. The EEG shows generalized spike–wave and polyspike that can correlate with the myoclonic jerks, with a normal background. Valproate is often first used, but other medication including ethosuximide, benzodiazepine, levetiracetam, and phenobarbital may be effective. Epilepsy is usually self-limited, and most infants can discontinue medication early in the toddler years. Despite seizure remission, intellectual and behavioral disability occurs in a substantial minority. This entity must be distinguished from West syndrome, myoclonic–atonic epilepsy, Dravet syndrome, and underlying neurometabolic disorders.

### ☝ CAUTION!

The diagnosis of myoclonic epilepsy in infancy should be made cautiously. It is important to exclude other conditions such as West syndrome, Dravet syndrome, myoclonic–atonic epilepsy of Doose, and neurometabolic disorders.

### Childhood onset

#### Generalized epilepsy with febrile seizures plus (GEFS+)

Generalized epilepsy with febrile seizures plus (GEFS+) is a common syndrome, presenting between 4 months and 10 years of age. The family history is characteristically positive for febrile and afebrile seizures, as the inheritance is autosomal dominant with incomplete penetrance (60–90%). GEFS+ is genetically heterogeneous with several loci now identified, including *SCN1A*, *SCN1B*, and *GABRG2*. The diagnosis is clinical – genetic testing is not required and does not alter clinical management. Children typically begin with febrile seizures that may continue beyond the age of usual remittance. Additionally, many develop afebrile seizures that can be generalized (generalized tonic–clonic, atonic, absence, myoclonic) or focal. Neuroimaging is normal and the EEG usually shows generalized interictal discharges, although focal and multifocal discharges may also be seen. Prophylactic antiepileptic medication should be considered for recurrent afebrile seizures and should be based on mode of onset. For children with generalized spike-wave, carbamazepine is best avoided as it may provoke absence seizures. Long-term epilepsy and intellectual outcome is variable. In most cases, epilepsy is pharmacoresponsive and self-limited. However, severe cases with associated epileptic encephalopathy and evolution to myoclonic–atonic epilepsy or Dravet syndrome occur.

#### Panayiotopoulos syndrome

This relatively common syndrome usually presents with infrequent focal autonomic seizures in healthy preschool-aged children. Two-thirds of seizures occur out of sleep – the child wakes with unilateral eye deviation, retching, vomiting, pallor or tachycardia, and possible confusion. Seizures may evolve to become hemiconvulsive or generalized tonic–clonic. Prolonged seizures longer than 30 min, often with ictus emeticus, occur in approximately one-third. Interictal EEG shows normal background with high-amplitude multifocal sharp waves significantly increasing wi drowsiness and sleep. Imaging is normal. Many children can be managed with abortive agents only and may not require prophylactic antiepileptic medication if seizure frequency is low. This epilepsy always remits in childhood, typically within 1–2 years of onset, with excellent long-term intellectual outcome.

### Benign epilepsy of childhood with centrotemporal spikes (BECTS)

Benign epilepsy of childhood with centrotemporal spikes is one of the most common epilepsy syndromes in childhood, accounting for approximately 15% of new-onset epilepsy. Etiology is unknown. However, a familial predisposition is likely, as family members frequently show similar EEG changes during the early school years. Seizures typically begin between 5 and 10 years and occur after falling asleep or in the 1–2 h before waking. Nocturnal seizures frequently manifest as drooling, dysarthria, tingling, or clonic activity of the unilateral lower face, which can spread to the ipsilateral upper extremity or become secondarily generalized. If seizures occur out of wakefulness, they typically involve motor or sensory symptoms of the unilateral lower face with intact awareness. The EEG shows characteristic high-amplitude sharp waves in the centrotemporal regions, increasing with drowsiness and sleep. Imaging is normal, although it is not needed in classic cases. If treatment is needed, most cases are pharmacoresponsive, and many antiepileptic agents are efficacious. Epilepsy is self-limited – most patients can discontinue medication after 1–2 years and remain seizure-free. Intellectual outcome is usually excellent, although rare cases evolve early in the course to show a continuous spike–wave pattern in sleep, with cognitive and language regression.

### ☝ CAUTION!

Benign epilepsy of childhood with centrotemporal spikes can occasionally have a more malignant course. Children present with cognitive and/or language regression in association with seizures. In this situation, a pattern of electrical status epilepticus in slow-wave sleep (ESES) can be seen on EEG. Occasionally, such a regression can be triggered by sodium channel agents such as carbamazepine. Children with this presentation should be aggressively treated for ESES (see succeeding text).

### Childhood absence epilepsy (CAE)

This common syndrome presents in healthy children between the ages of 3 and 10 with a peak at 6–7 years of age. Absence seizures are characteristically the only seizure type and occur 20–50 times per day. Hyperventilation will usually trigger an absence event in an untreated or undertreated child. Children are typically aware of missed time only with longer events. Untreated seizures may result in a decline in academic performance or in injury.

Imaging is not required and the EEG shows typical 3-Hz generalized spike–wave. A paroxysmal posterior delta rhythm is commonly seen, but otherwise the background is normal.

Antiepileptic drug (AED) therapy should be initiated given the frequent seizures. A comparative effectiveness study showed that ethosuximide and valproic acid were more effective than lamotrigine and that ethosuximide had fewer adverse attentional effects.

Childhood absence epilepsy is self-limited in approximately two-thirds of children. Patients who achieve seizure freedom for 2 years with resolution of the generalized EEG discharge should be considered for a trial off medication. A few children will continue to have absences into adulthood or will develop GTCS in their adolescent/young adult years and require ongoing antiepileptic therapy. Despite remission of epilepsy, a significant minority of young adults experience increased academic and social difficulties, suggesting comorbidities such as psychiatric disorders, attention problems, and academic difficulties that must be addressed.

### Autosomal dominant frontal lobe epilepsy

This autosomal dominant syndrome results from known mutations in the nicotinic acetylcholine receptor genes and has 80% penetrance. Affected family members may be undiagnosed, and a history of "parasomnias" or other "behavioral" problems in sleep should be sought. Nocturnal seizures, with brief dystonic posturing, hypermotor activity, complex behaviors, and moaning, typically begin in childhood to early adolescence. Ictal EEG may be normal but more commonly shows bifrontal, high-voltage sharp and slow waves or low-amplitude, fast frontal activity with the clinical seizure. Imaging is normal. Genetic testing is available commercially and should be considered in cases where a family history is found. Most patients respond well to antiepileptic medication such as carbamazepine. The long-term remission rate has not been well studied. However, seizures may persist through life.

### Focal epilepsy of unknown cause

Focal epilepsy of unknown cause accounts for a significant minority of pediatric epilepsy, nearly 30% in one study. Many cases had a favorable long-term outcome, with 81% being seizure-free at last follow-up (68% of whom had discontinued antiepileptic medication) and only 7% developing medically intractable epilepsy. However, this group is heterogeneous and comprises other etiological categories that are, as yet, unrecognized. Further investigation will likely identify specific genes or other etiologies that determine prognosis.

### Adolescent onset

#### Juvenile absence epilepsy

Juvenile absence epilepsy (JAE) presents in healthy patients, 10–16 years of age, slightly later than CAE. Absences are usually the initial seizure type, although 80% develop GTCS within 2 years. Absences are less frequent than in CAE, being seen up to 2–3 times per day. The EEG shows a normal background with 3.5–4-Hz generalized spike–wave discharge, at times polyspike and wave. First-line therapy should include medication active against both absence and GTCS, such as lamotrigine or valproic acid. Seizures are usually pharmacoresponsive, but most patients require lifelong therapy.

#### Juvenile myoclonic epilepsy

Juvenile myoclonic epilepsy (JME) accounts for 4–10% of all epilepsies, presenting between 12 and 18 years in neurologically normal patients. The most common initial seizure type is myoclonic seizures, frequently not recognized as significant, being attributed to early morning "clumsiness" or "the jitters." Most present to medical attention after their first GTCS. Approximately 40% have coexisting absence seizures, although these are often infrequent, brief, and without complete loss of awareness. Seizures tend to occur in the early morning, particularly following sleep deprivation, and often begin with a shower of myoclonus culminating in a generalized tonic–clonic event. Photic stimulation may also be a trigger. The EEG is abnormal in most untreated patients showing 4–6-Hz generalized

atypical polyspike-and-wave discharges. Up to 30% may also show focal discharges and 30–90% show photosensitivity.

Valproate has been traditionally a first-line therapy. Given its potential side effects including weight gain, teratogenicity, and polycystic ovarian syndrome, other agents such as lamotrigine, topiramate, or levetiracetam are often used first line, particularly in women of childbearing age. JME is pharmacoresponsive, with 85–90% achieving seizure control on appropriate medication. Remission is rare – only 10% of patients successfully discontinue antiepileptic medication and remain seizure-free.

> ### ★ TIPS AND TRICKS
>
> While JAE and JME are usually pharmacoresponsive to low doses of medication, they are markedly aggravated by sleep deprivation. Patients who continue to have breakthrough seizures and suboptimal control should be queried about sleep, and lifestyle issues should be addressed.

### Idiopathic generalized epilepsy with pure grand mal

This condition is less common than JME but presents at a similar age, with GTCS as the only seizure type. The EEG shows 3–5-Hz generalized spike–wave discharge and is abnormal in most untreated patients. Therapeutic recommendations and outcome are as for JME.

### Familial temporal lobe epilepsy

Familial temporal lobe epilepsy is classified by predominant seizure semiology into mesial and lateral subgroups, both of which are rare.

Familial mesial temporal lobe epilepsy begins in adolescence to early adulthood. Seizure semiology involves prominent déjà vu, fear, nausea, and altered awareness, rarely secondarily generalizing. Febrile seizures are antecedent in 9.8%. EEGs are nonspecific and can be normal and show minor slowing or focal temporal discharges. MRIs are typically normal, although some series report mesial temporal sclerosis in up to 30–57% of cases. While most respond well to medication, medically refractory cases occur, and surgery can be successful in these rare cases. The genetics of this syndrome are not yet clear and complex inheritance is likely.

The lateral subgroup usually presents between 10 and 30 years of age with focal seizures, often triggered by external noises, consisting of prominent auditory auras of ringing or humming, early ictal aphasia, and occasional evolution to secondarily generalized seizures. Febrile seizures are unusual.

The lateral subgroup of familial temporal lobe epilepsy is autosomal dominant, although penetrance may be low, and approximately half of cases have documented mutations in the leucine-rich glioma-inactivated gene 1 (*LGI1*) on chromosome 10. MRI is normal and EEGs show nonspecific temporal discharges. Seizures are usually pharmacoresponsive and intellectual outcome is good.

## "Malignant" childhood epilepsies

The "malignant" epilepsies are pharmacoresistant epilepsy syndromes that are often associated with an epileptic encephalopathy (Table 21.2).

### Infantile onset

*West syndrome*

West syndrome is a triad of epileptic spasms, EEG hypsarrhythmia, and intellectual disability, although this intellectual disability may be absent at presentation. This is the most common epileptic encephalopathy, presenting typically at age 3–7 months. Seizures are characterized by brief contraction of the trunk, neck, and extremities, followed by a brief tonic component. Spasms can be flexor, extensor, or mixed, occurring in clusters, multiple times per day, often shortly after awakening. Asymmetric spasms or coexisting focal seizures suggest a focal cortical lesion. Irritability associated with spasm clusters may lead to misdiagnosis of infantile colic.

The background EEG demonstrates hypsarrhythmia, characterized by high-voltage, poorly organized slowing with multifocal epileptiform discharges and periodic generalized electrodecrement. Hypsarrhythmia may be seen during non-REM sleep only, emphasizing the importance of a sleep recording. Not all children with spasms have hypsarrhythmia. If the clinical history is suggestive of spasms, but hypsarrhythmia is not present, prolonged video–EEG recording should be considered. The EEG during a seizure typically shows a high-voltage generalized sharp wave followed by electrodecrement. Focal discharges before, during, or after a spasm also suggest a focal lesion.

West syndrome is often due to an underlying structural, genetic, or metabolic etiology, such as tuberous sclerosis; preexisting brain injury due to ischemia, infection, or trauma; Down syndrome; *ARX* or *CDKL5* mutations; mitochondrial disease; or Menkes disease. In 15–30% no etiology is found.

The preferred treatments for infantile spasms are ACTH, high-dose oral steroids, or vigabatrin. For optimal developmental outcome, treatment must be initiated early with the goal to control spasms and hypsarrhythmia. There is poor consensus regarding the dose and duration of ACTH or steroid therapy. Vigabatrin appears to be most effective in children with tuberous sclerosis or cortical dysplasia. In children with spasms of unknown etiology, pyridoxine is also given in addition to one of the preferred treatments, to exclude pyridoxine dependency.

Although spasms often resolve within the first 2 years, developmental and epilepsy prognosis is poor. Other seizure types may be concurrent with spasms or develop later. Furthermore, motor delay and intellectual disability occur in up to 84% of children.

---

> ☆ **TIPS AND TRICKS**
>
> Focal lesions in infants and young children can manifest as generalized epilepsies. To improve seizure and cognitive outcome, children with West syndrome due to a focal lesion should be promptly evaluated for surgical resection.

---

*Dravet syndrome*

Dravet syndrome is a rare epilepsy syndrome that presents in healthy infants before 18 months of life with recurrent prolonged generalized or focal seizures associated with fever, infection, vaccination, or bathing. This is then followed by recurrent unprovoked seizures, stagnation of development, and intellectual disability. Hemiconvulsive, generalized convulsive, focal, myoclonic, and atypical absence seizures are common. The initial EEG is typically normal. Over time, there develops slowing of the background activity and emergence of multifocal and generalized potentially epileptiform discharges with increased activation during photic stimulation and drowsiness.

**Table 21.2.** Pharmacoresistant childhood epilepsies.

| Syndrome | Typical age at onset | Seizure types | Self-limited | Pharmaco-responsive | Associated epileptic encephalopathy | EEG | Etiology | Initial treatment |
|---|---|---|---|---|---|---|---|---|
| West syndrome | First year | Epileptic spasms | Usually | Usually | Yes | Hypsarrhythmia | Structural, genetic, and metabolic causes | ACTH, oral steroids, vigabatrin |
| Dravet syndrome | First 18 months | Febrile status epilepticus, then focal, myoclonic, absence | No | No | Yes | Multifocal and generalized spike–wave discharges with photic sensitivity | SCN1A mutation in 80% | Stiripentol, valproic acid, clobazam |
| Malignant migrating partial epilepsy in infancy | First 6 months | Multifocal seizures, often with apnea and cyanosis | No | No | Yes | Multifocal discharges, multifocal seizures arising concurrently | Unknown | No effective treatment; bromides, stiripentol, benzodiazepines |
| Lennox-Gastaut syndrome | Preschool aged | Generalized and focal, nocturnal tonic | No | No | Yes | Generalized slow spike and wave, paroxysmal fast | Structural, genetic, and metabolic causes | Valproic acid, benzodiazepines, topiramate, rufinamide, felbamate, ketogenic diet |
| Myoclonic–atonic epilepsy | Preschool aged | Myoclonic–atonic | Usually | Occasionally | Yes | Generalized slow spike and wave | Unknown, possibly genetic | Valproic acid, benzodiazepines, ketogenic diet |
| CSWS | Early school aged | Focal and generalized | Yes | Possibly | Yes | ESES, maximal frontal | Structural, unknown | Diazepam, oral corticosteroids |
| Landau-Kleffner | Early school aged | Nocturnal hemiclonic | Yes | Yes, but relapse is common | Yes | ESES, maximal temporal | Unknown | Diazepam, oral corticosteroids |

| Syndrome | Age | Seizure types | | | | EEG findings | Etiology | Treatment |
|---|---|---|---|---|---|---|---|---|
| Myoclonic–absence | School aged | Myoclonic–absence | No | No | No | Generalized 3-Hz spike and wave, generalized atypical spike and wave | Genetic (GLUT1), metabolic | Valproic acid, ethosuximide, benzodiazepines, ketogenic diet |
| Eyelid myoclonia with and without absence | School aged | Absence with eyelid myoclonia | No | No | No | Generalized 3-Hz spike and wave, generalized atypical spike and wave | Genetic (GLUT1), metabolic | Valproic acid, ethosuximide, benzodiazepines, ketogenic diet |
| Febrile infection-related epilepsy syndrome (FIRES) | School aged | Refractory convulsive status epilepticus with fever but without intracranial infection | No | No | Yes | Recurrent multifocal seizures and status epilepticus | Unknown | No effective treatment |
| Rasmussen's syndrome | Early childhood to young adulthood | Focal seizures that increase in frequency to become nearly continuous | No | No | Yes | Hemispheric slowing, hemispheric epileptiform discharges, may be bilateral | Likely immune mediated | Immunotherapy, most require hemispherectomy |
| Progressive myoclonic epilepsy | Infancy to adulthood | Worsening myoclonus, multiple seizure types | No | No | Yes | Generalized background slowing, generalized spike–wave with photosensitivity | Metabolic and genetic neurodegenerative conditions, including Tay–Sachs, NCL, Alpers' Lafora, and Unverricht–Lundborg diseases | No effective treatment |

CSWS, continuous spikes and waves during slow sleep; ESES, electrical status epilepticus in slow-wave sleep; NCL, neuronal ceroid lipofuscinosis.

Dravet syndrome occurs as a result of a mutation in the sodium channel α-1 subunit gene (*SCN1A*) in 80% of children. Most are spontaneous mutations. However, family members may also have *SCN1A* mutations but a milder phenotype such as GEFS+.

The seizures in Dravet syndrome are refractory to all treatments. Lamotrigine and carbamazepine worsen seizures. However, stiripentol, which has orphan drug status in the USA, reduces tonic–clonic seizures when used in combination with valproic acid or clobazam. Over time, prolonged seizures decrease, but refractory seizures and intellectual disability persist. Furthermore, the mortality rate in Dravet syndrome is 15%, with most deaths occurring due to status epilepticus and SUDEP.

---

### ⚠ CAUTION!

Dravet syndrome should be suspected in children presenting in their first year of life with recurrent hemiconvulsive or generalized convulsive febrile status epilepticus. Lamotrigine, carbamazepine, and phenytoin can worsen seizures in Dravet syndrome.

---

*Malignant migrating partial epilepsy in infancy*

This syndrome presents during the first 6 months of life with multifocal seizures, commonly with autonomic components including apnea, cyanosis, or flushing. Over time, these increase in frequency and become nearly continuous. The seizures occur in clusters followed by seizure-free periods lasting days to weeks. With time, evolution to generalized seizures also occurs. The children are typically normal at onset but show progressive delay in development and hypotonia. The EEG demonstrates slowing of the background activity with multifocal epileptiform discharges. During seizures, rhythmic theta frequency discharges arise from multiple areas, and several focal seizures can arise concurrently.

There is no known cause for malignant migrating partial epilepsy in infancy and no effective treatments. Some improvement has been reported with stiripentol, clonazepam, vigabatrin, bromides, rufinamide, and the ketogenic diet. The prognosis is poor. Over time, the seizures decrease, but there are profound intellectual disability, poor language development, and acquired microcephaly. Early mortality is high due to respiratory complications of the underlying disease.

## Childhood onset

*Lennox–Gastaut syndrome (LGS)*

Lennox–Gastaut syndrome presents in preschool-aged children, usually with previously abnormal development. Initially, the seizures can be subtle – atypical absence seizures and myoclonic seizures. Over time, they evolve to include atonic, generalized tonic–clonic, and nonconvulsive status epilepticus. The most characteristic seizure is the nocturnal tonic seizure, although these can be subtle and difficult to detect without video–EEG monitoring. As seizures evolve, development plateaus and may regress. Ultimately, over 80% of children with LGS have intellectual disability.

The triad of LGS consists of the multiple seizure types, cognitive dysfunction, as well as an interictal EEG with 1.5–2.5-Hz slow-spike and polyspike-and-wave discharges on a slow background. This pattern may not be seen upon initial presentation. Low-voltage, anteriorly predominant generalized paroxysmal fast activity seen during slow-wave sleep suggests the diagnosis. Two-thirds of children with LGS have a prior history of brain abnormality including perinatal insults, malformations of cortical development, neurocutaneous disorders, or metabolic/genetic disorders. One-third will also have a history of infantile spasms.

Seizures are typically pharmacoresistant. Valproic acid is commonly used, and lamotrigine, topiramate, rufinamide, clobazam, and felbamate have also been shown to reduce seizure burden. Felbamate should not be used first line due to the risk of aplastic anemia and hepatotoxicity. The ketogenic diet should be considered early, with nearly half of children having a significant seizure reduction. Corpus callosotomy should be considered to treat intractable generalized drop seizures. Vagus nerve stimulator can also be helpful.

Children with LGS continue to have seizures throughout life, although they often decrease with age. Most of these children have intellectual disability. Children with delayed development prior to seizure onset, a history of infantile spasms, early age at onset, frequent seizures, and recurrent nonconvulsive status epilepticus are more likely to have a poor cognitive outcome.

*Myoclonic–atonic epilepsy (Doose syndrome)*

Children with myoclonic–atonic epilepsy, or Doose syndrome, also present during early preschool age with multiple seizure types and developmental plateauing. Generalized slow-spike-and-wave discharges and background slowing are present on EEG. However, in contrast to LGS, development prior to seizure onset is normal, and there is often a family history of epilepsy. Myoclonic–atonic seizures and GTCS are prominent, but nocturnal tonic seizures typically do not occur.

Seizures in Doose syndrome can also be difficult to treat. However, a positive response to the ketogenic diet is often seen, so it should be introduced early. Unlike LGS, Doose syndrome does not always have a poor developmental outcome. Some children can have normal development, especially if seizures are controlled.

### Electrical status epilepticus in slow-wave sleep (ESES)

Electrical status epilepticus in slow-wave sleep, an EEG pattern in which epileptiform discharges become nearly continuous during slow-wave sleep, is seen in continuous spikes and waves during slow sleep (CSWS) syndrome and Landau–Kleffner syndrome (LKS). Both syndromes present in early school years with developmental and behavioral regression.

In CSWS, the epileptiform discharges are maximal over the frontal regions and the regression is global. CSWS can be seen in children with prior brain insult, and development prior to onset of regression may already be delayed. Seizures, including focal with and without dyscognitive features, unilateral or bilateral clonic, tonic–clonic, absence, and atonic seizures, are common and can be difficult to treat. Tonic seizures do not occur.

In LKS, the epileptiform discharges are maximal over the frontotemporal and temporal regions, and the children present with acquired auditory agnosia. Unlike children with CSWS, children with LKS have no history of prior brain insult, and early development is normal. The seizures in LKS are typically nocturnal hemiclonic and are rarely intractable.

While the seizures in CSWS and LKS may respond to antiseizure medications, the ESES and developmental regression do not. Carbamazepine, phenobarbital, and phenytoin often worsen ESES. While there is no consensus for treatment of ESES, corticosteroids and 3–4-week cycles of high-dose diazepam are often used with success, although relapses are common.

Electrical status epilepticus in slow-wave sleep and the seizures resolve in adolescence. However, the delays in development incurred during childhood do not resolve completely, and most children are left with decreased language and intellectual functioning.

### Atypical absence epilepsies

While childhood and juvenile absence epilepsies are typically pharmacosensitive with good outcome, this is not so for all absence epilepsy syndromes. Absence seizures accompanied by rhythmic myoclonic jerking of the limbs or head are suggestive of myoclonic–absence seizures or Tassinari syndrome. Non-suppressible eyelid myoclonia can also be present with and without absence seizures (Jeavons syndrome). Both of these atypical absence epilepsy syndromes typically present in previously healthy children. Other seizures, most often GTCS, also occur. While school performance can be affected by frequent seizures, there typically is no cognitive decline. The EEG demonstrates a normal background with generalized 3-Hz spike-and-wave discharges, similar to other absence epilepsies.

The cause of atypical absence epilepsies often is not known. However, glucose transporter 1 (GLUT1) deficiency is associated with early-onset atypical absence seizures and must be excluded. Unlike the typical absence epilepsies, the atypical absence epilepsies are often pharmacoresistant, and seizures are unlikely to spontaneously remit. Treatment typically includes combinations of valproic acid, ethosuximide, topiramate, levetiracetam, and benzodiazepines. The ketogenic diet should be considered early and must be considered for those with GLUT1 deficiency.

## Childhood and adolescent onset

### Progressive myoclonic epilepsies

The progressive myoclonic epilepsies present with multiple seizure types, worsening myoclonus, cerebellar dysfunction, and developmental regression. The baseline EEG demonstrates generalized background slowing. The myoclonus correlates with a generalized spike–wave discharge on EEG. Photosensitivity is often present.

These are rare disorders that are due to various metabolic and neurodegenerative conditions. During infancy, Tay–Sachs is due to deficiency in hexosaminidase A and presents with exaggerated startle reflex and developmental regression. During infancy and childhood, Alpers' disease, which is due to a *POLG1* mutation, presents with recurrent status epilepticus, hepatic failure, and progressive cognitive decline. In adolescence, causes include neuronal ceroid lipofuscinosis, Lafora disease, and Unverricht–Lundborg disease. The long-term outcome of the progressive myoclonic epilepsies is variable, but often there is progression of seizures and cognitive decline associated with high mortality.

## All ages

### Intractable focal epilepsies

Focal epilepsies, especially those due to structural etiology, are often pharmacoresistant and do not remit. Common structural etiologies in children include malformations of cortical development; encephalomalacia due to previous trauma, strokes, and infection; mesial temporal sclerosis; and vascular malformations. Malformations of cortical development may be focal, multifocal, hemispheric, or diffuse, and intractability occurs in up to 83% of children. Mesial temporal sclerosis may occur due to frequent or prolonged seizures, including febrile seizures, which may occur in conjunction with a focal brain malformation. Focal brain lesions also occur due to genetic disorders, such as tuberous sclerosis complex (TSC). Children with TSC may present with infantile spasms or later with focal seizures. For children with focal epilepsy due to structural lesions, only approximately one-third can be rendered seizure-free with medication alone, whereas up to two-thirds can be seizure-free with surgical intervention. Therefore, surgery should be considered early if medications fail.

Rarely, focal epilepsy occurs due to autoimmune disorders. Rasmussen's syndrome has variable age of onset but often presents in a previously healthy child with unilateral focal seizures without dyscognitive features. The seizures progressively increase in frequency and duration, eventually culminating in epilepsia partialis continua (EPC) and acquired hemiparesis. Immunotherapy is often initiated, although most children require hemispherectomy or modified hemispherotomy for seizure control.

## Bibliography

Camfield CS, Camfield PR, Gordon K, Wirrell E, Dooley JM. Incidence of epilepsy in childhood and adolescence: A population-based study in Nova Scotia from 1977 to 1985. *Epilepsia* 1996; **37**:19–23.

Chiron C, Dulac O. The pharmacologic treatment of Dravet syndrome. *Epilepsia* 2011; **52**(Suppl. 2):72–75.

Dhamija R, Moseley BD, Cascino GD, Wirrell EC. A population-based study of long-term outcome of epilepsy in childhood with a focal or hemispheric lesion on neuroimaging. *Epilepsia* 2011; **52**:1522–1526.

Dravet C, Bureau M, Dalla Bernardina B, Guerrini R. Severe myoclonic epilepsy in infancy (Dravet syndrome) 30 years later. *Epilepsia* 2011; **52**(Suppl. 2):1–2.

Glauser TA, Cnaan A, Shinnar S, et al. Ethosuximide, valproic acid, and lamotrigine in childhood absence epilepsy. *N Engl J Med* 2010; **362**:790–799.

Huang CC, Chang YC. The long-term effects of febrile seizures on the hippocampal neuronal plasticity – clinical and experimental evidence. *Brain Dev* 2009; **31**:383–387.

Pellock JM, Hrachovy R, Shinnar S, et al. Infantile spasms: A U.S. consensus report. *Epilepsia* 2010; **51**:2175–2189.

Wirrell EC, Grossardt BR, So EL, Nickels KC. A population-based study of long-term outcomes of cryptogenic focal epilepsy in childhood: Cryptogenic epilepsy is probably not symptomatic epilepsy. *Epilepsia* 2011; **52**:738–745.

Wirrell EC, Grossardt BR, Wong-Kisiel LC, Nickels KC. Incidence and classification of new-onset epilepsy and epilepsy syndromes in children in Olmsted County, Minnesota from 1980 to 2004: A population-based study. *Epilepsy Res* 2011; **95**:110–118.

# Epilepsy: When to Perform a Genetic Analysis

**Heather E. Olson and Annapurna Poduri**

Department of Neurology, Boston Children's Hospital, Boston, MA, USA
Department of Neurology, Harvard Medical School, Boston, MA, USA

## Introduction

Genetic mechanisms play an important role in the pathophysiology of epilepsy. Mechanisms include genomic rearrangements (e.g., ring chromosomes, translocations, monosomies, and trisomies), copy number variants (CNVs; deletions or duplications involving one or more genes), and single-nucleotide alterations, resulting in missense, frameshift, or nonsense mutations. Methylation defects or uniparental disomy may also affect one region of DNA (e.g., Prader–Willi and Angelman syndromes), resulting in gain or loss of function of genes typically expressed only from the maternal or paternal copy. Modes of inheritance vary depending on the type of genetic abnormality.

Many single-gene models of epilepsy have been identified for both lesional and nonlesional epilepsy. The most notable are the channelopathies (e.g., *SCN1A*-associated Dravet syndrome [DS]). Other mechanisms include modulation of synaptic vesicle docking and release (e.g., *STXBP1*), cell signaling (e.g., *CDKL5*), and transcription factors (e.g., *ARX*). In other cases, the genetics are thought to be more complex, involving multiple genes or susceptibility loci with incomplete penetrance and phenotypic variability likely due to gene–gene interactions and environmental and epigenetic factors (e.g., the idiopathic generalized epilepsies).

## Tools for genetic testing in epilepsy

There are a number of genetic testing techniques that can be used to evaluate patients for genetic causes of epilepsy. Table 22.1 outlines these tests and provides suggestions for when they are to be ordered.

## When to perform genetic testing in epilepsy

### Epilepsy in defined genetic syndromes

It is important to be able to recognize genetic syndromes in which epilepsy is a prominent feature, as the diagnosis may impact treatment and monitoring for other medical conditions (e.g., monitoring for long QT syndrome in Rett syndrome). Table 22.2 describes syndromes in which epilepsy is a prominent feature.

> ☆ **TIPS AND TRICKS**
>
> Gene testing for *TSC1* and *TSC2* is especially helpful in unclear cases of possible tuberous sclerosis complex (TSC) at onset, as it allows for confirmation of the diagnosis and appropriate clinical monitoring and treatment. It also helps with genetic counseling for the patient and family.

*Epilepsy*, First Edition. Edited by John W. Miller and Howard P. Goodkin.
© 2014 John Wiley & Sons, Ltd. Published 2014 by John Wiley & Sons, Ltd.

**Table 22.1.** Toolkit for genetic testing in epilepsy.

| Testing method | Description | Suggestions of when to use this test |
|---|---|---|
| Chromosomal microarray | Uses either single-nucleotide polymorphism (SNP) array or array-comparative genomic hybridization (using oligonucleotide probes). Evaluates targeted regions throughout the chromosomes for CNVs | Especially when epilepsy is seen in association with developmental delay, autism, and/or dysmorphisms. Can also be helpful in other idiopathic epilepsy syndromes |
| Single-gene sequencing | Evaluates for sequence alterations and whether they cause amino acid changes | When a specific genetic abnormality is suspected. For example, test *SLC2A1* when GLUT1 deficiency is suspected. |
| Single-gene duplication/deletion analysis | Evaluates for CNV in a targeted gene | When sequencing is negative and abnormality in a specific gene is suspected. More sensitive than microarray in this case |
| Targeted mutation analysis | Sequencing looking for a specific mutation | • Parental testing to help determine significance of a mutation of unknown significance<br>• Carrier testing |
| Panels of genes associated with a disorder | Sequencing ± duplication/deletion testing for a panel of genes of interest | In disorders with many associated genes, such as the EOEEs |
| Methylation studies | Evaluates for methylation abnormalities in a specific chromosomal region | Suspected methylation disorders such as Prader–Willi and Angelman syndromes |
| Fluorescent in situ hybridization (FISH) | Fluorescently labeled probes identify specific chromosomal regions | • Confirmation of a deletion/duplication<br>• Evaluate for deletion of a specific region (i.e., 22q11) |
| Karyotype | A photographic representation of all of the chromosomes in a single cell, arranged in pairs based on size and banding pattern | Consider in patients with dysmorphisms or multiple congenital anomalies. May be helpful in the case of large CNVs to evaluate for rearrangements |
| Whole exome or whole genome sequencing | Evaluates for sequence changes and CNVs throughout the genome | Consider when known clinical testing is not revealing and a genetic diagnosis is strongly suspected |

CNVs, copy number variants; EOEEs, early-onset epileptic encephalopathies.

**Table 22.2.** Key genetic syndromes with frequently associated epilepsy (not comprehensive).

| Syndrome | Genetics | Brief summary | EEG features |
|---|---|---|---|
| Classic Rett syndrome | *MECP2* deletions or mutations (autosomal dominant, most *de novo*)<br><br>Early-onset seizure variant is associated with *CDKL5* mutations/deletions<br><br>Congenital variant is associated with *FOXG1* mutations/deletions | Progressive microcephaly, loss of purposeful hand skills, stereotypic hand movements, partial/complete loss of language, gait abnormalities. Majority develop epilepsy in childhood | Frontocentral theta slowing<br><br>Loss of phase II sleep features<br><br>Focal or multifocal epileptiform activity |
| Angelman syndrome | Maternal deletion (majority) or uniparental disomy of 15q11-q13, methylation defect of this region (deletion of the imprinting center), or *UBE3* mutation or deletion (inheritance pattern varies by defect) | Severe DD or ID, severe speech impairment, gait ataxia and/or tremulousness of limbs, unique behavior of inappropriate happy demeanor. Microcephaly and seizures common | Intermittent rhythmic delta<br>Epileptiform activity |
| TSC | Mutation or deletion of *TSC1* or *TSC2* (autosomal dominant) | DD, typical skin findings, epilepsy, ± autism.<br>Also often involves the renal, cardiac, and other organ systems | Multifocal epileptiform activity ± slowing, associated with tubers. Not specific |
| Hypomel-anosis of Ito | Heterogeneous, frequently with mosaic chromosomal abnormalities/rearrangements including translocations, abnormal ploidy, trisomies, CNVs, or mosaicism for sex chromosomes. Most often found in cells from skin lesions | Hypopigmented skin lesions (whorls, streaks, patches) following the lines of Blaschko ± extracutaneous manifestations. ID and epilepsy common. Often associated with malformations including hemimegalencephaly, pachygyria, cortical dysplasia, and heterotopias | Not specific |
| Menkes disease | Mutation or deletion of *ATP7A* (X-linked recessive) | Males with hypotonia, failure to thrive, and seizures with onset at approximately 1–3 months. Typical sparse, coarse, twisted, lightly pigmented hair. Low copper/ceruloplasmin | Epileptiform activity and seizures initially posterior predominant<br><br>May develop hypsarrhythmia<br><br>Late multifocal epileptiform activity and slowing |
| 1p36 deletion syndrome | Deletion in the 1p36 region | DD, ID, hypotonia, craniofacial abnormalities, congenital heart defects, precocious puberty, obesity.<br>Epilepsy in approximately 50–60%. Spasms and apneic seizures are common | Multifocal and/or generalized spikes and slowing<br><br>Some develop hypsarrhythmia |

DD, developmental delay; ID, intellectual disability; TSC, tuberous sclerosis complex.

There are other syndromes that are suspected to be genetic in origin but for which we do not yet have an identified genetic etiology (e.g., myoclonic-atonic epilepsy).

### Epilepsy in association with features that suggest a genetic syndrome

If there are dysmorphic features or congenital anomalies that do not fit a well-described syndrome, consider initiating genetic testing with a broad screen such as a chromosomal microarray and referring to a pediatric geneticist.

In addition, there are an increasing number of identified genetic causes of epilepsy with brain malformations with or without other syndromic features (Table 22.3). In lissencephaly and double cortex syndrome, testing does not directly affect treatment but confirms a diagnosis and can help with prognosis and genetic counseling. For polymicrogyria, identification of DiGeorge syndrome or Zellweger syndrome would affect other medical management, and the other genes would provide an explanation. For periventricular nodular heterotopia (PVNH), a *FLNA* mutation helps predict prognosis and suggest the need for screening for vascular defects. In the case of

**Table 22.3.** Clinically testable genes associated with malformations.

| Type of malformation | Associated genetic abnormalities |
| --- | --- |
| Lissencephaly or pachygyria | *LIS1, ARX* (males), *DXC* (males), *RELN, TUBA1A* |
| Double cortex | *DXC* (females) |
| Polymicrogyria | *TUBA1A, TUBB2B, TUBB3, GPR56,* DiGeorge syndrome (22q11.2 deletion), Zellweger syndrome (*PEX1* and other *PEX* genes) |
| PVNH | *FLNA, ARFGEF2* |
| Microcephaly | *CDKL5, FOXG1* (duplication), *WDR62, ASPM, SLC25A22, PNKP* (recessive mutations) |
| Macrocephaly | *PTEN, NSD1* |
| TSC with tubers and subependymal nodules | *TSC1, TSC2* |

PVNH, periventricular nodular heterotopia.

microcephaly and macrocephaly, each of the genes listed in Table 22.3 has a well-described phenotype, and knowing the diagnosis could be helpful for prognosis and management.

### Epilepsy syndromes

There are an increasing number of identified genetic causes of defined epilepsy syndromes including benign familial neonatal–infantile seizures (Table 22.4; see Chapter 20 for additional details on neonatal epilepsy syndromes), idiopathic generalized epilepsies, and benign focal epilepsies. For example, there are several "hot spots" for CNVs in idiopathic generalized or idiopathic focal epilepsies (e.g., 15q11.2, 15q13.3, 15q11-q13, 16p11.2, 16p13.11, 1q21.1). At times CNVs contain known epilepsy genes.

Mutations in *SLC2A1* (Table 22.5) are associated with glucose transporter 1 (GLUT1) deficiency. Though typically early onset, it can be associated with other idiopathic generalized epilepsies. In addition to *SCN1A* and *PCDH19*, mutations or deletions in *SCN1B, SCN2A,* and *GABRG2* are associated with genetic epilepsy with febrile seizures plus (GEFS+). Genes identified as susceptibility factors for generalized epilepsies include *CACNA1H, CACNB4, CHRNA7, CLCN2,* and *EFHC1. CACNA1A* is a gene associated with absence epilepsy and episodic ataxia.

Genetic testing for autosomal dominant nocturnal frontal lobe epilepsy has a fairly low yield (<10% for *CHRNA4* and <5% for *CHRNB2*). Genetic testing for autosomal dominant partial epilepsy with auditory features (*LGI1*) may confirm the diagnosis, though if the family history is strongly suggestive it may not significantly affect management. It is not widely tested. *De novo* cases are rare. Indications to test for *SYN1* are not fully developed. Genetic testing for benign rolandic epilepsy and for the other benign focal epilepsies is not typically indicated.

In these situations, the decision of whether or not to pursue genetic testing depends on a balance of clinical suspicion and benefit to the family. In some cases, a genetic diagnosis may be helpful in predicting outcome (such as with the benign familial neonatal–infantile seizures) or in genetic counseling for the family.

### Early-onset epileptic encephalopathies (EOEEs)

The early-onset epileptic encephalopathies (EOEEs) include Ohtahara syndrome (OS), early myoclonic epilepsy (EME), nonspecific early-onset epileptic encephalopathy with burst–suppression (EOEE-BS), malignant migrating partial seizures in infancy

**Table 22.4.** Genes associated with benign familial neonatal–infantile seizures.

| Gene | Full gene name | Locus | Phenotype |
|------|----------------|-------|-----------|
| *KCNQ2* | POTASSIUM CHANNEL, VOLTAGE-GATED, KQT-LIKE SUBFAMILY, MEMBER 2 | 20q13.33 | Benign familial neonatal seizures or EOEE |
| *KCNQ3* | POTASSIUM CHANNEL, VOLTAGE-GATED, KQT-LIKE SUBFAMILY, MEMBER 3 | 8q24.22 | Benign familial neonatal seizures |
| *SCN2A* | SODIUM CHANNEL, VOLTAGE-GATED, TYPE II, ALPHA SUBUNIT | 2q24.3 | Benign familial neonatal–infantile convulsions, GEFS+ |

EOEE, early-onset epileptic encephalopathy; GEFS+, genetic epilepsy with febrile seizures plus. Another gene, *PRRT2* (pyridoxamine 5′-phosphate oxidase), has recently been associated with familial infantile convulsions and paroxysmal kinesigenic dyskinesia but is not yet clinically testable in the USA.

**Table 22.5.** Non-malformation-associated epilepsy genes identified in EOEE.

| Gene | Full gene name | Locus | Phenotype |
|------|----------------|-------|-----------|
| *ALDH7A1* | ALDEHYDE DEHYDROGENASE 7 FAMILY, MEMBER A1 | 5q23.2 | EOEE, EOEE-BS, or OS, pyridoxine-dependent epilepsy |
| *ATP7A* | COPPER-TRANSPORTING P-TYPE ADENOSINE TRIPHOSPHATASE | Xq21.1 | EOEE, Menkes disease |
| *ARX* | ARISTALESS-RELATED HOMEOBOX, X-LINKED (transcriptional repressor and activator) | Xp21.3 | EOEE, EOEE-BS, OS, or WS, especially if corpus callosal and/or genital abnormalities present, can be associated with lissencephaly |
| *CDKL5* | CYCLIN-DEPENDENT KINASE-LIKE 5 (serine–threonine kinase) | Xp22.13 | EOEE, often WS, rare EOEE-BS, especially with microcephaly, hypotonia, Rett-like features |
| *GAMT* | GUANIDINOACETATE METHYLTRANSFERASE | 19p13.3 | EOEE, creatine deficiency, epilepsy most prominent in GAMT mutations |
| *GATM* | L-ARGININE:GLYCINE AMIDINOTRANSFERASE | | |
| *SLC6A8* | SOLUTE CARRIER FAMILY 6, MEMBER 8 | | |
| *GLDC* | GLYCINE DECARBOXYLASE | 9p24.1 | EME, NKH/glycine encephalopathy |
| *AMT* | AMINOMETHYLSTRANSERASE | 3P21.31 | |
| *KCNQ2* | POTASSIUM CHANNEL, VOLTAGE-GATED, KQT-LIKE SUBFAMILY, MEMBER 2 (potassium channel) | 20q13.33 | Benign familial neonatal seizures or EOEE (rarely) |
| *MAGI2* | MEMBRANE-ASSOCIATED GUANYLATE KINASE INVERTED-2 (synaptic scaffolding protein) | 7q11.23-q21.1 | EOEE or WS |
| *PCDH19* | PROTOCADHERIN 19 | Xq22.1 | DS, epilepsy with ID in females |
| *PLCB1* | PHOSPHOLIPASE C, BETA-1 (enzyme involved in cellular signaling) | 20p12.3 | OS, WS, MMPEI |

*(Continued)*

**Table 22.5.** (*Continued*)

| Gene | Full gene name | Locus | Phenotype |
|------|----------------|-------|-----------|
| *PNKP* | POLYNUCLEOTIDE KINASE 3′-PHOSPHATASE (enzyme involved in DNA repair) | 19q13.33 | OS, WS, especially with microcephaly |
| *PNPO* | PYRIDOXAMINE 5′-PHOSPHATE OXIDASE | 17q21.32 | EOEE, EOEE-BS, or OS, PLP-DE |
| *POLG* | DNA POLYMERASE GAMMA | 15q26.1 | EOEE, Alpers' syndrome |
| *SCN1A* | SODIUM CHANNEL, NEURONAL TYPE I, ALPHA SUBUNIT (subunit of voltage-gated sodium channel) | 2q24.3 | GEFS+, DS, MMPEI |
| *SLC25A22* | SOLUTE CARRIER FAMILY 25 (MITOCHONDRIAL CARRIER, GLUTAMATE), MEMBER 22 (mitochondrial glutamate/H+ symporter) | 11p15.5 | OS, EOEE, especially with microcephaly present and in the case of consanguinity |
| *SLC2A1* | SOLUTE CARRIER FAMILY 2 (FACILITATED GLUCOSE TRANSPORTER), MEMBER 1 | 1p34.2 | EOEE, GLUT1 deficiency, early-onset absence seizures or other idiopathic generalized epilepsies, often with DD |
| *SPTAN1* | SPECTRIN, ALPHA, NONERYTHROCYTIC 1 (cytoskeletal protein) | 9q34.11 | OS?, WS |
| *STXBP1* | SYNTAXIN-BINDING PROTEIN 1 (modulator of synaptic vesicle release) | 9q34.11 | EOEE, OS, especially if movement disorder and severe DD |

MMPEI, malignant migrating partial seizures in infancy; NKH, non-ketotic hyperglycinemia; PLP-DE, pyridoxal-5′-phosphate-dependent epilepsy; WS, West syndrome.

(MMPEI), DS, and West syndrome (WS). With the exception of DS, which is most often associated with a mutation in *SCN1A*, the other syndromes are heterogeneous in etiology. OS is frequently associated with structural brain malformations but has also been associated with deletions or point mutations of the genes *STXBP1* and *SPTAN1*. EME is often associated with metabolic etiologies, which are typically genetic in origin. Additional details of the EOEEs are provided in Chapters 20 and 21.

The genes associated with the EOEEs are listed in Table 22.5. As more specific genetic etiologies are identified, the phenotypic spectrum may expand for each gene. Not included in the table are the genes for metabolic disorders, such as urea cycle disorders, organic acidurias, aminoacidopathies other than non-ketotic hyperglycinemia (NKH), and mitochondrial disorders other than *SLC25A22*.

These are typically identified through standard clinical screening methods.

In general, for EOEEs, the first step is to evaluate for a structural or metabolic etiology and then to consider genetic testing. If the patient fits the phenotype of a specific gene, then start by testing that gene. If the patient's presentation is not suggestive of a specific etiology, then consider testing a panel of genes associated with early-onset epilepsy. A chromosomal microarray may be helpful to identify potentially pathogenic CNVs.

### Progressive myoclonic epilepsies

Multiple genes associated with the progressive myoclonic epilepsies (PMEs) are identified and clinically testable. In addition to the genetic causes (Table 22.6), the differential diagnosis for PME also includes genetic disorders, sialidosis, and mitochondrial disorders, typically identifiable by ophthalmologic

**Table 22.6.** Genes associated with progressive myoclonic epilepsies.

| Gene | Full gene name | Locus | Phenotype |
|---|---|---|---|
| CSTB | CYSTATIN B | 21q22.3 | Unverricht–Lundborg disease |
| PRICKLE1 | REST-INTERACTING LIM DOMAIN PROTEIN | 12q12 | Unverricht–Lundborg-like PME |
| SCARB2 | SCAVENGER RECEPTOR CLASS B, MEMBER 2 | 4q21.1 | Unverricht–Lundborg-like PME |
| EPM2A | LAFORIN | 6q24.3 | Lafora disease |
| NHLRC1 (EPM2B) | MALIN | 6p22.3 | Lafora disease |
| PPT1/CLN1, TPP1/ CLN2, CLN3, CLN5, CLN6, MFSD8/ CLN7, CLN8, CLN10 | PALMITOYL-PROTEIN THIOESTERASE 1, TRIPEPTIDYL PEPTIDASE, BATTENIN, CEROID LIPOFUSCINOISIS, NEURONAL, 5–8 AND 10 | 1p34.2 11p15.4 16p11.2 13q22.3 15q23 4q28.2 8p23.3 11p15.5 | Neuronal ceroid lipofuscinosis, multiple subtypes |

examination and metabolic markers rather than single-gene testing. Genetic testing for myoclonic epilepsy with ragged red fibers (MERRF) can be done via mitochondrial gene sequencing or targeted mutation analysis. Genetic testing is recommended if a PME is suspected, as it would significantly affect prognosis for the patient. Clinical features and serum markers may guide testing in a stepwise manner.

### Genetic testing for potentially treatable conditions or those for which medication choices would change with treatment

Treatable genetic causes of epilepsy include those involving a metabolic pathway that is treatable (e.g., creatine disorders, GLUT1 deficiency, vitamin-responsive epilepsies, aminoacidopathies, and mitochondrial disorders). Inherited metabolic disorders are discussed in more detail in Chapter 23.

Currently, the effect of genetic diagnosis on treatment is illustrated by the following examples:

1. Use of vigabatrin for infantile spasms in patients with TSC.
2. Avoidance of AEDs that block sodium channels in patients with sodium channel mutations such as SCN1A. For example, lamotrigine often worsens seizures in patients with DS and SCN1A mutations.
3. Testing of patients of Asian descent for HLA-B*1502 and if positive, avoidance of carbamazepine, oxcarbazepine, phenytoin, and lamotrigine due to increased risk for Stevens–Johnson syndrome.
4. Specific treatments are indicated for GLUT1 deficiency (ketogenic diet), pyridoxine-dependent/folinic acid-responsive epilepsy (pyridoxine + folinic acid), pyridoxal-5′-phosphate-dependent epilepsy (PLP-DE) (pyridoxal-5′-phosphate), creatine disorders (creatine), and mitochondrial disorders (treatment recommendations vary).

### ✋ CAUTION!

1. Don't miss treatable metabolic epilepsies such as GLUT1 deficiency or pyridoxine-dependent epilepsy. These conditions are discussed in Chapter 23.
2. Avoid sodium channel blockers in patients with SCN1A mutations.

### Genetic counseling in epilepsy

With the rapidly expanding field of epilepsy genetics, involvement of genetic counselors and physicians knowledgeable in the field is increasingly important. They can help guide a stepwise approach to diagnosis and educate families about types of genetic testing and risks and benefits to the testing. When a genetic diagnosis is made, genetic counseling is critical to giving the family a sense of prognosis and an understanding of modes of inheritance that can be helpful for family planning.

## Conclusion and future perspectives

This field is rapidly evolving. Many more genes are likely to be identified, and incorporation of whole exome and whole genome sequencing may soon be common in clinical practice. As the genetics of epilepsy unfolds, there is hope that more gene-specific treatments will be discovered.

## Bibliography

Andrade DM. Genetic basis in epilepsies caused by malformations of cortical development and in those with structurally normal brain. *Hum Genet* 2009; **126**:173–193.

Cavalleri GL, McCormack M, Alhusaini S, Chaila E, Delanty N. Pharmacogenomics and epilepsy: The road ahead. *Pharmacogenomics* 2011; **12**(10):1429–1447.

Chiron C, Dulac O. The pharmacologic treatment of Dravet syndrome. *Epilepsia* 2011; **52**(Suppl. 2): 72–75.

Helbig I, Scheffer I, Mulley J, Berkovic S. Navigating the channels and beyond: Unraveling the genetics of the epilepsies. *Lancet Neurol* 2008; **7**:231–245.

Khwaja OS, Sahin M. Translational research: Rett syndrome and tuberous sclerosis complex. *Curr Opin Pediatr* 2011; **23**:633–639.

Mastrangelo M, Leuzzi V. Genes of early-onset epileptic encephalopathies: From genotype to phenotype. *Pediatr Neurol* 2012; **46**:24–31.

Mefford HC, Muhle H, Ostertag P, et al. Genome-wide copy number variation in epilepsy: Novel susceptibility loci in idiopathic generalized and focal epilepsies. *PLoS Genet* 2010; **6**(5):e1000962.

Michelucci R, Pasini E, Riguzzi P, Volpi L, Dazzo E, Nobile C. Genetics of epilepsy and relevance to current practice. *Curr Neurol Neurosci Rep* 2012; **12**:445–455.

Nicita Fa, De Liso P, Danti FR, et al. The genetics of monogenic idiopathic epilepsies and epileptic encephalopathies. *Seizure* 2012; **21**:3–11.

Olson HE, Poduri A. *CDKL5* mutations in early onset epilepsy: Case report and review of the literature. *J Pediatr Epilepsy* 2012; **1**:151–159.

Ottman R, Hirose S, Jain S, et al. Genetic testing in the epilepsies – Report of the ILAE Genetics Commission. *Epilepsia* 2010; **51**(4):655–670.

Paciorkowski AR, Thio LL, Bodyns WB. Genetic and biologic classification of infantile spasms. *Pediatr Neurol* 2011; **45**:355–367.

Poduri A, Lowenstein, D. Epilepsy genetics – Past, present, and future. *Curr Opin Genet Dev* 2011; **21**(3):325–332.

Sheidley BR, Poduri A. Genetics in clinical epilepsy: Issues in genetic testing and counseling. *J Pediatr Epilepsy* 2012; **1**:135–142.

Striano P, Coppola A, Paravidino R, et al. Clinical significance of rare copy number variations in epilepsy: A case–control survey using microarray-based comparative genomic hybridization. *Arch Neurol* 2012; **69**(3):322–330.

# Metabolic Disorders Not to Miss

**Phillip L. Pearl[1,2] and Yuezhou Joe Yu[1,3]**

[1]Department of Child Neurology, Children's National Medical Center, Washington, DC, USA
[2]Departments of Neurology and Pediatrics, School of Medicine and Columbian College of Arts and Sciences, The George Washington University, Washington, DC, USA
[3]Department of Neurology, Children's National Medical Center, Washington, DC, USA

## Introduction

Metabolic epilepsies are rare but important disorders that, in aggregate, are the subject of a significant proportion of child neurology. This chapter presents treatable metabolic epilepsies. Emphasis is given to entities in which prognoses are closely linked to early diagnosis and in which timely and targeted treatment is potentially crucial to avoid an otherwise catastrophic outcome.

## Specific treatable metabolic epilepsies

### Biopterin synthesis defects

Disorders of synthesis or recycling of tetrahydrobiopterin ($BH_4$), a vital cofactor in the synthesis of the monoamine neurotransmitters (e.g., dopamine, norepinephrine, epinephrine, and serotonin; Figure 23.1), can result in intellectual disability, epilepsy (typically myoclonic seizures with childhood onset), and extrapyramidal manifestations, including rigidity and dystonia. Notably, neuroimaging may show basal ganglia calcifications in this group of disorders, which may be reversible with folinic acid therapy. Biopterin disorders can usually be identified by hyperphenylalaninemia on newborn screening, although some variants are associated with a normal blood phenylalanine. Thus, evaluation for disorders in the $BH_4$ pathway should be

performed in infants with unexplained neurological disease. Treatment options include $BH_4$ supplementation, 5-hydroxytryptophan as a precursor to serotonin, L-dopa, and monoamine oxidase or catechol-O-methyltransferase (COMT) inhibitors.

> **✋ CAUTION!**
>
> Some biopterin synthesis disorders, including Segawa syndrome, which causes dopa-responsive dystonia, and sepiapterin reductase deficiency, associated with myoclonic epilepsy, require cerebrospinal fluid (CSF) screening for detection. Peripheral hyperphenylalaninemia is absent, and standard newborn screens will be blind.

### Cerebral folate deficiency

Cerebral folate deficiency is not a strictly defined syndrome but may represent a common final pathway of different neurological and genetic conditions. One underlying cause of cerebral folate deficiency involves autoantibodies that affect the folate FR1 receptor, which is required to transport folate from plasma to CSF. The phenotypes associated with cerebral folate deficiency involve epilepsy, intellectual disability, developmental regression,

*Epilepsy*, First Edition. Edited by John W. Miller and Howard P. Goodkin.

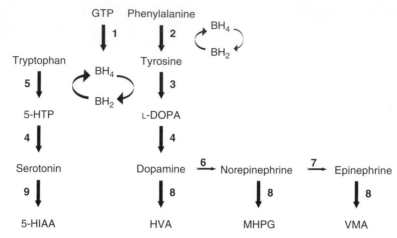

**Figure 23.1.** Monoamine and serotonin synthesis pathway. Reproduced with permission from Pearl, PL. *Inherited Metabolic Epilepsies*. New York: Demos Medical Publishing, 2013.

dyskinesias, and autism. Optic atrophy and cortical visual loss have been observed. Clinical diagnosis is based on low CSF 5-methyltetrahydrofolate, with normal peripheral folate levels. Treatment with folinic acid, which has better blood–brain barrier entry than folate, has been reported to improve seizures and other neurological dysfunction.

### Biotinidase deficiency

Biotinidase deficiency can present with intermittent metabolic acidosis and an organic acid profile of lactic and propionic acidemia. The phenotype is developmental delay, hypotonia, seizures, ataxia, and rash. Signs and symptoms usually appear between 3 and 6 months after birth, when the prenatal supply of biotin is exhausted. If left untreated, the deficiency can lead to cerebral edema and permanent injury. Treatment with 10 mg/day of biotin has resulted in gratifying outcomes, although sensorineural hearing loss and optic atrophy with vision loss, once present, tend to persist. Early and sustained therapy can prevent the onset of symptoms and subsequent neurological deficits.

---

### ⚗ SCIENCE REVISITED

The fundamental defect in this disorder is an inability to cleave biocytin using the enzyme biotinidase. This leads to an impaired ability to form free biotin or catalyze holocarboxylase synthetase, causing a biochemical scenario of multiple carboxylase deficiency. There are variants with partial deficiency and variable penetrance.

---

### ✋ CAUTION!

There are pitfalls and traps pertaining to biotinidase deficiency for even an experienced clinician. Cases of biotinidase deficiency have been misdiagnosed as "atypical" or "childhood" multiple sclerosis. Patients have presented in adolescence with spastic paraparesis. The dermatologic manifestations have been misdiagnosed as acrodermatitis enteropathica or anhidrotic ectodermal dysplasia. Furthermore, seizures (generalized, myoclonic, and infantile spasms) occur in the majority of patients and may be the *only obvious symptom*. Newborn screening will detect biotinidase deficiency but is not always obtained, especially in international patients.

---

### Serine synthesis defects

Disorders of serine synthesis present with a phenotype of congenital microcephaly and psychomotor retardation, which may be nonspecific, likely leading practitioners to suspect in utero processes such as a TORCH infection (infection with toxoplasmosis, syphilis, rubella, cytamegalovirus or herpes simplex virus) or other causes of perinatal, static difficulties. Yet a treatable metabolic disorder would be important to consider. While rare, there are disorders of serine biosynthesis that may be amenable to supplemental serine and glycine, in which prenatal intervention can prevent manifestations in newborns. Diagnosis of serine synthesis disorders can be confirmed by amino acid analysis of plasma or CSF for low serine.

## Creatine synthesis and transport deficiencies

Metabolic disorders of creatine were first described in 1994 with the discovery of guanidinoacetate methyltransferase (GAMT) deficiency. The phenotype includes failure to thrive and early developmental delay, neurological regression, intellectual disability, autistic behavior, hypotonia, epilepsy, movement disorders, and abnormal pallidal signal on MRI. MR spectroscopy may suggest the diagnosis by detection of a low creatine peak. Creatine disorders resulting from GAMT or arginine:glycine amidinotransferase (AGAT) deficiency can be treated with creatine supplementation, along with arginine restriction and ornithine supplementation in the case of GAMT deficiency. Some individuals will need complementary antiepileptics, although others may respond to creatine supplementation alone.

## Developmental delay, epilepsy, and neonatal diabetes (DEND) syndrome

A syndrome has been recently elucidated that combines the problems of developmental delay, epilepsy, and neonatal diabetes, acronymized as DEND. Neonatal diabetes, characterized by severe hyperglycemia within the first 6 months of life, is associated with gain-of-function mutations in a variety of potassium channel and sulfonylurea receptor genes in the pancreas and brain. About 3% of patients with neonatal diabetes will exhibit neurodevelopmental disabilities including generalized epilepsy. Treatment with sulfonylureas bypasses the defective potassium channel regulation, controlling diabetes in more than 90% of patients, and may ameliorate seizures and improve the encephalopathy. Insulin administration may correct systemic hyperglycemia but has no effect on the otherwise poorly understood CNS effects of the disorder.

## Hyperinsulinism/hyperammonemia

Hyperinsulinism/hyperammonemia (HI/HA) is a syndrome of congenital hyperinsulinism and hyperammonemia associated with activating mutations of glutamate dehydrogenase (GDH), a member of the insulin secretion pathway. Concurrent with hyperinsulinism is a plasma ammonia concentration two to five times the normal concentration. A constellation of generalized epilepsy, learning disorders, and behavior problems is characteristic.

An important indication of HI/HA is the occurrence of hypoglycemic seizures, particularly postprandially (after protein intake), rather than only in a fasting state. Elevated plasma ammonia within this context may indicate a diagnosis. Some patients, however, may have seizures unrelated to hypoglycemia. Typical symptoms associated with either chronic or acute hyperammonemia may also be absent. The condition is manageable with a combination of dietary protein restriction, antiepileptic medications, and diazoxide, a $K_{ATP}$ channel agonist that inhibits insulin release.

<table><tr><td>⚕ CAUTION!</td></tr></table>

The use of valproate for seizures can mask a diagnosis of HI/HA due to hyperammonemia misattributed to valproate rather than HI/HA.

## Glucose transporter 1 deficiency

The presence of seizures and developmental delay associated with hypoglycorrhachia, which is indicative of glucose transporter 1 (GLUT1) deficiency, has emerged as the leading metabolic indication for the ketogenic diet. The full clinical spectrum of this disorder is wide and includes early-onset refractory seizures, microcephaly, ataxia, and psychomotor delay. The majority of affected children will have epilepsy, although patients may present without any accompanying motor or cognitive deficits. Prognosis depends on the timeliness of diagnosis and treatment. Early-onset typical absence seizures should trigger suspicion of this disorder.

The signature of GLUT1 deficiency is hypoglycorrhachia in the context of normal plasma glucose and low-to-normal CSF lactate, measured in a fasting state. Seizures may often be refractory to standard antiepileptic drugs (AEDs), but response to the ketogenic diet is typically rapid and marked. A comprehensive approach to the diagnosis and treatment of GLUT1 deficiency is outlined in Table 23.1.

<table><tr><td>⚗ SCIENCE REVISITED</td></tr></table>

The ketogenic diet is an established therapy that restricts glucose intake, allowing ketone bodies, acetoacetate, and beta-hydroxybutyrate to act as alternative fuels.

<table><tr><td>⚕ CAUTION!</td></tr></table>

Valproate, phenobarbital, benzodiazepines, theophylline, and methylxanthines should be avoided with glucose transporter deficiency because these agents themselves can inhibit any residual transporter activity.

**Table 23.1.** Flowchart for diagnosis and treatment of GLUT1 deficiency syndrome.

| |
|---|
| *Clinical features* |
| ± epilepsy refractory to standard AEDs |
| ± paroxysmal movement disorder |
| ± acquired developmental delay |
| ± acquired microcephaly |
| ± ataxia |
| *Fasting lumbar puncture and bloodwork* |
| Hypoglycorrhachia (<40, possibly <60 mg/dL) with normoglycemia |
| CSF/plasma glucose < 0.4 |
| Low or normal CSF lactate (<2.2 mM) |
| *Confirmatory genetic testing* |
| Molecular analysis |
| Erythrocyte glucose uptake assay |
| *Treatment* |
| Ketogenic diet (maintain beta-hydroxybutyrate levels at approximately 5 mM) |
| Avoid inhibitors of GLUT1 transporter: barbiturates, valproate, phenobarbital, theophyllines, and methylxanthines |

Adapted with permission from Pong AW, De Vivo DC. Glucose type I transporter deficiency and epilepsy. In Pearl PL, ed. *Inherited Metabolic Epilepsies*. New York: Demos Publishers, 2013.

## Pyridoxine-dependent epilepsy

Pyridoxine-dependent epilepsy (PDE) is the prototype of a metabolic epilepsy unresponsive to standard anticonvulsants but specifically treated with a vitamin or cofactor. Clinical diagnosis has traditionally been based on an EEG with concomitant administration of intravenous pyridoxine (an updated comprehensive approach is outlined in Table 23.2). Laboratory diagnosis can be established by detecting increased levels of aminoadipic semialdehyde (AASA) or pipecolic acid in urine or plasma or mutations in the *ALDH7A1* or *PNPO* genes.

Atypical PDE cases have been described in which there are asymptomatic periods without pyridoxine supplementation and diagnoses are discovered later in infancy after apparently being ruled out in the neonatorum. Neurodevelopmental disability may be improved by early diagnosis and treatment

**Table 23.2.** Proposed diagnostic and treatment steps for pyridoxine-related responsive seizures.

| Diagnostic studies | • Blood for α-AASA or pipecolic acid<br>• Urine for AASA<br>• DNA mutation testing for either *ALDH7A1* or *PNPO* genes |
|---|---|
| Therapeutic trials | • Pyridoxine 100–500 mg intravenously<br>• PLP 30 mg/kg/day divided in three or four doses enterally, for 3–5 days<br>• Folinic acid 3–5 mg/kg/day enterally, for 3–5 days |
| Chronic therapy | • For confirmed PDE: pyridoxine 15–30 mg/kg/day (maximum daily dose of 500 mg) and folinic acid 3–5 mg/kg/day<br>• For confirmed PNPO deficiency: PLP 30–50 mg/kg/day divided in four to six doses |

Adapted with permission from Gospe, SM. Pyridoxine-related responsive seizures. In Pearl PL, ed. *Inherited Metabolic Epilepsies*. New York: Demos Publishers, 2013. AASA, aminoadipic semialdehyde; PDE, pyridoxine dependent epilepsy; PLP, pyridoxal-5-phosphate; PNPO, pyridoxamine 5′-phosphate oxidase.

(including in utero), and affected patients should receive regular, lifetime pharmacological doses of the vitamin or cofactor. Folinic acid dependency has been identified as allelic with PDE, and patients have been documented that responded to folinic acid (either alone or together with pyridoxine). In addition, patients with PNPO deficiency require pyridoxal-5-phosphate (PLP), the biologically active form of pyridoxine.

### ⚠ CAUTION!

Pyridoxine-dependent epilepsy may mimic neonatal hypoxic-ischemic encephalopathy and should be considered and reconsidered in cases of refractory epilepsy and status epilepticus in neonates and infants.

### Urea cycle disorders

Urea cycle disorders can present in the first days of life with lethargy and hyperammonemia, progressing to seizures, cerebral edema, coma, and death. The survival rate for acute neonatal hyperammonemia due to urea cycle defects is about 75%, compared to better prognoses with later presentation or incomplete deficiency. Males typically present as neonates and with higher mortality. Female heterozygotes can become symptomatic, with the severity and timing dependent on the extent of hepatic lyonization.

Early recognition and aggressive supportive and anticonvulsant treatment are the key elements of intervention. Once a patient is in crisis, management includes a combination of hemodialysis, pharmacological scavenging using sodium benzoate and sodium phenylacetate, and reversal of the catabolic state. The latter management method emphasizes the use of intravenous fluids with a high dextrose concentration and a lipid source for caloric support. Other modalities include temporary withholding of protein to prevent muscle breakdown and provision of essential amino acids to stimulate protein synthesis, an effective sink for excess nitrogen. While orthotopic liver transplant may be curative, this will not reverse neurological injury.

### ⚠ CAUTION!

When managing seizures in the context of urea cycle dysfunction, valproate and systemic steroids should be avoided. These may lead to further elevation of plasma ammonia and precipitate metabolic crises.

### Hyperekplexia

Hyperekplexia, or stiff baby syndrome, can appear in a major form with significant hypertonia and symptoms of infantile falling, shaking, hyperreflexia, and unsteady gait. There also appears to be a more common minor form with isolated but excessive startle reactions. Both forms may involve frequent difficulty with swallowing and choking, which are likely responsible for the known tragic complication of sudden death. Attacks have been described as preventable with sudden flexion of the head and limbs, and clonazepam is recommended. While this condition would be considered an epilepsy mimic, the notion that sudden death could be prevented

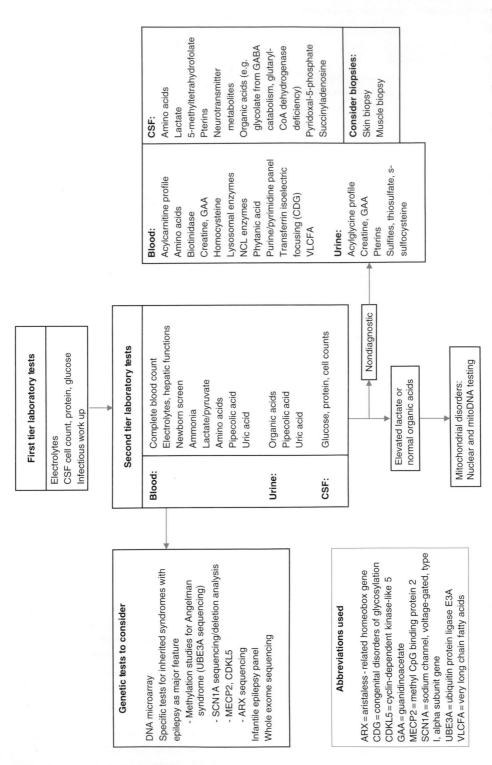

**Figure 23.2.** Epileptic encephalography: Laboratory approach. Adapted from Pinto A, Pearl PL. Clinical approach to inherited metabolic epilepsies. In: Pearl PL, ed. *Inherited Metabolic Epilepsies.* New York: Demos Medical Publishing, 2013, with permission.

with an inexpensive benzodiazepine in a condition that may be misdiagnosed as epilepsy is compelling.

---

### ☆ TIPS AND TRICKS

A helpful bedside test for hyperekplexia is the nose tap: use the finger to tap the nose in search of a prominent and dramatic startle response.

---

### ⚖ SCIENCE REVISITED

Hyperekplexia is due to impairment in glycine-mediated inhibition at the brainstem and spinal cord levels. Whereas GABA is the major inhibitory neurotransmitter of the brain, glycine is the major inhibitory transmitter of the brainstem and cord. In hyperekplexia, mutations may be seen in glycine inhibitory receptor GLRA1 or glycine transporters.

---

## Summary and conclusions

Metabolic disorders are a concern in patients with epilepsy with suggestive neurological signs and symptoms, especially in children and patients who do not respond to standard epilepsy management. The prognosis of many of the conditions we describe depends on early diagnosis and treatment (Figure 23.2).

## Bibliography

Brusilow SW, Danney M, Waber LJ, et al. Treatment of episodic hyperammonemia in children with inborn errors of urea synthesis. *N Engl J Med* 1984; **310**:1630–1634.

De Vivo DC, Trifiletti RR, Jacobson RI, Ronen GM, Behmand RA, Harik SI. Defective glucose transport across the blood–brain barrier as a cause of persistent hypoglycorrhachia, seizures, and developmental delay. *N Engl J Med* 1991; **325**(10):703–709.

Gospe, SM. Pyridoxine-related responsive seizures. In Pearl PL, ed. *Inherited Metabolic Epilepsies*. New York: Demos Publishers, 2013.

Hunt AD, Stokes J, McCrory WW, Stroud HH. Pyridoxine dependency: Report of a case of intractable convulsions in an infant controlled by pyridoxine. *Pediatrics* 1954; **13**(2):140–145.

Mills PB, Struys E, Jakobs C, et al. Mutations in antiquitin in individuals with pyridoxine-dependent seizures. *Nat Med* 2006; **12**:307–309.

Mineyko A, Whiting S, Graham GE. Hyperekplexia: Treatment of a severe phenotype and review of the literature. *Can J Neurol Sci* 2011; **38**:411–416.

Palladino AA, Stanley CA. The hyperinsulinism/hyperammonemia syndrome. *Rev Endocr Metab Disord* 2010; **11**(3):171–178.

Pearl PL. *Inherited Metabolic Epilepsies*. New York: Demos Publishers, 2013.

Pearl PL, Gospe SM. Pyridoxal phosphate dependency a newly recognized treatable catastrophic epileptic encephalopathy. *J Inherit Metab Dis* 2007; **30**(1):2–4.

Pearson ER, Flechtner I, Njølstad PR, et al. Switching from insulin to oral sulfonylureas in patients with diabetes due to Kir6.2 mutations. *N Engl J Med* 2006; **355**(5):467–477.

Pinto A, Pearl PL. Clinical approach to inherited metabolic epilepsies. In: Pearl PL, ed. *Inherited Metabolic Epilepsies*. New York: Demos Medical Publishing, 2013.

Pong AW, De Vivo DC. Glucose type I transporter deficiency and epilepsy. In Pearl PL, ed. *Inherited Metabolic Epilepsies*. New York: Demos Publishers, 2013.

Ramaekers VT, Rothenberg SP, Sequeira JM, et al. Autoantibodies to folate receptors in the cerebral folate deficiency syndrome. *N Engl J Med* 2005; **352**(19):1985–1991.

Schubiger G, Caflisch U, Baumgartner R, Suormala T, Bachmann C. Biotinidase deficiency: Clinical course and biochemical findings. *J Inherit Metab Dis* 1984; **7**(3):129–130.

Schulze A, Battini R. Pre-symptomatic treatment of creatine biosynthesis defects. *Subcell Biochem* 2007; **46**:167–181.

Stöckler S, Holzbach U, Hanefeld F, et al. Creatine deficiency in the brain: A new, treatable inborn error of metabolism. *Pediatr Res* 1994; **36**(3):409–413.

Summar ML, Dobbelaere D, Brusilow S, Lee B. Diagnosis, Symptoms, frequency and mortality of 260 patients with urea cycle disorders from a 21-year, multicentre study of acute hyperammonaemic episodes. *Acta Paediatr* 2008; **97**(10):1420–1425.

Tabatabaie L, Klomp LW, Berger R, de Koning TJ. L-serine synthesis in the central nervous system: A review on serine deficiency disorders. *Mol Genet Metab* 2010; **99**:256–262.

# Part V

# Special Topics in Adult Epilepsy

# Juvenile Myoclonic Epilepsy and Other Primary Generalized Epilepsies

**Shahin Hakimian**

Department of Neurology, UW Regional Epilepsy Center, University of Washington, Seattle, WA, USA

## Introduction

Myoclonic, absence, and primary generalized tonic-clonic seizures (GTCSs) commonly occur in a group of overlapping epilepsy syndromes in otherwise neurologically intact patients. These constitute the idiopathic primary generalized epilepsies (IGEs), which in adults include juvenile myoclonic epilepsy (JME), juvenile absence epilepsy (JAE), and primary generalized tonic–clonic seizures upon awakening (PGTC, also known as *idiopathic generalized epilepsy with pure grand mal*) (see Chapters 2 and 21). In practice, symptoms and features among IGE syndromes overlap. IGEs can be distinguished from other forms of epilepsy based on history, neurological examination, and EEG. Recognizing IGEs affects treatment choices and helps with prognosis. The features of IGEs in adults and their differential diagnosis and treatment choices are discussed here.

## Clinical features

Idiopathic primary generalized epilepsy syndromes in adults are common, representing 10–30% of new-onset epilepsy. Both genders are equally affected. "Idiopathic" in IGE implies a suspected genetic cause. A family history is frequently present (in up to 40%), but seizure manifestations may differ among family members. The genetic causes appear heterogeneous and polygenic. Autosomal dominant inheritance and autosomal recessive inheritance have been reported. In practice, a single causative genetic mutation is rarely identifiable.

> **SCIENCE REVISITED**
>
> Some of the identified genes in IGEs are widely distributed ion channels. This gives credence to the idea that their etiology is "general" cortical excitability.

Typically, seizures present in the teens to late 20s. However, age of onset can vary. Some 10–20% of children diagnosed with childhood absence epilepsy are later classified as having an adult IGE. Presentation after the third decade of life, while uncommon, is not entirely rare. Late presentation as the result of a GTCS may be the first *recognized* manifestation of an IGE whose earlier signs (e.g., jerks or absence) went unnoticed. Late presentation of a severe syndrome, however, should prompt consideration for other diagnoses such as symptomatic generalized epilepsy (SGE), particularly a progressive form. The bedside neurological examination is typically normal. Careful neuropsychological studies, however, have identified subtle frontal executive dysfunction in many patients with IGE.

*Epilepsy*, First Edition. Edited by John W. Miller and Howard P. Goodkin.
© 2014 John Wiley & Sons, Ltd. Published 2014 by John Wiley & Sons, Ltd.

The presence and relative frequency of absence, myoclonic, and GTCSs differ among patients and characterize the individual syndromes of JAE, JME, or PGTC. The seizures are typically stereotyped for an individual. Yet, occurrence and provocation of another generalized seizure type is possible.

*Absence seizures* (common in JAE but also seen in JME) show the typical brief interruptions of sensorium also found in classic childhood absence. Patients may report these as "losing time," "spacing out," dizziness, or light-headedness. These are sometimes reported as "auras," which may mislead the practitioner. In adults, prolonged absence seizures (absence status) occur occasionally. During these, patients are somewhat interactive although they may appear forgetful, inattentive (spacey), or slow to respond.

> ### ✋ CAUTION!
>
> Absence seizures and absence status in adults can sometimes be subtle. Recognizing absence status can be particularly challenging in acute care settings.

*Myoclonic seizures* are most common in JME, although not every patient recognizes them. The jerks are brief, sudden muscle contractions occurring singly or repetitively in a burst. Myoclonus usually involves upper extremities, often synchronously and typically early in the morning upon awakening. Patients usually retain some awareness during brief bursts of myoclonus and can recall an experience of body jerks or "electrical jolts." Involuntary twitches in arms disrupt activities such as writing, eating, applying makeup, shaving, and brushing teeth. The jerks are frequently dismissed as nervousness or clumsiness, however, until specifically exposed during medical history. Facial and vocal involvement is possible but uncommon. Lower limbs and torso may also suddenly contract, resulting in falls. Violent jerks are less common in IGE than SGE, although injuries can still occur from falls, dropping objects, mishandling motorized tools, etc. Bursts of myoclonus may "build up," leading to a GTCS.

> ### ☆ TIPS AND TRICKS
>
> Carefully obtaining a history of myoclonus (and distinguishing it from benign sleep myoclonus) is a key to making a diagnosis of JME.

*Generalized tonic–clonic seizures* are the defining feature of PGTC but also commonly occur in JME and even JAE. Like the myoclonus, they preferentially occur early in the day. They are sometimes preceded by absence or myoclonic seizures. Lateralized semiology such as forced head version, unilateral tonic extension, or asymmetric myoclonus can occur in IGE, but stereotyped lateralization is less common. Injuries, falls, car accidents, and even unexpected death are possible with more severe seizures.

## Differential diagnosis for idiopathic primary generalized epilepsy

The differential diagnosis for IGE is quite broad, encompassing precipitated seizures (such as alcohol-related seizures), focal epilepsy, and SGE syndromes. Some of these are discussed later in this chapter. Other nonepileptic causes are psychogenic events (see Chapter 6), subcortical myoclonus, syncope, narcolepsy, benign sleep myoclonus, and even periodic limb movement disorder. Nonepileptic causes can all be distinguished from IGE through a careful neurological history and examination confirmed by video–EEG recording.

Among focal onset epilepsies, frontal seizures may be mistaken for PGTC because both can present in the early-morning hours. The high-amplitude frontal discharges found on the EEG can be similar to the generalized spike-and-wave complexes found in IGE. If clinically warranted, the syndromes can be distinguished by careful EEG review and video–EEG monitoring to characterize semiology and ictal EEG. Focal motor seizures (including focal cortical myoclonus) may resemble myoclonus in JME. In focal motor seizures, epileptiform discharges are exclusively contralateral to the involved limb, and other typical IGE features are lacking. Multifocal epilepsy can be difficult to differentiate from IGE by history or interictal EEG alone. Ictal EEG patterns and semiology separate the two. Epileptogenic MRI abnormalities should be absent in IGE.

Symptomatic generalized epilepsies are defined as epilepsies caused by another neurological disorder. SGEs are distinguished from IGEs based on neurological history and an abnormal neurological examination. Multiple seizure types may be present.

Occasionally in adults, generalized seizures are an early manifestation of an SGE due to a neurodegenerative disorder. These are labeled progressive myoclonic epilepsies (PMEs). Because patients may initially appear neurologically intact, a PME may be misclassified as idiopathic. Over time PMEs more clearly resemble other SGEs: seizure becomes more severe; EEG shows background slowing; and neurological signs such as ataxia, cognitive impairment, dysarthria, tremors, and hearing loss develop. PMEs presenting in adults and teens include Unverricht–Lundborg disease, myoclonic epilepsy with ragged red fibers (MERRF), Lafora body disease, adult neuronal ceroid lipofuscinosis (type 4), dentato-rubral–pallidoluysian atrophy (DRPLA), and Gaucher disease (subacute neuronopathic form, type 3). PME should be considered in the differential diagnosis of patients with unusual clinical findings who deteriorate or fail to respond to antiepileptic drugs (AEDs). Repeat diagnostic evaluation may be necessary, including MRI examination of the brain. The genetics of several of the PMEs are reviewed in Chapter 22.

## EEG in primary generalized epilepsy

The classic EEG findings in JME are 3–5-Hz frontally maximum generalized spike-and-wave discharges (Figure 24.1). The discharges may be overtly symptomatic (associated with myoclonic seizures), subtle (associated with absence or subtle twitches), or without overt manifestations, even in the same patient at different times. Focal fragments of epileptiform discharges or some shifting asymmetry of discharges on EEG (Figure 24.1B) are expected and part of the syndrome. Other common findings are multispikes, generalized paroxysmal fast discharges, and photoparoxysmal responses. Figure 24.2 shows an ictal EEG recording for PGTC.

In practice, distinguishing generalized discharges and high-amplitude frontal spikes can be challenging. Therefore, frontal midline focal epilepsy should be considered in the differential diagnosis of IGE syndromes. Other EEG findings that overlap with IGE include multifocal discharges, benzodiazepine or alcohol withdrawal, and SGEs.

## Imaging

Brain MRI appears normal in IGE. Nevertheless, imaging is recommended (e.g., by the American Academy of Neurology quality standards) for all cases of new onset of epilepsy in adults. The guidelines do not make a distinction between focal onset epilepsy and IGE. Prospective data for making an imaging exception for IGE solely based on history or EEG is lacking. Given the differential diagnosis, initial imaging with either CT or MRI is warranted in all patients. When there are atypical features, an abnormal neurological exam, seizures refractory to common AEDs, or evidence of progression, careful imaging with modern MRI scanners is necessary.

## Treatment and prognosis

Fewer AED trials for IGE than for focal onset epilepsies have been performed. The data is particularly incomplete for the latest drugs and for myoclonic and absence seizures (Chapter 11). Valproate has clear efficacy for all three seizure types. Levetiracetam, lamotrigine, and topiramate have all shown efficacy primarily for GTCSs. Their efficacy for absence seizures is accepted but not supported by well-done trials. Lamotrigine in particular may paradoxically exacerbate myoclonus. Zonisamide has some incomplete evidence supporting its use. Benzodiazepines such as clonazepam (and probably clobazam) are helpful, particularly for eliminating myoclonic seizures and sometimes for GTCSs. Ethosuximide is a good choice for absence seizures but lacks efficacy for other seizure types seen in adults. Felbamate, phenobarbital, and primidone show efficacy but are best avoided as first- or second-line AEDs because of adverse effects.

By contrast, several drugs exacerbate absence and myoclonic seizures: carbamazepine, oxcarbazepine, vigabatrin, tiagabine, gabapentin, pregabalin, and probably eslicarbazepine acetate (Chapter 11). These should be avoided in IGE. These AEDs may change the manifestation of epilepsy. For example, carbamazepine may unmask absence seizures in PGTC epilepsy. Phenytoin, although effective for GTCSs, can also exacerbate absence or myoclonic seizures. Adequate data on lacosamide, rufinamide, and ezogabine are lacking. When there is uncertainty about the diagnosis, broad-spectrum AEDs should be favored over drugs that can exacerbate IGEs.

### ⚠ CAUTION!

Avoid carbamazepine, oxcarbazepine, phenytoin, vigabatrin, tiagabine, gabapentin, pregabalin, and eslicarbazepine acetate in IGE because they can exacerbate absence or myoclonic seizures.

Due to the teratogenic risk of valproate, avoid it in women of childbearing age.

(A)

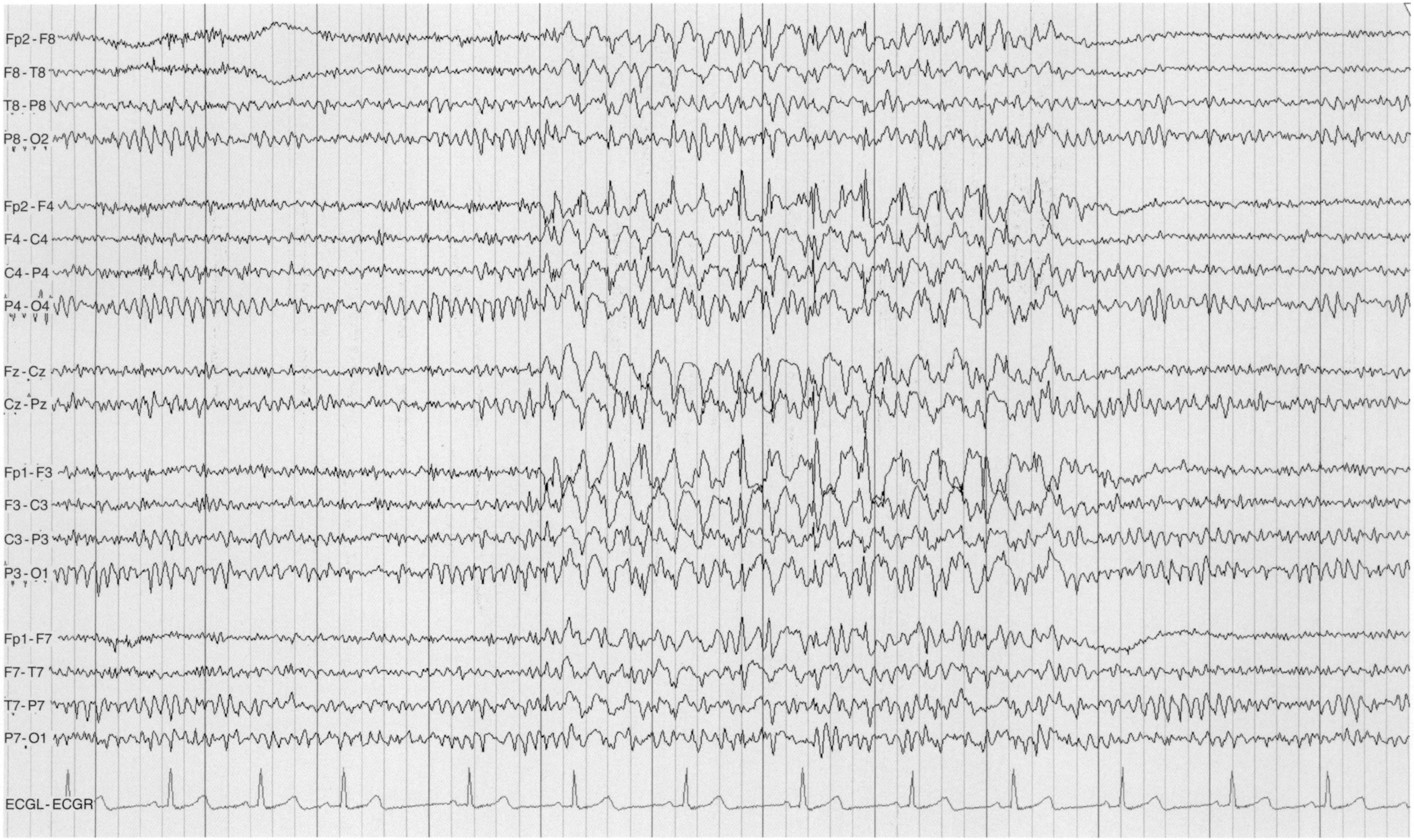

Fp2 - F8
F8 - T8
T8 - P8
P8 - O2
Fp2 - F4
F4 - C4
C4 - P4
P4 - O4
Fz - Cz
Cz - Pz
Fp1 - F3
F3 - C3
C3 - P3
P3 - O1
Fp1 - F7
F7 - T7
T7 - P7
P7 - O1
ECGL - ECGR

**Figure 24.1.** Examples of generalized spike-and-wave discharges in idiopathic generalized epilepsy. (A) 3.5- to 4-Hz generalized discharges in JME. (B) Shifting asymmetry of discharges in the same patient as in (A).

(B)

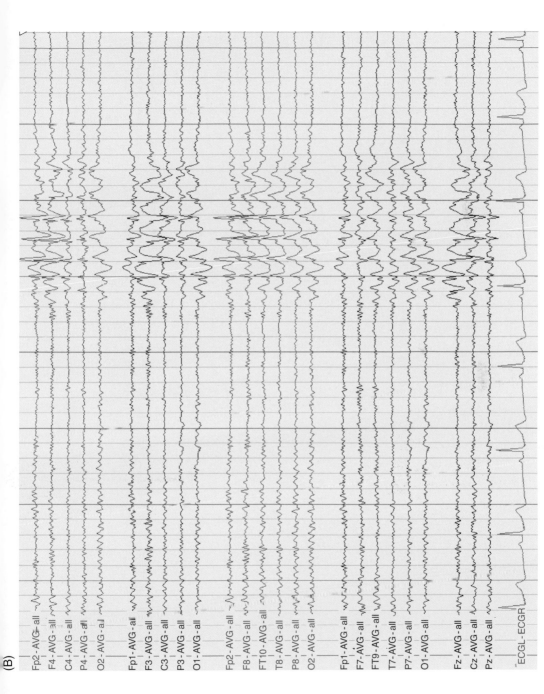

**Figure 24.1.** (*Continued*)

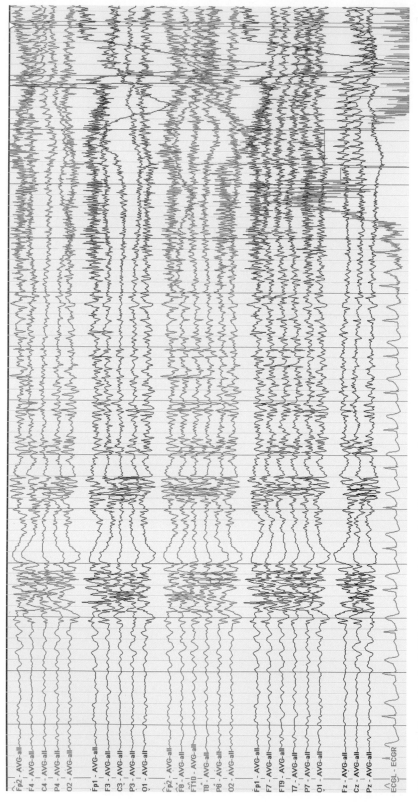

**Figure 24.2.** Example of a GTCS with generalized multispikes arising from sleep.

Appropriate head-to-head trials of the AEDs for combined efficacy and tolerability are done infrequently. Still, randomized trials can reveal only short-term efficacy and toxicity. Long-term toxicity, a concern for drugs taken over a lifetime, may take decades to decipher, particularly in select vulnerable populations. Valproate, for example, has excellent efficacy for JME and was *the* drug of choice for all IGEs until its high teratogenic risk was recognized. Valproate should be avoided in women of childbearing age. Other long-term toxicities concern weight gain, cognitive functioning, reproductive well-being, bone health, and overall longevity. Data for these effects are lacking, making AED selection challenging.

A minority of IGE patients have difficult-to-control epilepsy. Polytherapy may be necessary, particularly if valproate is excluded. Vagus nerve stimulation (VNS) efficacy for IGE has been reported in case series, but VNS is not FDA approved for this use. Ketogenic, Atkins, or low glycemic index diets, while promising, are not supported by good trials. Thalamic and other subcortical stimulators are investigational methods of unproven value for IGE. Corpus callosotomy is a palliative surgical treatment used for akinetic seizures in Lennox–Gastaut syndrome, but it is of unproven value for IGE.

## Patient counseling

Nearly all patients with juvenile onset IGE require life-long AED treatment, although cases of remission off of AEDs have been reported. Most patients (but certainly not all) achieve seizure freedom on appropriate treatment, often with monotherapy. Severe status epilepticus and SUDEP occur less frequently in IGE than with intractable focal epilepsy syndromes. Standard mortality ratios are only slightly elevated in IGEs.

In all three syndromes, seizures are particularly prone to exacerbation by precipitating factors such as alcohol, sleep deprivation, menstrual cycle, several prescribed medications, and illicit drug use. Patients should be counseled to avoid such precipitants.

## Conclusion

Idiopathic primary generalized epilepsy syndromes are common conditions. The key to their appropriate treatment is recognizing the clinical features, confirming the diagnosis with EEG (if possible), and providing the appropriate medication and counseling for the patient. Overall, with appropriate diagnosis and treatment, most patients do well, leading mostly normal lives.

## Bibliography

Boylan LS, Labovitz DL, Jackson SC, Starner K, Devinsky O. Auras are frequent in idiopathic generalized epilepsy. *Neurology* 2006; **67**:343–345.

Durón RM, Medina MT, Martínez-Juárez IE, et al. Seizures of idiopathic generalized epilepsies. *Epilepsia* 2005; **46**(Suppl. 9):34–47.

Faught E. Clinical presentations and phenomenology of myoclonus. *Epilepsia* 2003; **44** (Suppl. 11): 7–12.

Geithner J, Schneider F, Wang Z, et al. Predictors for long-term seizure outcome in juvenile myoclonic epilepsy: 25–63 years of follow-up. *Epilepsia* 2012; **53**(8):1379–1386.

Jallon P, Latour P. Epidemiology of idiopathic generalized epilepsies. *Epilepsia* 2005; **46**(Suppl. 9):10–14.

Kostov H, Larsson PG, Røste GK. Is vagus nerve stimulation at treatment option for patients with drug-resistant idiopathic generalized epilepsy? *Acta Neurol Scand* 2007; **115**(Suppl. 187):55–58.

Leutmezer F, Lurger S, Baumgartner C. Focal features in patients with idiopathic generalized epilepsy. *Epilepsy Res* 2002; **50**:293–300.

Marson AG, Al-Kharusi AM, Alwaidh M, et al. The SANAD study of effectiveness of valproate, lamotrigine, or topiramate for generalised and unclassifiable epilepsy: An unblinded randomised controlled trial. *Lancet* 2007; **369**:1016–1026.

Mohanraj R, Brodie MJ. Outcomes of newly diagnosed idiopathic generalized epilepsy syndromes in a non-pediatric setting. *Acta Neurol Scand* 2007; **115**:204–208.

Oguni H. Symptomatic epilepsies imitating idiopathic generalized epilepsies. *Epilepsia* 2005; **46**(Suppl. 9):84–90.

Reichsoellner J, Larch J, Unterberger I, et al. Idiopathic generalised epilepsy of late onset: A separate nosological entity? *J Neurol Neurosurg Psychiatry* 2010; **81**:1218–1222.

Seneviratne U, Cook M, D'Souza W. The electroencephalogram of idiopathic generalized epilepsy. *Epilepsia* 2012; **53**(2):234–248.

Shorvon S, Walker M. Status epilepticus in idiopathic generalized epilepsy. *Epilepsia* 2005; **46**(Suppl. 9):73–79.

Sozmen V, Baybas S, Dirican A, Koksal A, Ozturk M. Frequency of epilepsies in family members of patients with different epileptic syndromes *Eur Neurol* 2011; **65**:4–9.

Zupanc ML, Legros B. Progressive myoclonic epilepsy. *Cerebellum* 2004; **3**:156–171.

# Epilepsy in Women of Childbearing Age

## Autumn Klein

Department of Neurology, UPMC Presbyterian/Magee Women's Hospital of UPMC, Pittsburgh, PA, USA

## Introduction

Throughout their reproductive lives, women with epilepsy (WWE) face challenges that place them and their unborn offspring at risk of adverse events. The estimated epilepsy prevalence in women of childbearing age is 0.3–0.5%. Juvenile absence epilepsy and juvenile myoclonic epilepsy are particularly common in women of this age. While it is important to choose an antiepileptic drug (AED) that is appropriate for the patient's particular epilepsy syndrome, this chapter will also review considerations for AED choice that are specific to WWE.

## Catamenial epilepsy

Catamenial epilepsy is defined as a twofold increase in daily seizure frequency during specific phases of the menstrual cycle. This may occur during (1) menses (perimenstrual), (2) ovulation (periovulatory), or (3) the entire second half of the cycle (luteal phase). Approximately one-third of women with temporal lobe epilepsy have a catamenial pattern. Diagnosis of catamenial epilepsy requires careful documentation of seizure patterns related to the menstrual cycle.

The perimenstrual pattern is the most common. During this phase, the estrogen to progesterone balance favors estrogen, which has pro-convulsant properties. Fluctuations in metabolism of certain AEDs around the time of menses might also predispose patients to seizures if levels fall, although this theory is not strongly substantiated.

Treatment options include targeted AED therapy at the most vulnerable times of the cycle; select use of contraception; and use of medroxyprogesterone acetate, natural progesterone, or other hormonal treatments such as the investigational agent ganaxolone or clomiphene citrate. The use of natural progesterone lozenges for perimenstrual catamenial epilepsy has the best evidence of efficacy.

## Contraception

The choice of contraception for a WWE prescribed AED therapy can be challenging. As the best AED and oral contraceptive pill (OCP) combination is not known, many physicians and WWE choose alternate contraceptive options, some not as reliable as OCPs.

> ☆ **TIPS AND TRICKS**
>
> Ethinyl estradiol induces the uridine-diphosphate glucuronosyltransferase metabolism of lamotrigine. Therefore, when a WWE is prescribed or discontinues a combined estrogen–progesterone OCP, lamotrigine dosing may need to be adjusted to account for the change in clearance.

*Epilepsy*, First Edition. Edited by John W. Miller and Howard P. Goodkin.
© 2014 John Wiley & Sons, Ltd. Published 2014 by John Wiley & Sons, Ltd.

The cytochrome P450 system, specifically CYP3A4, is the primary metabolic pathway of ethinyl estradiol and other sex hormones. Because AED induction of this pathway will accelerate hormone clearance, it will also reduce OCP efficacy. Some enzyme-inducing AEDs may also lead to an increase in sex hormone-binding globulin, which reduces free levels of reproductive hormones. Therefore, when using an enzyme-inducing AED, an OCP containing 30 µg or more of estrogen should be used, although there is no direct evidence supporting this suggestion. The CDC Medical Eligibility Criteria for contraception classifies phenytoin, carbamazepine, phenobarbital, primidone, topiramate, and oxcarbazepine as increasing the risk of birth control failure in individuals who use OCPs.

### EVIDENCE AT A GLANCE

There has been only one pharmacokinetic study looking at true pregnancy risk related to an AED. In the study, women took carbamazepine and a low-dose estrogen-containing OCP for 2 months. Hormone levels decreased dramatically, and there was ovulation in half of the cycles, with increased breakthrough bleeding, all suggesting the decreased contraceptive efficacy of this combination.

## Preconception counseling

As up to a half of pregnancies are unplanned, WWE of reproductive age should be prescribed an AED with low risk to offspring.

### ★ TIPS AND TRICKS

Management of epilepsy in women of childbearing age is based on the answers to these questions:

1. Are there active seizures?
2. Is an AED necessary?
3. Does the AED used have a low rate of malformations and will it control the specific seizure type?

Consider stopping AEDs in WWE who are entering their reproductive years. Factors to be considered when deciding whether to stop AEDs are discussed in Chapter 17. For those who need to be maintained on an AED, one with the lowest possible rate of

major congenital malformations should be used, at the lowest dose necessary for seizure control. In addition, all WWE of childbearing age should take a daily prenatal vitamin and additional folic acid. Although the ideal dose of folic acid is not actually known, a total daily dose of about 5 mg/day is frequently recommended. In the USA, this equals four 1 mg folic acid tablets and one prenatal vitamin, which typically has 800 µg of folic acid.

Once it has been determined that a WWE is on the best AED for childbearing and seizure control, a baseline AED level will be helpful for medication titration during pregnancy. Patients should be attentive to the earliest signs of pregnancy (missed menses, nausea, fatigue) and notify their neurologist immediately if they conceive. Serum blood levels can change dramatically within the first trimester, prior to the first obstetrical visit, so immediate monitoring and adjusting may be needed.

## Infertility

Infertility is the inability to conceive after 1 year of regular unprotected sexual intercourse in women younger than 35 years of age and for 6 months in women older than 35 years. The national infertility rate is estimated at 10–15% of all couples. The infertility rate is higher in WWE, with a pregnancy rate approximately 60–75% of that of the general population.

The reasons for this lower pregnancy rate are multiple. In the past, WWE might not have been allowed to marry or have children. Recently, lower marriage rates have also been documented. Some WWE may have cognitive impairment, which leads to a lower chance of living independently. They may also not be as socially engaged as their peers. Understandably, they can be concerned about the effects of medications on their offspring, the inheritance of disease, and the difficulty of raising children. In addition to depression, WWE frequently have impaired sexual function and lower self-reported arousal; those on enzyme-inducing medications are usually the most affected.

There is some evidence that WWE have endocrine abnormalities at a higher rate than the general population, which may contribute to infertility. These endocrine abnormalities include polycystic ovarian syndrome (PCOS), hyperprolactinemia, and premature menopause. PCOS, characterized by polycystic ovaries, hirsutism, obesity, and infertility, occurs in about 5% of the general population but in approximately 20% of women with temporal lobe epilepsy.

Seizures themselves, especially convulsions, can lead to prolonged increases in prolactin levels. Prolactin at sustained high levels is known to suppress ovulation and therefore may affect fertility in women with frequent seizures. Finally, for unknown reasons, WWE have higher rates of premature ovarian failure, defined as primary gonadal failure, high gonadotropin levels, and amenorrhea before 40 years of age.

## Antiepileptic drugs

Antiepileptic drug choice is critical for pregnancy outcome but should really be determined before conception. Most choices are governed by the rates of major congenital malformations associated with first-trimester exposure. Several large international pregnancy and pharmaceutical company registries track these malformations. Unfortunately, studies are underpowered for many AEDs. These registries agree that first-trimester valproic acid exposure is associated with an increased rate of major congenital malformations, while lamotrigine and levetiracetam are associated with some of the lowest rates of malformations. The American Academy of Neurology (AAN) guidelines recommend avoiding use of valproic acid during the first trimester to reduce risk of malformations. In addition, they suggest avoiding polytherapy of any AED and, if possible, avoiding phenytoin and phenobarbital to prevent reduced cognitive outcomes.

A recent publication by the North American Antiepileptic Drug Pregnancy Registry reviewed findings on malformations and monotherapy AED exposure in pregnancy (Table 25.1). In this study, valproate was associated with neural tube defects, hypospadias, cardiac defects, and oral clefts, while phenobarbital had a higher risk of cardiac defects and oral clefts. In addition, a prospective investigation of AED exposure during pregnancy confirmed a high rate of fetal malformation with valproate exposure and also demonstrated a lower IQ measured at age six. Given the findings from these studies, lamotrigine and levetiracetam are becoming more commonly used AEDs in women of childbearing age.

### ☝ CAUTION!

If at all possible, valproic acid should be avoided in women of childbearing age. Try alternate AEDs; only if they fail should valproic acid be considered. If valproic acid must be used, try the lowest possible dose, ideally <1000 mg/day.

### EVIDENCE AT A GLANCE

Children exposed to valproic acid as monotherapy in utero have significantly lower IQs than offspring of women using carbamazepine, lamotrigine, or phenytoin as monotherapy.

## Pregnancy

Management of AEDs during pregnancy requires frequent monitoring because of increased hepatic and renal clearance of medications. The AAN guidelines recommend monitoring of lamotrigine, carbamazepine, and phenytoin during pregnancy, with monitoring of levetiracetam and oxcarbazepine also being considered. Although there was insufficient

**Table 25.1.** Malformation rates associated with select antiepileptic drugs.

| Antiepileptic drug | Pregnancies enrolled | Total malformations | Prevalence of malformations (%) |
|---|---|---|---|
| Lamotrigine | 1562 | 31 | 2.0 |
| Carbamazepine | 1033 | 31 | 3.0 |
| Phenytoin | 416 | 12 | 2.9 |
| Levetiracetam | 450 | 11 | 2.4 |
| Topiramate | 359 | 15 | 4.2 |
| Valproate | 323 | 30 | 9.3 |

Source: Hernandez-Diaz S, Smith CR, Shen A, et al. Comparative safety of antiepileptic drugs during pregnancy. *Neurology* 2012; **78**(21):1692–1699, with permission.

evidence to recommend monitoring levels of other AEDs, such testing nonetheless seems reasonable.

The risk of seizures during pregnancy reflects prepregnancy seizure control. Many WWE will not have a change in seizures during pregnancy, while similar portions of pregnant WWE will experience an increase or decrease. Those treated with oxcarbazepine and lamotrigine are at risk for increased seizures during pregnancy, presumably due to pharmacokinetic changes.

The effect of seizures on the fetus is not entirely clear. Convulsions probably lead to a decrease in blood flow to the placenta, whereas focal seizures probably do not, as long as blood pressure and perfusion are maintained. If a woman has repeated convulsions in pregnancy, aside from the potential for physical injury, the repeated episodes of lack of blood flow might restrict fetal growth.

Currently, many women in the USA get a detailed anatomic ultrasound between weeks 16 and 20 to look for major malformations. All WWE should receive this screening, and delivery at a high-level neonatal center should be considered if there is a malformation. No other special obstetrical monitoring is needed except for frequent AED monitoring. If a WWE has a convulsion, then she should be seen soon by an obstetrician, and an ultrasound should be considered.

There is insufficient evidence to know whether WWE have higher rates of preeclampsia or are more likely to undergo Caesarean delivery. It is likely that WWE who smoke have a higher risk of premature contractions and labor.

There is increased seizure risk at the time of delivery due to lack of sleep, physical stress, and discomfort. This risk can be minimized by maintaining proper AED dosing, minimizing pain, and allowing rest where possible. If there is a concern for seizure with either an aura or a typical prodrome, then lorazepam 0.5–1 mg intravenously can be administered preventatively. If a WWE has a seizure around the time of delivery, lorazepam and magnesium should be administered in case the patient may be developing preeclampsia or eclampsia.

### EVIDENCE AT A GLANCE

Only about 2–3% of WWE have a seizure around the time of delivery. If seizures are well controlled in the 9 months prior to pregnancy, there is almost a 90% chance that the WWE will be seizure-free during the pregnancy.

Older AEDs were thought to increase bleeding risk in WWE and their newborns, so WWE were given vitamin K supplementation in the last month of pregnancy. The AAN guidelines found insufficient evidence to comment on this. Supplemental oral vitamin K is probably not needed during pregnancy, because all newborns routinely receive it at birth.

Given the psychological stress that comes with pregnancy, there is an increased risk of nonepileptic seizures during it. Careful history and video–EEG can help to identify these events and avoid unnecessary AED exposure. It is also important to remember that pregnant women have a nadir in blood pressure in the second trimester, putting them at risk for loss of consciousness and convulsive syncope.

## Postpartum

The postpartum period is a time of physical, emotional, and financial stress for any new mother but particularly for WWE. These concerns are not fully appreciated by many providers.

Sleep deprivation is a great concern in new mothers with epilepsy. WWE should obtain at least 8 h of sleep per day, even if somewhat disrupted, to maintain seizure control. A spouse or family member can help with child care during the night, reducing sleep disruption for the WWE. In addition, the risk of seizures when holding or caring for a newborn should be discussed.

Antiepileptic drug levels should be checked within a few weeks postpartum. Some AEDs, like lamotrigine, can rise over a few days postpartum, leading to toxicity shortly after delivery, so rapid reduction in dose postpartum is recommended. Women should be warned of symptoms of toxicity. Most AEDs will be increased throughout the pregnancy and will need postpartum reduction. Eventually, the goal is to return to the prepregnancy dose.

Breastfeeding has short-term and long-term benefits for mother and child, yet many WWE are hesitant to breastfeed because of concern about medication exposure in the child. Many factors, including family, work, and healthcare provider support, are influential in this decision.

Primidone and levetiracetam get into breast milk in potentially clinically important amounts, while valproic acid, phenobarbital, phenytoin, and carbamazepine probably do not. Gabapentin, lamotrigine, and topiramate are possibly excreted into breast milk in clinically significant amounts. It is concluded in the AAN practice parameters that "the clinical consequences for the newborn of ingesting AEDs via breast milk remain sorely underexplored and will continue to produce anxiety in WWE bearing children and all who care for these clinical dyads." Despite this lack of information, many epileptologists feel that the benefits of breastfeeding probably outweigh the risks of exposure to most AEDs.

## Bone effects

Women with epilepsy are at an increased risk of osteoporosis and fractures. While many individual medical factors contribute to one's risk for osteoporosis, adolescent girls and menopausal WWE exposed to AEDs are at the highest risk for later-life osteoporosis. Seizures themselves also lead to falls, putting the individual at increased risk of injury. AEDs themselves are associated with a two to sixfold increase in risk of fracture, presumably due to the effects of the AED on bone turnover.

The specific AEDs associated with higher bone turnover and an increased rate of fractures include carbamazepine, gabapentin, oxcarbazepine, phenytoin, and phenobarbital. The effects of the newer AEDs and some older AEDs, including valproic acid, on bone mineral density (BMD) are unclear. If a WWE is at risk for osteoporosis, then dual-energy X-ray absorptiometry (DEXA) scanning should be considered. While several treatments are used to reduce bone loss in WWE, only high-dose vitamin D has been shown to be effective. Therefore, WWE should be counseled about exercise as well as adequate vitamin D and calcium intake. If they are on an AED that induces hepatic enzymes, consideration should be given to switching to one that does not.

## Menopause

Little is known about the effect of menopause on seizure control. Menopause, defined as 1 year after the last menstrual cycle, occurs on average at an age of 50–51 in the USA. The years just before menopause (perimenopause) may be a tumultuous time due to the effects of hormonal fluctuations. While this is not clearly a time for new-onset epilepsy, there can be changes in seizure patterns. Two-thirds of WWE surveyed showed an increased seizure frequency around menopause. For women with catamenial epilepsy, there can be a seizure exacerbation around perimenopause, with subsequent improvement in seizures during and after menopause. Altered sleep patterns and vasomotor symptoms around this time may also predispose women to seizure activity.

Women with epilepsy have a higher rate of premature ovarian failure. In one study, 14% of 50 WWE had premature ovarian failure, compared to 3.7% of healthy control women. Interestingly, WWE with more seizures reported a significantly earlier age of menopause (46–47 vs 50–51). While the mechanisms for this are unknown, it suggests an effect of epilepsy, seizures, or AEDs on hypothalamic function.

Finally, it is important to note that hormone replacement therapy after menopause has been associated with an increase in seizure frequency.

## Conclusion

When treating WWE of childbearing age, choose an AED that can control seizures, does not interfere with contraception, and has a low association with fetal malformation. Pregnant women need folic acid, prenatal vitamins, frequent medication management, and careful obstetrical monitoring. Postpartum WWE should be monitored for postpartum depression and advised to get enough sleep. With proper counseling and attentive care, WWE can maintain seizure control and deliver healthy babies.

## Bibliography

Christensen J, Kjeldsen MJ, Andersen H, Friis ML, Sidenius P. Gender differences in epilepsy. *Epilepsia* 2005; **46**:956–960.

Harden CL, Koppel BS, Herzog AG, Nikolov BG, Hauser WA. Seizure frequency is associated with age at menopause in women with epilepsy. *Neurology* 2003; **61**:451–455.

Harden CL, Pennell PB, Koppel BS, et al. Management issues for women with epilepsy – focus on pregnancy (an evidence-based review): III. Vitamin K, folic acid, blood levels, and breast-feeding: Report of the Quality Standards Subcommittee and Therapeutics and Technology Assessment Subcommittee of the American Academy of Neurology and the American Epilepsy Society. *Epilepsia* 2009; **50**:1247–1255.

Hernandez-Diaz S, Smith CR, Shen A, et al. Comparative safety of antiepileptic drugs during pregnancy. *Neurology* 2012; **78**(21):1692–1699.

Klein P, Serje A, Pezzullo JC. Premature ovarian failure in women with epilepsy. *Epilepsia* 2001; **42**:1584–1589.

Meador KJ, Baker GA, Browning N, et al. Fetal antiepileptic drug exposure and cognitive outcomes at age 6 years (NEAD study): A prospective observational study. *Lancet Neurol* 2013 January; **12**(3):244–252.

# Epilepsy After Sixty

**Edward Faught**

Department of Neurology, Emory University, Atlanta, GA, USA

## Introduction

After age 60, the incidence of new-onset seizures rises steeply. Surveys in varied populations revealed incidence rates of about 100/100,000 per year at age 70 and 150/100,000 per year at age 80 (Figure 26.1). Based on nationwide Medicare diagnostic coding data, there is an incidence of 108/100,000 of new-onset seizures for patients 65 and older, translating to over 60,000 new cases per year in the USA. These figures are striking and will increase with an aging population and greater longevity. Prevalence is less than the expected accumulated incidence, suggesting that death rates among elderly patients with seizures are high. Important differences from epilepsy in younger adults are summarized in Table 26.1.

## Diagnosis

Focal seizures with altered awareness (complex partial seizures) are the most common seizure type in the elderly (Figure 26.2). Unfortunately, these brief staring spells may go unnoticed or be dismissed as inattention or forgetfulness. Automatisms become less prominent with aging, so the seizures may be manifested merely by bland staring.

Therefore, a high index of suspicion coupled with a careful eyewitness description is essential. Routine EEG is helpful if abnormal, but the yield of epileptiform abnormalities, 28%, is less than in younger adults. Continuous video–EEG monitoring either at home or in the hospital is a reasonable option, though expensive. Home cell phone video is surprisingly helpful, though seizure onset is usually missed.

Another factor that contributes to the underdiagnosis of seizures in the elderly is that the differential diagnosis is long and difficult. Included in this differential list are transient cerebral ischemia (TIA), syncope (vasovagal, orthostatic, cardiac dysrhythmia, aortic stenosis, etc.), migraine, metabolic conditions, and psychogenic events.

It is common for seizures to be misdiagnosed as TIAs. It should be noted that TIAs usually produce negative motor phenomena such as weakness. In contrast, motor phenomena during seizures, if present, are positive, as with increased tone or clonus. Transient loss of consciousness is uncommon with TIA. Transient global amnesia usually lasts much longer than does a complex partial seizure.

Syncope is heralded by premonitory symptoms followed by the loss of body tone and a quick recovery. The premonitory symptoms of light-headedness, visual change, and nausea are uncommon for seizures. Syncope may involve some clonic jerking or even a full tonic–clonic sequence—this is "convulsive syncope," not epilepsy.

*Epilepsy*, First Edition. Edited by John W. Miller and Howard P. Goodkin.
© 2014 John Wiley & Sons, Ltd. Published 2014 by John Wiley & Sons, Ltd.

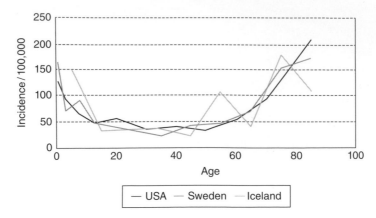

**Figure 26.1.** Incidence of unprovoked seizures in developed countries. From Cloyd J, Hauser W, Towne A, et al. Epidemiological and medical aspects of epilepsy in the elderly. *Epilepsy Res* 2006; **68**(Suppl. 1):S39–S48, with permission.

**Table 26.1.** Major features of epilepsy in older adults.

| |
|---|
| Seizures are very common; incidence increases with age over 60 |
| Cerebrovascular disease is the most likely cause |
| Complex partial seizures predominate and are difficult to diagnose |
| A first seizure is likely to recur |
| Drugs must be used at lower dosages |
| The seizures are often easy to control |

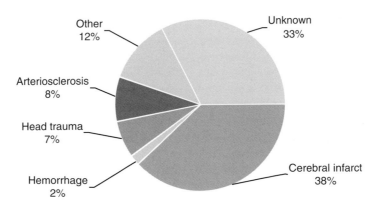

**Figure 26.2.** Etiology of seizures in patients over the age of 60 (VA Cooperative Study). From Ramsay RE, Rowan AJ, Pryor FM. Special considerations in treating the elderly patient with epilepsy. *Neurology* 2004; **62**(5 Suppl. 2):S24–S29, with permission.

## Etiology

The most common identifiable cause of new-onset seizures after age 60 is cerebrovascular disease (Figure 26.3). Embolic, hemorrhagic, large, or cortical strokes are most likely to cause seizures.

About 10% of strokes are followed by seizures, with about half occurring "early" (often defined as within 2 weeks) and half "late." This differentiation has prognostic significance and therefore influences decisions about treatment.

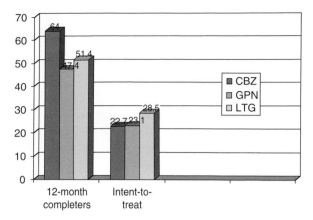

**Figure 26.3.** Percentage of patients seizure-free at 12 months, VA new-onset geriatric epilepsy study. From Rowan AJ, Ramsay RE, Collins JF, et al. New onset geriatric epilepsy: A randomized study of gabapentin, lamotrigine, and carbamazepine. *Neurology* 2005; **64**:1868–1873, with permission.

### ⚛ SCIENCE REVISITED

It is not known why certain strokes lead to seizures. In fact, the mechanisms of epileptogenesis are murky for all types of cortical lesions. Early strokes may be precipitated by compounds from blood-contacting neurons such as thrombin. Thrombin was recently shown to facilitate a "persistent" sodium current, thus keeping neurons in a slight state of depolarization. These seizures are often focal motor. Late seizures may be generated by different mechanisms, such as the effects of iron, glial proliferation, or aberrant reinnervation. These late seizures tend to be complex partial, suggesting that different brain areas may vary in terms of relative susceptibility to immediate and delayed seizure-generating factors.

Alzheimer's disease is a risk factor for seizures, with up to 10% incidence, usually late in the course. Of the metabolic causes, hyperglycemia can cause partial as well as generalized-onset seizures. Hypoglycemia more often produces syncope or other symptoms recognizable by the patient as low-sugar related. Many prescription drugs carry warnings of seizures, but in practice this association is infrequent. Occasionally bupropion, maprotiline, tramadol, theophyllines, thorazine, fluoroquinolones, or other drugs can be implicated, usually in association with large doses. Other antibiotics, neuroleptics, and antidepressants rarely cause trouble, and if indicated, they should not be withheld. Alcohol or benzodiazepine withdrawal is suspected if heavy consumption and then abstention is followed in 24–72 h by seizure.

### ✋ CAUTION!

Patients >50 or with vascular risk factors who have a first seizure should be evaluated for a stroke and be prescribed aspirin unless contraindicated.

### ✋ CAUTION!

Be skeptical of drug and environmental explanations for a seizure. Do not let your or a patient's reluctance to diagnose epilepsy interfere with judgment.

### ✋ CAUTION!

It should be noted that enzyme-inducing antiepileptic drugs (AEDs) reduce the efficacy of some statins.

Despite the multitude of insults common to the aging brain, many new-onset seizures remain unexplained (Figure 26.3). There is something unknown about the aging process that may make neurons more excitable.

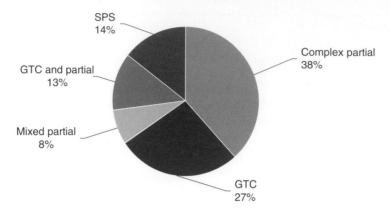

**Figure 26.4.** Frequency of seizure types in patients 60+ years old. CPS, complex partial seizure; GTCS, generalized tonic–clonic seizure; SPS, simple partial seizure. From Ramsay RE, Rowan AJ, Pryor FM. *Special considerations in treating the elderly patient with epilepsy. Neurology* 2004; **62**(5 Suppl. 2):S24–S29, with permission.

## Prognosis

Most neurologists do not treat a first seizure in an otherwise healthy child or young adult with a normal EEG, normal neuroimaging, and no history of a probable remote symptomatic cause, because the chance of recurrence is believed to be less than half. However, recurrence rates after a first seizure in the elderly may reach 70%, and many authorities recommend treatment after the first seizure. On the other hand, for "early" poststroke seizures, the recurrence rate is only 6%, compared to 48% for "late" poststroke seizures. Although treatment of early seizures may be indicated in the acute setting, there is no evidence that it prevents the later development of epilepsy. Ongoing seizures should be suspected after stroke and trauma when mental status fluctuates or is worse than expected based on lesion size; experience with continuous video–EEG monitoring indicates a high rate of subclinical seizures.

New-onset seizures in the elderly are thought to be more easily treatable than those in younger groups, with high seizure-free rates, from 60% to 75% for several common drugs as first monotherapy. In the largest controlled study, the Veterans' Administration (VA) Cooperative Study of Geriatric Epilepsy, seizure-free rates for those able to tolerate their first drug ranged from 47% to 64% at 1 year (Figure 26.4).

## The decision to treat

Both treatment and withholding of treatment may have more negative consequences in the elderly. Drug side effects are common. Only 22–28% of participants in the VA study completed a year's treatment seizure-free without stopping or changing their initial drug, mostly because of side effects (Figure 26.4). Ataxia, tremor, somnolence, and mental confusion—all common side effects—can exacerbate preexisting problems.

Not treating is also risky. Seizures cause falls, burns, fractures, head injuries, sudden death, and status epilepticus. Status epilepticus is particularly dangerous for older people, with mortality approaching one out of three. On balance, drug treatment is usually a better option than waiting for a second seizure. Exceptions are early poststroke seizures and those clearly attributable to correctible metabolic or drug-related factors.

## Treatment: Specific drugs

In the VA study, *gabapentin* and *lamotrigine* were better tolerated than *carbamazepine*, with no differences in efficacy. However, *carbamazepine timed-release* at low doses, for example, 400 mg/day, may be well tolerated by older people. These drugs cannot be started quickly. Carbamazepine and its less interacting cousin, *oxcarbazepine*, may precipitate hyponatremia, especially with concomitant diuretics. However, oxcarbazepine can be titrated to a therapeutic dose more quickly.

*Levetiracetam* can be started quickly and has no drug interactions because of almost complete renal elimination. However, sedation, fatigue, agitation, irritability, or depression may occur, and the dose is difficult to manage in cases of renal failure.

*Valproic acid* can be started quickly, causes little ataxia, and may have calming effects in agitat

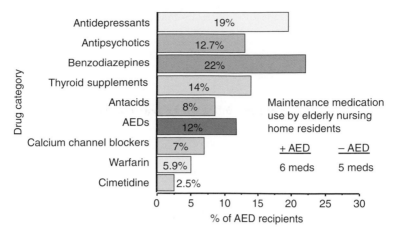

**Figure 26.5.** Comedication use in elderly nursing home residents taking AEDs. From Lackner TE, Cloyd JC, Thomas LW, Leppik IE. Antiepileptic drug use in nursing home residents: Effect of age, gender, and comedication on patterns of use. *Epilepsia* 1998; **39**:1083–1087, with permission.

**Table 26.2.** Drugs of choice for new-onset seizures in the elderly.

| Source | 1st | 2nd | 3rd |
|---|---|---|---|
| Rivlin et al. (2006) | Lamotrigine | Gabapentin | Carbamazepine XR[a] |
| Daily dose[b] | 100–150 mg | 900–1200 mg | 400 mg |
| Stephen and Brodie (2000) | Lamotrigine | Valproate | Carbamazepine XR |
| Daily dose[b] | 100 mg | 1000 mg | 400 mg |
| Author's choice (2013) | Lamotrigine | Levetiracetam | Oxcarbazepine |
| Daily dose[b] | 200 mg | 1000 mg | 600 mg |

[a]Unless bone health or interactions are an issue.
[b]Maintenance doses; initial doses should be lower.

geriatric persons. Its use may be hampered by drug interactions, as with aspirin, and it may cause bone loss (as do the enzyme-inducing drugs) and essential tremor. Valproate encephalopathy can develop subtly.

*Phenytoin* is frequently used for emergency loading, but it is a bad choice for chronic therapy. Not only does it display nonlinear kinetics, making proper dosing excruciatingly difficult, but phenytoin and other hepatic enzyme inducers (barbiturates, carbamazepine) are fraught with potentially serious drug interactions, such as with warfarin. The average older person takes five other medications (Figure 26.5).

*Topiramate* is mostly renally excreted. It is useful for concomitant migraine prophylaxis and aids weight loss. However, it may be more likely to cause cognitive side effects in the elderly.

*Lacosamide* is a renally excreted, sodium channel–blocking drug with a relatively good cognitive profile. Dizziness limits dosage.

*Pregabalin* shares a mechanism of action with gabapentin. Dosing is easier because it is absorbed more predictably and is also renally excreted. Drowsiness limits dosing.

*Ezogabine* is a renally excreted potassium channel facilitator that may be problematic in older men because it has bladder muscle-inhibiting properties. Dizziness limits dosing.

## Treatment: General principles

Suggested doses in Table 26.2 are relatively low because of the high incidence of adverse effects and because as the livers and kidneys age, they become less capable of metabolizing and excreting drugs. The overriding principle of AED treatment in the elderly is gentleness. Doses producing seizure freedom in older adults are surprisingly low (Table 26.3).

**Table 26.3.** Daily monotherapy doses in seizure-free elderly patients with newly diagnosed epilepsy.

| Antiepileptic drug | π | Median dose (mg) | Range of dose (mg) |
|---|---|---|---|
| Carbamazepine | 24 | 400 | 200–700 |
| Lamotrigine | 20 | 100 | 50–400 |
| Valproate | 20 | 800 | 300–1500 |
| Oxcarbazepine | 5 | 300 | 100–600 |
| Phenytoin | 3 | 200 | 100–600 |
| Gabapentin | 1 | 1800 | NA |

NA indicates not applicable.
From Leppik IE. Epilepsy in the elderly. *Epilepsia* 2006; **47**(Suppl. 1):S65–S70, with permission.

This principle does not apply when rapid onset of action is needed. Oral drugs that can be started quickly are levetiracetam, oxcarbazepine, valproate, and phenytoin – in that order of preference, in my opinion. Treatment of status epilepticus is another issue, and principles do not differ greatly from those for younger adults.

★ **TIPS AND TRICKS**

If the starting dose, titration rate, and initial target dose of AEDs in patients over age 65 are about *half* of those usually chosen for younger adults, tolerability will increase and there will be a good chance of seizure control.

⬡ **SCIENCE REVISITED**

Many physiological changes accompany drug disposition with aging. The major pharmacokinetic changes affecting the use of AEDs are as follows:

1. Decreased activity of hepatic cytochrome P450 and thus slower metabolism of phenytoin, phenobarbital, carbamazepine, and valproate.
2. Decreased serum albumin levels, resulting in relatively more free (unbound, active) drug. Only unbound drug crosses the blood–brain barrier. Thus, stronger neurological effects, wanted and unwanted, ensue for highly protein-bound drugs such as phenytoin and valproate. It may be useful to measure unbound (free) serum levels for these drugs.

3. Decreased creatinine clearance and thus slower excretion of levetiracetam, topiramate, gabapentin, pregabalin, lacosamide, and ezogabine.
4. Minor loss of activity of hepatic glucuronidation, so that lamotrigine metabolism decreases little with age.

**Choice of therapeutic program**

Initial drug choice and sequence are still largely a matter of physician preference. Factors to be considered include cost, concomitant drugs, weight effects, gait stability, comorbidities, and ease of use. Seizure type is a lesser issue, since nearly all seizures in the elderly are either focal onset or generalized tonic–clonic. One size does not fit all, but Table 26.4 lists a suggested order of preference for chronic oral therapy of epilepsy in patients over age 65.

✋ **CAUTION!**

Do not choose a drug that may worsen a preexisting problem: no valproate with essential tremor or obesity, no topiramate with aphasia, no phenytoin with ataxia, and no levetiracetam with aggressive behavior.

Monitoring therapeutic efficacy requires vigilance by family or others, since complex partial seizures in particular often go unrecognized by the patient. An accurate seizure count using a calendar is essential. The effect of dose changes takes time to evaluate; statistically at least five times the average interseizure interv

**Table 26.4.** Chronic oral therapy of epilepsy in patients over age 65.

| Good choices | Lamotrigine | Levetiracetam | Oxcarbazepine | Valproate | Gabapentin |
|---|---|---|---|---|---|
| Less good choices | Carbamazepine | Topiramate | Phenytoin | Phenobarbital | |
| Insufficient data | Pregabalin | Lacosamide | Ezogabine | | |

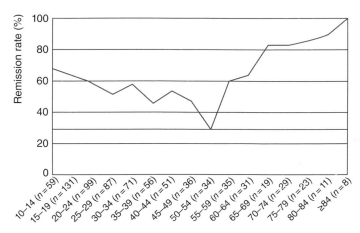

Age (years) and cohort size

**Figure 26.6.** Remission rate as function of age. From Brodie MJ, Kwan P. Epilepsy in elderly people. *BMJ* 2005; **331**: 1317–1322, with permission.

is necessary to conclude that there has been at least a 20% improvement. Serum levels may be helpful. "Standard" dosing can cause unexpectedly high levels. Levels are imperfect in assessing adherence but are one tool. Other aids to adherence, especially weekly pill trays, cannot be overemphasized.

How long should patients be treated? Those with early poststroke seizures may reasonably be tapered off drug after the acute phase of illness has resolved, especially if the EEG is not epileptiform. Whether this should be after 1 week, 6 months, or some other interval is unproven. For other patient groups, lifelong therapy is probably in store. Recurrence rates are high in this age group if therapy is stopped (Figure 26.6).

## Conclusion

Seizures in older adults are common, must be looked for actively, and can be treated effectively, and relatively low doses of medications work well. Better drugs are those without interactions and without side effects likely to exacerbate common

problems. Cerebrovascular disease is a frequent etiology, but the cause is often undiscoverable. Onset of seizures in late life can be socially and psychologically devastating because of the associated loss of independence, and they are at least as dangerous for the elderly as for younger adults. For these reasons, complete seizure control is just as important as it is for a person of any age.

## Bibliography

Berg AT. Epilepsy in the elderly is common, but where does it go? *Neurology* 2012; **78**:444–445.

Brodie MJ, Kwan P. Epilepsy in elderly people. *BMJ* 2005; **331**:1317–1322.

Brodie MJ, Elder T, Kwan P. Epilepsy in later life. *Lancet Neurol* 2009; **8**:1019–1030.

Cloyd J, Hauser W, Towne A, et al. Epidemiological and medical aspects of epilepsy in the elderly. *Epilepsy Res* 2006; **68**(Suppl. 1):S39–S48.

Faught E, Richman J, Martin R, et al. Incidence and prevalence of epilepsy among older US Medicare beneficiaries. *Neurology* 2012; **78**:448–453.

Isaeva E, Hernan A, Isaev D, Holmes GL. Thrombin facilitates seizures through activation of persistent sodium current. *Ann Neurol* 2012; **72**:192–198.

Lackner TE, Cloyd JC, Thomas LW, Leppik IE. Antiepileptic drug use in nursing home residents: Effect of age, gender, and comedication on patterns of use. *Epilepsia* 1998; **39**:1083–1087.

Lambrakis CC, Lancman ME. The phenomenology of seizures after stroke. *J Epilepsy* 1998; **11**:233–240.

Leppik IE. Epilepsy in the elderly. *Epilepsia* 2006; **47**(Suppl. 1):S65–S70.

Mendez MF, Lim GTH. Seizures in elderly patients with dementia. *Neurology* 2003; **20**(11):791–803.

Ramsay RE, Rowan AJ, Pryor FM. Special considerations in treating the elderly patient with epilepsy. *Neurology* 2004; **62**(5 Suppl. 2):S24–S29.

Rivlin P, Montavont A, Nighoghossian N. Optimizing therapy of seizures in stroke patients. *Neurology* 2006; **67**(Suppl. 4):S3–S9.

Rowan AJ, Ramsay RE, Collins JF, et al. New onset geriatric epilepsy: A randomized study of gabapentin, lamotrigine, and carbamazepine. *Neurology* 2005; **64**:1868–1873.

Stephen LJ, Brodie MJ. Epilepsy in elderly people. *Lancet* 2000; **355**(9213):1441–1446.

Stephen LJ, Brodie. *Special problems: Adults and elderly. Epilepsia* 2008; **49**(Suppl. 1):45–49.

Part VI

# What Can Be Done When Medication Doesn't Work?

# When Should Epilepsy Neurosurgery Be Considered, and What Can It Accomplish?

**Paul A. Garcia**

Clinical Epilepsy Services, Department of Neurology, University of California San Francisco, San Francisco, CA, USA

A substantial minority of people with epilepsy continue to have seizures despite appropriate medical management. Although surgical techniques have been shown to reduce or eliminate seizures in this circumstance, epilepsy surgery remains underutilized, with only a small fraction of potential candidates referred to comprehensive epilepsy surgery programs. Because surgery for these patients often provides the only realistic possibility for seizure control, it is important that practitioners identify and refer these patients. Recognizing a surgical candidate requires knowing when further medication changes are not likely to be beneficial. It also requires an understanding of the various types of surgical treatment available as well as the expected risks and benefits of these treatments.

## When are medication changes unlikely to bring seizures under control?

Pivotal, community-based studies demonstrate that half of all people with newly diagnosed epilepsy will be seizure-free with their initial anticonvulsant treatment. Of those who continue having seizures, only 10% come under complete control with the next medicine. Even after treatment with multiple medications or combinations of medicines, roughly a third of patients will continue to have at least some seizures.

From these findings, we can reasonably infer that medication trials quickly reach a point of diminishing returns, at least for the prospect of eliminating seizures. Does this mean that it is futile to try new medicines when initial trials have failed? No, a small number of patients with uncontrolled epilepsy (approximately 4% per year) achieve a 6-month or greater seizure remission with ongoing medical trials. Furthermore, additional patients will have their seizure control improved, so we should not "give up" on medical treatments. However, the low chance for seizure freedom when initial anticonvulsant trials have not been effective should serve as a "red flag," indicating that a patient is unlikely to gain seizure control except through seizure surgery.

> **☝ CAUTION!**
>
> Persistence of seizures after a second adequate anticonvulsant trial should serve as a "red flag," indicating that medications alone are unlikely to provide complete seizure control.

*Epilepsy*, First Edition. Edited by John W. Miller and Howard P. Goodkin.
© 2014 John Wiley & Sons, Ltd. Published 2014 by John Wiley & Sons, Ltd.

## What constitutes "seizure control"? Is it ok if my patient still has some seizures?

For the most part, even occasional seizures are associated with significant risks and a profound impact on quality of life. In the USA, this negative effect is best illustrated by driving. Patients experiencing just a few "breakthrough" seizures each year are not allowed to drive. Except for people living in certain metropolitan areas, this loss may limit employment, educational, and social opportunities. In fact, the lives of people with "nearly complete" seizure control often resemble those of people with poor control more closely than those of people with complete control.

Nevertheless, seizures vary widely in physical manifestations and predictability, and these factors can mitigate the impact of seizures on a patient's life. For example, focal seizures that do not result in a loss of consciousness or motor control don't expose the person to a risk for accidents, and they usually don't interfere with driving or working. Most patients and their physicians don't consider surgery in this circumstance. An intermediate situation would be seizures occurring exclusively during sleep. The predictability allows patients to go about their daily activities (including working and driving) without fear of having a seizure. However, the ongoing nocturnal seizures still pose significant physical risks. While patients may not feel that the seizures are impacting their lives, they must be reminded that surgery can reduce the morbidity and mortality related to the ongoing seizures. Finally, seizures with prolonged premonitory symptoms may allow patients to get to safety, preventing accidents and injuries. When the pattern is consistent, people are sometimes allowed to drive. Although prolonged auras may lessen the impact of seizures, they don't stop seizures from occurring during important daily activities. Thus, they should rarely be a consideration in whether to refer a patient for surgery.

## Should my patient be referred for seizure surgery now? A bottom line

Over a decade has passed since a randomized trial of anterior temporal lobectomy (the most common resective surgery) highlighted the dramatically enhanced chance of seizure freedom in patients who undergo surgery over those those relying on medication alone. More recent studies suggest that successful epilepsy surgery results in prolonged life span, improved quality of life, and lower medical costs. Surprisingly, these findings have not led to increased utilization of seizure surgery. The reasons are not clear. Societal and healthcare system issues appear to play a role; patients are increasingly managed in regional centers (with lower surgical volumes and higher complication rates) rather than referral centers focused on surgical management. Also, surgery is less likely to be performed for ethnic minorities and those with Medicaid insurance, suggesting that economic barriers to surgery play a role.

While societal constraints and healthcare system issues contribute to surgical underutilization, physician and patient perceptions also affect the use of seizure surgery. Despite overwhelming evidence of surgical efficacy and strong recommendations from professional societies, many neurologists do not refer patients for epilepsy surgery. In response to the concern that many good candidates for surgery are not being referred, a panel of experts developed an online tool for identifying candidates for seizure surgery. This panel of epileptologists, neurosurgeons, and general neurologists reviewed thousands of clinical scenarios, reaching general agreement about surgical candidacy for patients who had tried appropriate medicines with incomplete control of disabling seizures.

> ☆ **TIPS AND TRICKS**
>
> Refer patients for surgical evaluation if (1) the underlying pathology otherwise requires surgical treatment (vascular malformations or tumors), (2) if seizures persist despite treatment with two or more medicines, and (3) if unsure whether your patient should be referred; an online tool for patients 12 years of age and older can be found at http://www.epilepsycases.com/.

## How will my patient be evaluated?

Video–EEG monitoring remains the cornerstone of the presurgical evaluation, serving several purposes. First, it eliminates the possibility that medication trials failed due to "mistaken identity." Seizure mimics such as syncope, parasomnias, and psychogenic nonepileptic events are a common finding on the epilepsy monitoring unit. They sometimes surprise us, especially in patients with coexistent well-controlled epilepsy. Second, video–EEG monitoring determines whether seizures begin from a single focus, from multiple foci, or diffusely. Often, prior evaluations have hinted at this outcome, but recordings obtained during the seizures are the "gold standard" for defining seizure physiology. Third, the recordings may be sufficient to localize the seizure onset zone, helping to define a "target" for resective surgery.

Referring physicians should ensure that prior studies are included with the referral packet, as these anatomic (MRI) and physiologic (EEG) data help to guide the video–EEG evaluation. For example, patients with a focal lesion on MRI may not need extensive video–EEG recording to "prove" that their seizures arise near the lesion. Conversely, a patient with an EEG showing independent spike discharges from the left and right temporal lobe may require more extensive monitoring before one can be confident that resection of a single focus will be of benefit.

Over the last two decades, high-resolution anatomic imaging with MRI has become a mainstay of the presurgical evaluation for patients who are candidates to undergo resection of the seizure focus. Even when a patient's initial MRI obtained at the time of diagnosis fails to reveal an abnormality, high-resolution scans often demonstrate subtle localizing abnormalities such as mesial temporal sclerosis or focal cortical dysplasia. In addition to refining the seizure localization, MRI often indicates the underlying pathology, hence the prognosis for complete seizure control after surgery.

When MRI fails to demonstrate a structural "target," nuclear medicine studies such as positron emission tomography (PET) and single-photon emission computed tomography (SPECT) may provide localizing information to confirm or refine the video–EEG localization. Both are low-resolution, functional studies that provide little anatomic information. SPECT measures blood flow at the time of injection (typically increased during a seizure) and thus is most useful when the radioisotope is injected at the onset of the seizure. 18-Fluorodeoxyglucose is the most commonly used PET tracer; it measures glucose uptake indicating tissue metabolism, which is typically reduced in the seizure focus (except during seizures), so PET should not be performed in the peri-ictal period. Functional and anatomic studies can be combined by co-registering (superimposing) MRI scans and physiological studies including EEG, magnetoencephalogram (MEG), or nuclear medicine studies. The combined information draws on the advantages of both modalities and can be especially useful in mapping out a surgical plan, especially in complex cases.

Neuropsychological studies remain critical in formulating a surgical plan. The Wada (intracarotid amobarbital) test is the conventional test for lateralizing language function. Many centers now use functional MRI for this purpose, and further evolution towards noninvasive studies seems likely. A full cognitive battery is administered before surgery and repeated at a defined time (usually a year) after surgery. This ensures that patients who undergo surgery can be counseled on subtle new deficits whether or not they recognize a problem.

Precise seizure focus localization and implementation of the final surgical plan requires the best possible EEG recordings. Sometimes this information can be obtained only by directly evaluating cortical tissue. Cortical EEG recording, known as electrocorticography (ECoG), is used to hone the surgical plan. ECoG can be performed during the operation or extraoperatively over the course of days to weeks. Following characterization of the seizure focus, the final surgical plan is implemented, balancing the need for eliminating seizure-producing tissue with the risk for affecting functional tissue identified by classical anatomy, electrical stimulation mapping, or both (Figure 27.1).

## What are the surgical options and expected outcomes?

### Resective surgery

When seizures can't be controlled with medicine, excision of seizure-producing tissue provides the best chance for gaining seizure control. These excisions range from simple removal of a focal lesion such as cavernous malformation to removal of all cerebral cortex of the hemisphere such as that performed during an anatomic hemispherectomy in patients with Rasmussen's syndrome. Despite considerable variation in technique and patient population, surgical series have consistently shown that most patients undergoing focal resections benefit from surgery. The prognosis for complete seizure control is largely based on the underlying pathology; patients with discrete lesions such as cavernous malformations or hippocampal sclerosis have an 80–90% chance that their seizures will be completely controlled 2 years after surgery. Patients with more diffuse pathologies such as cortical dysplasia are less likely to gain complete control. Nevertheless, experienced centers have developed strategies that provide complete seizure control for most patients undergoing surgery

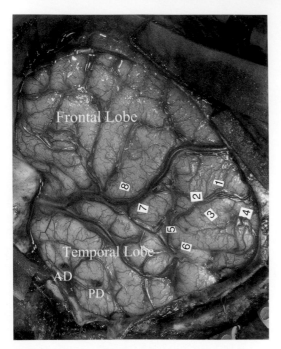

**Figure 27.1.** Intraoperative photograph showing a left hemispheric functional map in a young man with nonlesional temporal lobe epilepsy. Electrical stimulation mapping revealed sensory or motor responses at sites 1–4 and speech arrests at sites 5–8. ECoG revealed continuous epileptiform activity from anterior (AD) and posterior (PD) depth electrodes inserted through the middle temporal gyrus into the amygdala and hippocampus, respectively. Documentation of a medial temporal seizure focus along with a lack of anterior temporal language sites allowed for a successful, tailored anterior-medial temporal resection.

for cortical dysplasia. As expected, long-term outcomes reported using life table analyses are less favorable than those in which only the prior year or two are considered. Taken together, long-term follow-up studies indicate that roughly half of all patients who undergo an anterior temporal lobectomy stop having seizures altogether, while many others experience many seizure-free years after surgery, even if they have occasional relapses.

Patients whose seizures are caused by progressive or "unstable" lesions deserve special consideration. Specifically, surgical intervention for tumors or arteriovenous malformations may serve dual purposes of treating the underlying condition as well as improving seizure control. Standard neurosurgical

treatment focused exclusively on the lesion often improves seizure control in this situation. However, treatment at an epilepsy surgery program may provide an even better chance of seizure control, as epileptogenic cortex sometimes extends beyond the obvious structural abnormality.

While most patients undergoing seizure surgery benefit from the operation, the possibility of negative surgical outcomes must be considered in the decision-making process. The risk for complications depends upon many factors including the location of the seizure focus, the need for chronic intracranial EEG recordings, the patient's general medical condition, and the experience of the surgical team. Nationwide, perioperative mortality is less than one per thousand cases. Furthermore, seizure surgery is associated with a low (1%) risk for neurological complication (including stroke) at high-volume epilepsy surgery programs, though the risk is higher (4%) where less surgery is performed. Approximately 6% of patients (roughly double this number at low-volume centers) will have at least one complication such as local infection, venous thrombosis, or pulmonary embolism. Finally, we recognize that there are can be subtle cognitive changes that are often difficult for patients to appreciate. For example, a third of patients who undergo dominant anterior temporal resection will have measurable decrements in verbal list learning and naming tasks. The impact of these subtle changes (that typically go unnoticed by patients) is unclear because these patients often improve on other cognitive measures, exhibiting little change in day-to-day functioning.

As most of the expected complications from surgery are modest, reversible, or rare, it seems clear that the most common "bad outcome" from surgery is incomplete seizure control. In counseling candidates for surgery, it is often helpful to reiterate this for two reasons: it is reassuring that the most likely negative outcome is "no significant change from baseline," and it reinforces the ongoing risk of seizures in the present circumstance.

### Palliative operations

Vagus nerve stimulation (VNS) reduces seizure frequency and severity and will be described extensively in the following chapter. Since it is effective regardless of the epilepsy syndrome, patients who are not candidates for resection, including those with multifocal and generalized epilepsy, ma benefit. Though randomized controlled trials have demonstrated that VNS reduces seizure frequency, the efficacy is roughly comparable to that reported in trials with new anticonvulsants; that is, patients have roughly a 50% chance that their seizures will be reduced by half during the initial months of treatment. Treatment is not expected to render the patient seizure-free. Thus, this treatment will not have the impact on seizure-related morbidity and mortality anticipated with resective surgery.

While the most important reason to avoid VNS in candidates for resective surgery is that it consigns patients to ongoing seizures, it should also be noted that it may interfere with ongoing neurological management and future evaluation for resective surgery. Specifically, it limits subsequent MRI studies for the patient. The leads are designed for use with an MRI head coil, so it is still possible for patients to have head MRI scans after the device is implanted. Body MRI should not be performed for VNS patients, however. Furthermore, if the device is removed due to infection, lead breakage, or patient preference, the FDA and manufacturer recommend that no MRI scans (head or body) be performed due to the risk for heating of the lead remnants (the leads can rarely be removed completely from where they are wrapped around the nerve). Thus, serious deliberation is warranted before implanting VNS in patients who are likely to require brain MRI surveillance, including those with tumors or vascular malformations. Patients who may someday wish to have resective surgery should recognize that implantation of VNS may interfere with MRI and MEG studies required for optimal surgical planning. Finally, patients with medical conditions requiring body MRI should not have VNS.

### ☞ CAUTION!

Vagus nerve stimulation may limit optimal presurgical testing in patients who later decide to pursue resective surgery.

Corpus callosotomy involves sectioning part or all of the corpus callosum, the largest white matter structure connecting the hemispheres. In contrast to VNS, callosotomy has only one clear indication: palliation of generalized tonic or atonic seizures. These seizures result in sudden, devastating falls and consequent injuries. Patients with these seizures are often wheelchair bound as a precaution for their seizures, though they are fully capable of walking. Though there are variations on the approach, all involve a standard craniotomy.

Callosotomy series consistently demonstrate outstanding results in reducing or eliminating tonic and atonic seizures. Other seizures types are sometimes improved, though less consistently. Though patients continue to have seizures after surgery, control of the "drop attacks" often allows them to ambulate safely without wearing helmets.

Cortical disconnection syndromes have been reported after callosotomy. The risk is clearly highest in high-functioning patients. Patients who have prominent cognitive dysfunction seem to have a very low risk for this complication. Callosotomy should be considered when patients have significant disability or risk related to tonic or atonic seizures as well as prominent cognitive disability.

## What should my patient expect after seizure surgery?

In the days and weeks after surgery, patients may be discouraged by ongoing seizures or unexpected neurological complications. While seizures occurring during this time are a poor prognostic factor for complete seizure control, many patients will stop having seizures as postoperative inflammation and edema remit; others will be able to achieve seizure freedom with straightforward medication changes. Thus, patients should be encouraged to remain positive about their ongoing management. Similarly, postoperative neurological symptoms such as weakness or dysphasia typically remit as the perioperative cortical changes resolve. If symptoms persist longer than expected, referral for therapy may be helpful.

While studies consistently show that surgery leads to improved quality of life, the effect is modest compared to the effect on seizure control. Studies showing the greatest change typically look over a longer course as many chronic problems are not immediately improved when seizures abate. For example, patients who have been unemployed for years may require retraining or further education before entering the workforce, if they are able to do so at all. We typically counsel patients that surgery is an effective means of gaining seizure control but that a more holistic approach is necessary to address the effects of chronic seizures on their lives. Perhaps the strongest argument to be made for early identification of surgery candidates is the observation that surgery, though potentially life prolonging, is sometimes "too little, too late" for life quality measures.

Problems with mood and adjustment are common after surgery. Though it is more common for surgery to improve mood than worsen it, many patients remain depressed after surgery, and a small number develop depression for the first time. Though one might expect that postoperative mood status would be strongly related toseizure outcome, patients with both successful and unsuccessful surgeries can experience mood disorders. Depression should be aggressively treated as it is highly correlated with quality of life and patient perception of functional outcome.

Patients who gain seizure control are interested in knowing whether they can stop taking anticonvulsant medications. As might be expected in a group that has only gained seizure control through surgery, many are reluctant to risk medication withdrawal; therefore, randomized trials of medication discontinuation are limited. It seems that 50–80% of seizure-free patients who attempt to come off of medication are able to do so without seizures, though the number may be lower for patients who have diffuse pathologies such as cortical dysplasia. Most (but not all) who experience a seizure regain seizure control when the medication is restarted. Since many patients will require medication or will choose to continue anticonvulsants after surgery, surgery should be considered an effective means of achieving seizure control rather than a "cure." Given the risks associated with medication withdrawal, patient-specific factors often prove most decisive in the decision to taper medicines. Women planning a pregnancy will often try to come off of medicine. Parents will often choose to have their children come off of medicine to reduce the effect of medicine on learning. Finally, patients who have long been tolerating medication side effects are often eager to try tapering medicine.

## Conclusion

Epilepsy neurosurgery, while underutilized, often provides the best chance of seizure control when medicines aren't completely stopping seizures. Early recognition of patients with refractory epilepsy is now possible. Prompt referral of patients with refractory seizures for inpatient video–EEG monitoring allows for development of an individualized treatment plan and, if appropriate, surgery. The presurgical evaluation is aimed at minimizing surgical risks and maximizing the chance for a good outcome as successful epilepsy surgery can lead to longer, happier lives for many people with epilepsy.

## Bibliography

Choi H, Sell RL, Lenert L, et al. Epilepsy surgery for pharmacoresistant temporal lobe epilepsy: A decision analysis. *JAMA* 2008 December 3; **300**(21):2497–2505.

Engel J Jr., McDermott MP, Wiebe S, et al. Early surgical therapy for drug-resistant temporal lobe epilepsy: A randomized trial. *JAMA* 2012 March 7; **307**(9):922–930.

Englot DJ, Ouyang D, Garcia PA, Barbaro NM, Chang EF. Epilepsy surgery trends in the United States, 1990–2008. *Neurology* 2012 April 17; **78**(16): 1200–1206.

Englot DJ, Ouyang D, Wang DD, Rolston JD, Garcia PA, Chang EF. Relationship between hospital surgical volume, lobectomy rates, and adverse perioperative events at U.S. epilepsy centers. *J Neurosurg* 2013; **118**(1):169–174.

Jette N, Quan H, Tellez-Zenteno JF, et al. Development of an online tool to determine appropriateness for an epilepsy surgery evaluation. *Neurology* 2012 September 11; **79**(11):1084–1093.

Kwan P, Brodie MJ. Early identification of refractory epilepsy. *N Engl J Med* 2000 February 3; **342**(5):314–319.

McIntosh AM, Kalnins RM, Mitchell LA, Fabinyi GC, Briellmann RS, Berkovic SF. Temporal lobectomy: Long-term seizure outcome, late recurrence and risks for seizure recurrence. *Brain* 2004 September; **127**(Pt 9):2018–2030.

Park KI, Lee SK, Chu K, et al. Withdrawal of antiepileptic drugs after neocortical epilepsy surgery. *Ann Neurol* 2010 February; **67**(2):230–238.

de Tisi J, Bell GS, Peacock JL, et al. The long-term outcome of adult epilepsy surgery, patterns of seizure remission, and relapse: A cohort study. *Lancet* 2011 October 15; **378**(9800):1388–1395.

Wiebe S, Blume WT, Girvin JP, Eliasziw M, Effectiveness and Efficiency of Surgery for Temporal Lobe Epilepsy Study Group. A randomized, controlled trial of surgery for temporal-lobe epilepsy. *N Engl J Med* 2001 August 2; **345**(5):311–318.

# When Should Vagus Nerve Stimulation Be Considered, and What Can It Accomplish?

**Pearce J. Korb and Sandra L. Helmers**

Department of Neurology, Emory University School of Medicine, Atlanta, GA, USA

## Introduction

Approximately 70% of people with epilepsy can be successfully treated with one or two antiepileptic agents, but the remaining 20–30% have recurrent seizures and are considered refractory to medications. Although a proportion of these patients are resective epilepsy surgery candidates, many are not. It is this group of patients who may benefit from vagus nerve stimulation (VNS). VNS uses an implantable neuromodulatory device as adjunctive therapy for refractory epilepsy. The device (developed by Cyberonics in Houston, Texas) consists of a small, programmable pulse generator that is placed subcutaneously in the left upper thoracic area and connected by a bipolar lead to the left cervical vagus nerve trunk. The implanted generator delivers intermittent electrical stimulation or pulses to the left vagus nerve at programmed intervals and intensities. Additionally, it can be activated by a magnet that can be used by the patient or family member at the onset of a seizure to help stop or alter the seizure's natural course. This chapter describes who should be considered for VNS therapy and discusses its effectiveness, technical considerations, and common adverse reactions.

> ### ⚗ SCIENCE REVISITED
>
> The exact mechanism of seizure reduction is not known. A current hypothesis is that stimulation alters synaptic transmission in several thalamic and brainstem nuclei (e.g., nucleus tractus solitarius, locus coeruleus), leading to desynchronization of thalamocortical connections.

## Patient selection

Vagus nerve stimulation is an adjunctive treatment for patients with medically refractory epilepsy who are not resective surgery candidates. Therefore, patients with epilepsy who have failed adequate trials of several antiepileptic drugs (AEDs) should be considered for nonpharmacological therapies such as VNS – Chapter 14 suggests failure of five or six AEDs as the criterion. The evaluation to determine the appropriateness of VNS should consist of EEG, MRI, and in many cases long-term video–EEG monitoring. The goal of this evaluation is to ensure that the patient is not an appropriate candidate for epilepsy surgery.

Vagus nerve stimulation was initially approved in the USA by the FDA in 1997 for use in medically refractory *focal* onset (localization-related) epilepsy in people 12 years and older. However, it should also be considered in the treatment of refractory *generalized* epilepsies. In Lennox–Gastaut syndrome (LGS) and other symptomatic generalized epilepsies, seizure frequency is reduced by more than 50% in about half of the patients. The most dramatic reduction is with generalized tonic–clonic (GTC) and absence seizures. Although there is evidence, albeit from smaller studies, for a similar reduction in seizure frequency for patients with primary or idiopathic generalized epilepsies, VNS for these patients is not universally accepted. Additionally, patients who have undergone epilepsy surgery and have failed to obtain adequate response can be considered for VNS therapy.

In addition to the effectiveness of VNS for the broad spectrum of epilepsies, there is evidence for its effectiveness in the pediatric population younger than 12 years. Evidence shows significant seizure reduction in pediatric epilepsy populations equal to and in some cases better than reduction in the adult epilepsy population. In summary, many patients with refractory epilepsy who either are not good epilepsy surgery candidates or have failed epilepsy surgery can be considered for VNS implantation.

---

### ★ TIPS AND TRICKS

Because VNS therapy rarely makes patients seizure-free, it should not be considered in patients who are candidates for resective epilepsy surgery (Chapter 27).

---

## Effectiveness of VNS

Seizure freedom after placement of a VNS is rare (<10%). Almost all patients in whom a VNS is implanted still require continued AEDs to maintain seizure reduction. VNS typically produces a significant (>50%) reduction in seizure frequency for 20–65% of patients. At least 20–25% of patients will have little change in seizures. Other benefits reported with VNS in some patients include a decrease in seizure severity or in the duration of the postictal period. There is also potential for reduction in other severe epilepsy-related clinical events including convulsive status epilepticus, fractures, and traumatic head injuries.

The secondary benefits of VNS that have been shown to occur independent of seizure frequency reduction include a positive effect on mood and improved quality of life.

## Device and implantation

The device is titanium encased and small (about 4 cm across), comparable in size to a silver dollar or pocket watch. It includes the pulse generator and a lithium battery. There is an attached lead wire with a flexible spiral end that encircles the left cervical vagus nerve (Figure 28.1).

The surgery is performed under local or general anesthesia. The wires are connected to the left vagus trunk due to concern of the possibility of bradycardia with stimulation of the right vagus nerve. Usually two small incisions are made in the left neck and left upper chest area. The device is implanted superficially below the clavicle, and the tethering or coiling of the electrode around the left vagus nerve trunk is done via the neck incision. The operative time is about 60–90 min. Usually, patients will be discharged on the same day; however, some patients may be kept overnight for observation. Surgical complications such as infection (<~1.6%) are rare. One possible complication is vocal cord paresis or paralysis from temporary or permanent injury during surgery of the recurrent laryngeal nerve, a branch of the left vagus. If this untoward event is noted in the immediate postoperative period, the patient should be reassured that permanent paralysis is unusual (<0.2% of cases) and that the condition is likely to improve with time.

## Technical considerations

The VNS system consists of a handheld "wand" connected to a portable display device that can be made to interface with the generator simply by holding the interrogating "wand" over the left chest where the generator is implanted. The system can be turned on in the operating room immediately after the surgery or during the immediate postoperative office checkup. The display device has software for the detection and manipulation of the stimulation parameters. There are several stimulation parameters, five of which can be set and modified by a practitioner (usually a neurologist or supervised nurse practitioner or physician's assistant) during routine office visits to optimize activation of the

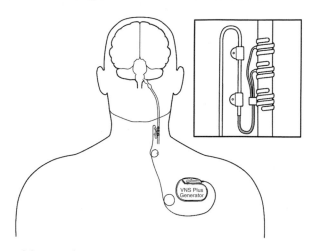

**Figure 28.1.** Schematic of the impulse generator placed in the superficial left infraclavicular chest with bipolar leads that terminate in spirals around the cervical trunk of the left vagus nerve in the neck. The pulse generator can be palpated and the programming wand placed over the area to interrogate the device. Figure modified from original drawing provided by Cyberonics, Inc., with permission.

**Table 28.1.** Overview of VNS stimulation parameters.

| Stimulation parameter | Description | Starting level | Range | Common increment | Usual range |
|---|---|---|---|---|---|
| *Normal mode* | | | | | |
| Amplitude/output current | Changes current in a single pulse | 0.25 mA | 0–3.50 mA | 0.25 mA | 0.75–2.0 |
| Pulse width | Changes duration of single pulse | 500 μs | 130–1000 μs | 250 μs | 250–500 ms |
| Signal frequency | Changes frequency of pulses | 30 Hz | 20–30 Hz (1–145 Hz) | Variable | 20–30 Hz |
| Signal ON time | Changes duration of the stimulation | 30 s | 7–270 s | Variable | 21–30 s |
| Signal OFF time | Changes duration of time between stimulations | 5 min | 0.2–180 min | 5 min (5–60); 30 min (60–180) | 1.1–5.0 min |
| *Magnet activation mode* | | | | | |
| Amplitude/output current | Changes current in a single pulse | 0.50 mA | 0–3.50 mA | 0.25 mA | 1–2.25 mA |
| Pulse width | Changes duration of single pulse | 500 μs | 130–1000 μs | 250 μs | 250–500 ms |
| Signal ON time | Changes duration of the stimulation | 30 s | 7–270 s | Variable | 21–30 s |

vagus nerve. The most common settings that are adjusted are the stimulation amplitude, signal frequency, pulse width, and signal ON and OFF times (duty cycle) (see Table 28.1).

Reprogramming of the parameters is done to increase effectiveness of nerve activation and to minimize stimulation-related side effects. The amplitude or current output is commonly adjusted by

0.25 mA in a stepwise fashion at intervals of 2–4 weeks up to approximately 1.5–2 mA to fully activate the vagus nerve. The pulse width, which is the duration of the individual pulses in a stimulation, also affects activation of the vagus nerve, with 250–500 µs recommended. The effects of changing the signal frequency are less understood, but the standard settings are 20–30 Hz. *Duty cycle* refers to the relative time the stimulation is on (signal ON time) and the time between the stimulations (signal OFF time). The signal ON time is usually set to 30 s but can be adjusted from 7 to 270 s. The signal OFF time is usually 5 min but can be adjusted from 0.2 to 180 min. Decreasing the pulse width to 250 µs or the frequency to 20–25 Hz can reduce many stimulation-induced adverse effects. As a last resort, one can lower the output current if the side effects persist.

### ✋ CAUTION!

To minimize the possibility of injury to the nerve, the VNS duty cycle (defined as signal ON time/(signal ON time + signal OFF time) should be set at less than 50%.

The current output, frequency, pulse width, and ON time are set separately for magnet-activated "on demand" stimulation. The magnet activation is used to abort or alter seizures. Patients, caregivers, and families should be counseled on its proper use.

## Complications and adverse effects

The most common adverse effects of VNS are dysphonia, coughing, and hoarseness during stimulation ON time. Other reported stimulation-related side effects include dyspnea and pharyngeal paresthesias. Although cardiac arrhythmias are much more associated with stimulation of the right vagus nerve, some reversible bradyarrhythmias have been reported in the operating room. Most side effects reported are tolerable and lessen over time.

### ★ TIPS AND TRICKS

Side effects are usually attenuated or eliminated with changes to the stimulation parameter settings, particularly pulse width or frequency.

The most common but infrequent complications associated with VNS implantation are infection around the lead or generator sites and vocal cord paresis or paralysis. Infection occurs in less than 2% of patients, usually with resolution with antibiotics. The system will rarely need to be removed.

## Conclusions

Vagus nerve stimulation therapy is an effective adjunctive treatment to improve seizure control in people with refractory epilepsy. The implantation is a minor procedure with very infrequent complications and minimal side effects. In addition to improved seizure control, improvement in quality of life can be seen. VNS rarely produces seizure freedom. It is a consideration when multiple AEDs have failed to control seizures and resective epilepsy surgery is not an option.

## Bibliography

Ardesch JJ, Buschman HPJ, Wagener-Schimmel LJJC, van der Aa HE, Hageman G. Vagus nerve stimulation for medically refractory epilepsy: A long-term follow-up study. *Seizure* 2007; **16**:579–585.

Ben-Menachem E, Hellström K, Waldton C, Augustinsson LE. Evaluation of refractory epilepsy treated with vagus nerve stimulation for up to 5 years. *Neurology* 1999; **52**:1265–1267.

DeGiorgio CM, Schachter SC, Handforth A, et al. Prospective long-term study of vagus nerve stimulation for the treatment of refractory seizures. *Epilepsia* 2000 September; **41**(9):1195–1200.

DeGiorgio CM, Thompson J, Lewis P, et al. Vagus nerve stimulation: Analysis of device parameters in 154 patients during the long-term XE5 study. *Epilepsia* 2001 August; **42**(8):1017–1120.

Elliott RE, Rodgers SD, Bassani L, et al. Vagus nerve stimulation for children with treatment-resistant epilepsy: A consecutive series of 141 cases. *J Neurosurg Pediatr* 2011; **7**:491–500.

Englot DJ, Chang EF, Auguste KI. Vagus nerve stimulation for epilepsy: A meta-analysis of efficacy and predictors of response. Review. *J Neurosurg* 2011 December; **115**(6):1248–1255.

Handforth A, DeGiorgio CM, Schachter SC, et al. Vagus nerve stimulation therapy for partial-onset seizures: A randomized active-control trial. *Neurology* 1998; **51**:48–55.

Helmers SL, Wheless JW, Frost M, et al. Vagus nerve stimulation therapy in pediatric patients with refractory epilepsy: Retrospective study. *J Child Neurol* 2001 November; **16**(11):843–848.

Helmers SL, Begnaud J, Cowley A, et al. Application of a computational model of vagus nerve stimulation. *Acta Neurol Scand* 2012 November; **126**(5): 336–343.

Holmes MD, Silbergeld DL, Drouhard D, Wilensky AJ, Ojemann LM. Effect of vagus nerve stimulation on adults with pharmacoresistant generalized epilepsy syndromes. *Seizure* 2004 July; **13**(5): 340–345.

Klinkenberg S, Majoie HJM, van der Heijden MMAA, Rijkers K, Leenen L, Aldenkamp AP. Vagus nerve stimulation has a positive effect on mood in patients with refractory epilepsy. *Clin Neurol Neurosurg* 2012 May; **114**(4):336–340.

Kostov H, Larsson PG, Røste GK. Is vagus nerve stimulation a treatment option for patients with drug-resistant idiopathic generalized epilepsy? *Acta Neurol Scand Suppl* 2007; **187**:55–58.

Ng M, Devinsky O. Vagus nerve stimulation for refractory idiopathic generalised epilepsy. *Seizure* 2004; **13**(3):176–178.

Schachter SC, Saper CB. Vagus nerve stimulation. Review. *Epilepsia* 1998 July; **39**(7):677–686.

# Ketogenic Diet and Alternative Therapies

**Dana Ekstein[1] and Steven C. Schachter[2]**

[1]Department of Neurology, Epilepsy Center, Hadassah-Hebrew University Medical Center, Jerusalem, Israel
[2]Department of Neurology, Center for Integration of Medicine and Innovative Technology, Beth Israel Deaconess Medical Center, Massachusetts General Hospital and Harvard Medical School, Boston, MA, USA

## Introduction

The ketogenic diets (KDs), including the classic KD, the medium-chain triglycerides (MCT) KD, the modified Atkins diet (MAD), and the low glycemic index treatment (LGIT), are nutritional therapies that increase the serum concentration of ketones and are efficacious for treating children with drug-resistant epilepsy. This chapter provides a practical guide to the implementation of these diets as well as a discussion of currently available complementary and alternative medications for the treatment of epilepsy.

## Ketogenic diets

The KD was developed at the Mayo Clinic in Rochester, Minnesota, in the early 1920s, at a time when the only other available drug therapies for epilepsy were bromides and phenobarbital. The KD was designed to mimic the metabolic effects of fasting, which had been commonly recommended for the treatment of epilepsy for centuries. While widely used initially in children and adults, the KD became less popular after the introduction of phenytoin and other antiepileptic drugs (AEDs) in the middle of the 20th century. As a result, its use became restricted almost exclusively to the treatment of very severe cases of epilepsy in children at a limited number of tertiary epilepsy centers. Since the 1990s, renewed interest has led to more frequent, mainstream use of the KD. During the past several years, there have been clinical trials supporting its efficacy, introduction of new modified protocols, and increasing use in the adult population, and surprisingly, extension to nonepileptic medical conditions.

The classic KD requires consumption of 4 g of fat for each gram of combined proteins and carbohydrates (ketone ratio 4:1). Often, although there is a lack of evidence for this practice, an overall calorie and fluid restriction is also implemented as part of the KD protocol. The net effect is that 90% of consumed energy is derived from fats. The fat consists of long-chain triglycerides (LCT) found in standard foods, such as butter and mayonnaise. The efficacy of this regimen has been reliably demonstrated.

> **EVIDENCE AT A GLANCE**
>
> In a recent randomized controlled trial of the KD composed of 145 children, the mean seizure frequency decreased by 38% in subjects treated with the KD for 3 months and increased by 37% in the control group. Overall, published studies have demonstrated seizure freedom in 3–33% of patients; 7–56% have more than a 90% reduction of seizure frequency and 19–38% experience seizure reductions of 50–90%.

*Epilepsy*, First Edition. Edited by John W. Miller and Howard P. Goodkin.

There have been attempts to introduce modifications to the classic KD protocol over the years. For example, a reduction of the ketogenic ratio to 3:1 was found to be as effective as the 4:1 ratio at 3 and 6 months; however, the onset of the effect may be faster with the classic protocol. MCT fat, available as coconut milk, oil, and emulsions, produces more ketones per gram than does LCT fat. Therefore, when MCTs are used as a substitute for LCTs, only 60% of energy has to be derived from fat, allowing a higher proportion of protein and carbohydrates to be consumed. The efficacy of this MCT KD variant was shown to be similar to that of the classic KD at 3 months and up to 1 year, although, again, the effect of the classic KD may be initiated more quickly. In practice, KD treatment is individualized by combining various proportions of MCT- and LCT-derived fat to achieve sufficient ketones and the best tolerance.

The MAD and the LGIT have also been adopted for the treatment of epilepsy in the last decade. These regimens do not restrict protein intake, calories, or fluids and are therefore more easily implemented and better tolerated. The MAD restricts carbohydrate consumption to 10 g initially and up to 20 g after 3 months, resulting in a ketogenic ratio of approximately 1:1. The LGIT is based on carbohydrates that produce only a minimal acute increase in blood glucose, allowing for a total of 40–60 g/day of carbohydrates. No randomized controlled trials that directly compare these diets and the KD have been performed. However, the reported efficacy of the MAD and the LGIT is not much lower than that of the classic KD, in particular after 6 months of treatment. Higher fat intake in the first month of the diet and lower carbohydrate consumption in the first 3 months lead to improved seizure control in patients treated with the MAD.

### Indications and preparations for treatment with the ketogenic diet

The KD is the first-line treatment of choice for glucose transporter 1 (GLUT1) and pyruvate dehydrogenase deficiency (PDHD) syndromes. In these diseases, characterized by the inability to use glucose as a metabolic substrate, ketones serve as the substitute fuel for the brain. KD should also be used in the treatment of people with epilepsy who are drug resistant, which means they have failed to achieve seizure freedom after two adequately chosen and implemented AED regimens (Chapter 14). Several epilepsy syndromes may respond particularly well to the KD, including Dravet, Doose, and Rett syndromes, as well as infantile spasms and other epileptic encephalopathies including Landau–Kleffner syndrome (conditions described in Chapter 21). In addition, beneficial effects have been reported in Lafora body disease, subacute sclerosing panencephalitis, selected mitochondrial disorders, and focal epilepsy secondary to lissencephaly. In these types of epilepsy, as well as in small children who are fed formula and patients using enteral nutrition, KD may be tried relatively early after diagnosis of AED intractability (see Chapter 14). Although the data on the use of KD in adults are still limited, growing evidence from small trials lasting 3–12 months suggests that 22–55% of this population may have more than 50% seizure reduction.

Another emerging indication for treatment with the KD is super-refractory status epilepticus (SE), defined as SE that continues for more than 24 h despite anesthesia. In the literature, there are 20 cases of patients who benefited from the diet in this setting, nine of them having febrile infection-related epilepsy syndrome (FIRES), a very severe epilepsy syndrome affecting previously healthy children. Further discussion of the initial management and intensive care unit (ICU) management of SE is provided in Chapters 31 and 32.

Patients in whom epileptic foci were identified and who are candidates for epilepsy surgery may have a less favorable response to KD. For them and for patients in whom adequate nutrition cannot be maintained due to their resistance or caregivers' noncompliance, the KD is relatively contraindicated. The KD is absolutely contraindicated in people with disorders of fat metabolism, although MCT fat–only diets may be given safely to individuals with carnitine deficiency. In search of these disorders, a thorough metabolic evaluation of blood, urine, and CSF should be obtained in patients in whom the precise etiology of epilepsy has not been determined and in individuals with developmental delay, hypotonia, cardiomyopathy, and exercise intolerance.

> ### ☆ TIPS AND TRICKS
>
> The ketogenic diet should not be tried in patients with disorders of fatty acid transport or oxidation, such as deficiencies of carnitine, carnitine palmitoyltransferase (CPT) I and II, carnitine translocase, pyruvate carboxylase, defects of

β-oxidation, and porphyria. Prior to initiation of the KD in eligible individuals, baseline growth data should be documented, consisting of weight, height, and growth percentile. Laboratory evaluations should also be obtained: a complete blood count, electrolytes (including calcium, magnesium, phosphate, zinc, selenium, bicarbonate, albumin, and total protein), kidney and liver functions, lipid profile, amino acid levels, and serum acylcarnitine profile. ECG should be performed, individuals with history of heart disease should have an echocardiogram, and patients with family history of kidney stones should undergo renal ultrasound.

## Initiating the ketogenic diet

In preparing to start the KD, counseling and education visits for the patient and caregivers are scheduled with the neurologist and the dietician. During these visits, nutritional habits and preferences are determined, and efficacy and adverse event expectations are discussed. The decision about the type of diet and its implementation is based on all the acquired clinical information, the nutritional needs of the patient, and the experience of the treating team.

Previously, the KD was initiated in the hospital after 12–48 h (depending on the rate of achieving a high ketone level) of fasting and fluid restriction. The meals were then advanced over about 3 days either by keeping the ketogenic ratio constant and gradually increasing the total daily calorie intake or by beginning with full calories and gradually increasing the ketogenic ratio. New studies have demonstrated that initial fasting does not influence the clinical outcome of the diet at 3 months. Therefore, and since fasting is associated with an increased risk for adverse events, present guidelines favor a gradual initiation of the KD. However, in instances when a rapid response is needed, such as in the treatment of super-refractory SE, fasting may be advantageous. In most centers, the KD is still initiated in the hospital for safety and to enable education of patients and caregivers under the team's close supervision. Beginning the KD as an outpatient is also possible if fasting is not implemented, good ambulatory services are available, and the patient has rapid access to a medical facility. The MAD and the LGIT are started at home under the guidance of a dietician.

## Adverse events of the ketogenic diet

When the patient is in experienced hands, the risk for serious adverse events of the KD is low, but the treating team should be aware of the possible side effects, and the caregivers should be counseled in this regard. Although adverse events rarely require discontinuation of the diet by themselves, they may lead to noncompliance and eventually to cessation of the KD treatment. At the initiation of the diet, with or without initial fasting, patients may develop hypoglycemia, acidosis, nausea, vomiting, dehydration, anorexia, and lethargy. There is also a small risk for increase in seizures.

The most frequently found chronic metabolic side effects of the KD are hyperuricemia (in 2–26% of the patients), hypocalcemia (2%), hypomagnesemia (5%), decreased amino acid levels and acidosis (2–5%), and hypercholesterolemia (14–59%). Carnitine deficiency has also been described. Gastrointestinal complaints are reported by 12–50% of the patients and include vomiting, constipation, diarrhea, and abdominal pain. Notably, because consumption of LCT fat is associated with constipation and excessive MCT fat induces diarrhea and abdominal pain, a rational combination of the two may significantly ameliorate gastrointestinal side effects. Pancreatitis, hepatitis, and gallstones have been reported along with cardiac abnormalities (cardiomyopathy and prolonged QT interval), mostly secondary to deficiency of selenium. Nephrolithiasis is discovered in 3–7% of individuals, but it only rarely requires lithotripsy or diet discontinuation. Long-term treatment is also associated with an increased risk of bone fractures.

Reduced growth in weight and height during the diet is to be expected, but the data on risk factors and long-term consequences are still inconclusive. One trial found that younger and ambulatory children may be more sensitive to this adverse event, but the type of fat used in the diet, whether LCT or MCT, does not influence growth. Another recent study demonstrated the reversibility of the diet's influence by showing that 1 year after KD discontinuation, most children caught up in growth. However, nonambulatory children and patients who did not achieve seizure freedom had a lower rate of improvement. The KD does not have chronic adverse cognitive effects, and it is well recognized that it improves attention. Confounding data exist concerning the influence of the KD on mood. In children, a detrimental effect was reported after 6 months, while improvement of mood and quality of life (QOL) measurements was described in adults.

**Followup of patients on the ketogenic diet**

All patients should receive supplementation with a carbohydrate-free multivitamin with minerals, calcium, and vitamin D. Some therapists also add zinc, magnesium, phosphorus, and selenium. Oral citrates should be administered to prevent kidney stones. Constipation and reflux should be treated symptomatically if they occur. Carnitine is supplemented in children who have low serum levels or are symptomatic (lethargy, muscle weakness). Caregivers are usually instructed to monitor urine ketones several times a week.

Patients receiving the KD should be followed up with at least once every 3 months and be provided with easy accessibility to members of the treating team in between visits. More frequent visits should be offered to children below 1 year of age and persons with cerebral palsy, low growth parameters (under fifth percentile), difficulty consuming the diet, or illness after its initiation. After the first year of the diet, followup visits may be spread apart to once every 6 months. At the time of followup, weight and height should be measured and blood tested for albumin and protein, cholesterol and triglycerides, complete blood count, liver and kidney function, magnesium, phosphate, calcium, bicarbonate, acylcarnitine, urinalysis, and urinary calcium and creatinine. Measurement of serum β-hydroxybutyrate (one of the ketone bodies) may be of value, especially if urine ketones are not in good correlation with epilepsy control. Kidney ultrasound and bone density scans are performed in patients on long-term treatment with the KD.

During the planned follow-up visits, the diet is reviewed and adjusted if needed, seizures are reviewed, and AEDs are adjusted or tapered. The diet's parameters may be altered to change the ketogenic index or the relative proportions of fat sources. The side effects are balanced against efficacy when decisions are made about continuation or discontinuation of the KD. There are no known interactions between the KD and AEDs, but patients treated with topiramate or zonisamide should be monitored for development of acidosis and kidney stones. While the KD and valproate may predispose patients to similar adverse events,

such as hepatotoxicity, pancreatitis, and carnitine deficiency, this combination is not contraindicated. If possible, only carbohydrate-free medications should be consumed. Otherwise, the carbohydrate content of the drugs should be counted in the diet. The combination of vagus nerve stimulation and the KD was shown to be especially beneficial to patients.

**Discontinuation of the ketogenic diet**

If there is worsening of seizures for more than a few days after the initiation of KD, the diet should be discontinued immediately. The diet is usually discontinued for inefficacy after about 3 months of treatment, although 75% of those who respond will do so after less than 2 weeks. In most cases, when the KD induces more than 50% seizure reduction, it is continued for at least 2 years. Patients with almost complete seizure control (>90% seizure reduction or seizure freedom) and those with GLUT1 deficiency, PDHD, or tuberous sclerosis (TS) may be left on the diet for longer. An EEG is usually performed prior to discontinuation. Of the patients who achieve seizure freedom, 80% will not relapse upon discontinuation of the diet. Recurrence of seizures is higher in those with EEG or imaging abnormalities or with TS.

The tapering of the KD is performed gradually over about 3 months, during which the ketogenic ratio is lowered in a stepwise manner from 4:1 to 3:1 and 2:1, after which proteins and fluids are allowed freely and carbohydrates are introduced once urinary ketosis is lost. This gradual wean allows return to the last effective step in the case of worsening of seizures, and in 58% of cases, seizure control is reached again. If cessation of the diet is made necessary by a medical emergency, the diet can be discontinued abruptly, but the patient should then be admitted to an ICU for a few days because severe exacerbation of seizures may occur.

## Alternative therapies

Complementary and alternative medicine (CAM) refers to a group of diverse medical and healthcare systems, practices, and products that are not generally considered part of conventional medicine as practiced in the West. Such therapies are widely used by people in Western countries in general and in particular by individuals with neurological conditions, including epilepsy.

Although they have a long tradition of use in various regions of the world, to date, the efficacy of different CAM interventions for epilepsy has not been adequately studied or proven in clinical trials. These modalities include relaxation techniques and yoga, biofeedback, traditional Chinese medicine practices in general, acupuncture, and natural products. However, relaxation techniques are effective in reducing depression and improving sleep, and acupuncture can treat pain and migraines.

While there are now abundantly available data on the efficacy of herbal-derived remedies in preclinical studies, published clinical trials of botanicals in epilepsy, especially well-designed ones, are at present extremely scarce. Furthermore, contrary to the popular belief that "natural is safe," these therapies can be harmful to people with epilepsy, posing a risk of side effects, interactions with AEDs, and seizure exacerbation, and many of them have not been thoroughly studied. For example, ginkgo biloba, often taken to enhance cognitive function, and St. John's wort, effective for the treatment of mild depression, are commonly consumed by people with epilepsy. However, they may interact with AEDs and increase the potential for seizures. Nonetheless, some natural products and their constituent compounds are undergoing further preclinical evaluation and in the future may prove to be efficacious and safe adjunctive treatments for epilepsy.

## Summary

Growing evidence exists for the use of KD, implemented by well-trained and experienced personnel, in patients with drug-resistant epilepsy. Future research will better determine the target patient populations and the best protocols for increased efficacy and tolerability of this treatment. On the other hand, there is not yet adequate evidence to support the use of complementary and alternative treatments for epilepsy.

## Bibliography

Ekstein D, Schachter SC. Natural products in epilepsy – the present situation and perspectives for the future. *Pharmaceuticals* 2010; **3**:1426–1445.

Kessler SK, Neal EG, Camfield CS, Kossoff EH. Dietary therapies for epilepsy: Future research. *Epilepsy Behav* 2010; **22**:17–22.

Kossoff EH, Cross JH. Ketogenic diets: Where do we go from here? *Epilepsy Res* 2012; **100**:344–346.

Kossoff EH, Zupec-Kania BA, Amark PE, et al. Optimal clinical management of children receiving the ketogenic diet: Recommendations of the International Ketogenic Diet Study Group. *Epilepsia* 2009; **50**:304–317.

Lambrechts DA, Bovens MJ, de la Parra NM, Hendriksen JG, Aldenkamp AP, Majoie MJ. Ketogenic diet effects on cognition, mood, and psychosocial adjustment in children. *Acta Neurol Scand* 2013 February; **127**(2):103–108.

Lee PR, Kossoff EH. Dietary treatments for epilepsy: Management guidelines for the general practitioner. *Epilepsy Behav* 2011; **21**:115–121.

Levy RG, Cooper PN, Giri P. Ketogenic diet and other dietary treatments for epilepsy. *Cochrane Database Syst Rev* 2012; **3**:CD001903.

Li Q, Chen X, He L, Zhou D. Traditional Chinese medicine for epilepsy. *Cochrane Database Syst Rev* 2009; **3**:CD006454.

Miranda MJ, Turner Z, Magrath G. Alternative diets to the classical ketogenic diet – can we be more liberal? *Epilepsy Res* 2012; **100**:278–285.

Neal EG, Chaffe H, Schwartz RH, et al. The ketogenic diet for the treatment of childhood epilepsy: A randomised controlled trial. *Lancet Neurol* 2008; **7**:500–506.

Ramaratnam S, Baker GA, Goldstein LH. Psychological treatments for epilepsy. *Cochrane Database Syst Rev* 2008; **3**:CD002029.

Schachter SC. Botanicals and herbs: A traditional approach to treating epilepsy. *Neurotherapeutics* 2009; **6**:415–420.

Williams E, Abrahams J, Maguire A, Harris G. A parent's perspective on dietary treatments for epilepsy. *Epilepsy Res* 2012; **100**:338–343.

# Part VII

# How are Acute Seizures and Status Epilepticus Evaluated and Treated in the Emergency Department and the Hospital?

# Acute Symptomatic Seizures in Children and Adults: Evaluation and Treatment

**J. Stephen Huff[1] and Jessica L. Carpenter[2]**

[1]Departments of Emergency Medicine and Neurology, University of Virginia, Charlottesville, VA, USA
[2]Department of Neurophysiology, Children's National Medical Center, George Washington University, Washington, DC, USA

## Introduction

The approach to any patient in the emergency department or hospital who has had an apparent seizure begins with assessment of airway integrity, ventilation, and circulatory support. If required, intervention may involve a variety of airway maneuvers such as repositioning the patient's head, suctioning, insertion of a nasopharyngeal airway, bag–valve-mask-assisted ventilations, or consideration of endotracheal intubation or a laryngeal mask airway if consciousness is impaired or respirations are deemed inadequate. For any patient with altered consciousness, intravenous access should be obtained. Rapid bedside determination of blood glucose should be performed, and if hypoglycemia is found, intravenous dextrose or intramuscular glucagon should be administered. If rapid glucose determination is not available and the possibility of hypoglycemia exists, intravenous dextrose should be administered. Intravenous thiamine should be given before or concurrently with dextrose infusion if there is the possibility of poor nutrition or a malabsorptive state.

The differential diagnosis for convulsive events includes syncope, convulsive concussion, movement disorder, sleep-related event, nonepileptic seizure, rigors, and other etiologies that are discussed in Chapter 5. In this chapter, we discuss patients diagnosed with acute symptomatic or provoked seizure(s). *By definition, an acute symptomatic seizure occurs at the time or within seven days of an acute neurological, systemic, metabolic, or toxic insult.* After patient stabilization, the clinician's task is to discriminate between provoked and unprovoked seizures.

Some basic groupings of patients readily become apparent. Has the patient had a single seizure and returned to a waking state and baseline neurological function, or has the patient had a series of seizures? Has the patient failed to regain consciousness now that the convulsion has stopped? Was the seizure associated with fever or intoxication? Is there a head injury present? Diagnostic evaluation and treatment decisions are guided by these groupings. Recognition of status epilepticus, including subclinical status epilepticus, is critical. Management of status epilepticus is considered in Chapter 31.

## Common causes

About 25–30% of first seizures are provoked or acute symptomatic seizures. Causes of acute symptomatic seizures may be grouped into primary central nervous system (CNS) etiologies such as hypoxia, stroke, trauma, infection, and inflammation and

*Epilepsy*, First Edition. Edited by John W. Miller and Howard P. Goodkin.

**Table 30.1.** Causes of acute symptomatic seizures.

| *Neurological* |
| --- |
| Stroke (e.g., ischemic, hemorrhage) |
| Hypoxic brain injury |
| Traumatic brain injury |
| Neoplasm (primary or metastatic) |
| CNS infection (e.g., meningitis, encephalitis, abscess) |
| Inflammatory (e.g., ADEM, lupus cerebritis, NMDAR Ab encephalitis) |
| *Systemic* |
| Sepsis |
| Fever (i.e., febrile seizures) |
| Toxic/metabolic |
| Electrolyte disturbance (e.g., hypoglycemia, hyponatremia, hypocalcemia) |
| Acute intoxications (e.g., antidepressants, theophylline) |
| Withdrawal syndromes (e.g., ethanol, benzodiazepines, barbiturates) |

ADEM, acute disseminated encephalomyelitis; CNS, central nervous system; NMDAR Ab, anti-$N$-methyl-$D$-aspartate receptor antibody.

systemic causes such as electrolyte abnormalities, toxins, infection/sepsis, and fever (Table 30.1). In emergency departments, ethanol-related seizures are likely the most commonly encountered provoked seizures in adults. Hypoglycemia and electrolyte disturbances, notably hyponatremia, are also relatively common. Other etiologies are less likely but may be vital to detect and treat.

### ☝ CAUTION!

"Don't miss" diagnoses for etiologies of acute symptomatic seizures include infection, hypoxia, trauma, neoplasms, electrolyte disturbances, and ingestions/toxins.

Common causes of acute symptomatic seizures in children are similar to those of seizures in adults, with infection representing a larger percentage. Febrile seizures are common, occurring in 2–5% of all children. A febrile seizure, by definition, is any convulsion in a child between the ages of 6 months and 5 years

**Table 30.2.** Febrile seizures.

| *Simple febrile seizures* |
| --- |
| <15 min in duration |
| Nonfocal (i.e., generalized, including onset) |
| Does not recur in a 24-h period |
| *Complex febrile seizures* |
| >15 min in duration |
| Focal (or postictal focal weakness) |
| Recurrent within a 24-h period |

associated with a fever ($T > 38°C$) at the time of illness, without a CNS infection. Febrile seizures can be classified as simple or complex (Table 30.2), with simple febrile seizures being associated with a good neurodevelopmental outcome (including only a slight increase risk of epilepsy later in life). Febrile seizures tend to run in families – recent studies have identified several genetic mutations (e.g., *SCN1A* in generalized epilepsy with febrile seizures plus [GEFs+]) associated with an increased risk for this type of provoked seizure. There has long been concern that children with febrile status epilepticus (FebSTAT) may be a specific subset of children with febrile seizures that are at increased risk of epilepsy later in life. This question is the focus of a large prospective study of children with prolonged FebSTAT. Thus far, the study has demonstrated an increased risk for hippocampal injury after prolonged febrile seizures, but the true risk for epilepsy is still to be determined.

### ☝ CAUTION!

While febrile seizures are common and typically occur in otherwise normal children, they can occasionally be the presentation of a more serious condition (i.e., Dravet syndrome, an epileptic encephalopathy most commonly associated with sodium channel mutations). History and physical examination are critical to distinguishing these outliers.

### Diagnostic evaluation

A detailed history is critical for determining the potential cause of a seizure. For example, a seizure occurring with a history of alcohol abuse or ingestion may direct specific therapies (Figure 30.1). If the event is associated with fever, the evaluation for concomitant infection is

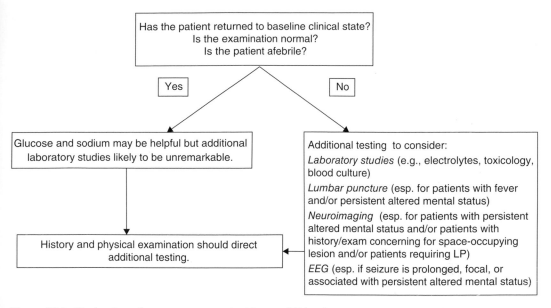

**Figure 30.1.** Evaluation of acute symptomatic seizures. LP, lumbar puncture.

steered by details of the illness as well as age of the patient. The diagnostic evaluation for a simple febrile seizure differs significantly from that for a seizure in a neonate with fever. A seizure occurring in conjunction with a head injury may prompt neuroradiological evaluation. A history of a metabolic disorder or use of a medication may suggest electrolyte disturbances in need of detection and correction. Significant medical history that includes a history of cancer or immunosuppression may guide diagnostic testing, which may include neuroimaging or cerebrospinal fluid analysis.

### ★ TIPS AND TRICKS

For the child at baseline at the time of presentation following a simple febrile seizure, the diagnostic studies should be focused on determination of the cause of fever. EEG, neuroimaging, or laboratory studies are not necessary for evaluation of the seizure itself.

If the history and/or physical examination is in any way concerning for a CNS infection, the clinician should perform a lumbar puncture (LP) and consider empiric antibiotics. Of particular concern are children less than 12 months of age who are at increased risk for bacterial meningitis, especially if they have not received their immunizations.

History and physical examination predict the majority of adult patients with a laboratory abnormality. Laboratory testing has a very low yield in patients with a single new-onset seizure who have returned to normal neurological status. Glucose abnormalities and hyponatremia are the most frequent electrolyte disturbances detected in adults and children. Though other laboratory testing is frequently performed, it will likely have little value for determining seizure etiology. Noncontrast cranial CT may be useful especially when there is an abnormal neurological examination, significant history, or focal onset of seizures. Patients with persistent altered mental status or fever require a more extensive evaluation.

A toxicology screen for frequently abused drugs is commonly obtained in patients with first-time seizures, but there is little data regarding its utility. Occasionally ECG may show abnormalities associated with preexcitation syndromes, Brugada syndrome, or long QT syndromes, suggesting that an arrhythmia has precipitated an episode of convulsive syncope. ECG is commonly obtained in patients with suspected toxic ingestion; for example, prolonged QRS complexes may suggest tricyclic antidepressant toxicity, or additional long QT intervals or other conduction abnormalities may be discovered.

In the patient with persistent altered mental status, fever, or a history of immunosuppression, performance of an LP should be considered. In children, an immunization history should be taken to assess for vulnerability to *Haemophilus influenzae* or *Streptococcus pneumoniae* infections. Empiric antibiotics should be considered when appropriate.

> ☆ **TIPS AND TRICKS**
>
> EEG is indicated when an acute symptomatic seizure is prolonged, focal, or associated with persistent altered mental status. EEG obtained on an emergency basis may be necessary to assess for nonconvulsive status epilepticus in patients with cessation of convulsive movements but persistent altered mental status.

## Treatment decisions

Axiomatic in the approach to provoked or acute symptomatic seizures is to detect and then treat any underlying cause. There is remarkably little literature from prospectively collected data to guide decision making. If a patient has had a single seizure and is at normal neurological baseline, likely no specific treatment is needed other than identifying and addressing any precipitating cause and assessing the risk for recurrence. However, if several seizures occur over a short period, treatment with benzodiazepines is generally initiated. In the hospital setting, lorazepam has become the favored benzodiazepine because of its relatively longer anticonvulsant effects (Chapter 18). There are no head-to-head comparisons with other benzodiazepines for treatment of provoked seizures. In general, for provoked seizures from toxins, benzodiazepines are also agents of choice.

With ethanol-related seizures, it has been shown that 2 mg of lorazepam decreased recurrent seizures over a 12-h period. Dosing of lorazepam for adults is often initiated with 2 mg intravenously to be repeated as necessary for a total dose of 4–8 mg (Chapter 18). Recommended dosages in children for lorazepam range from 0.05 to 0.1 mg/kg to a maximum of 4 mg. Side effects include respiratory depression, largely related to rate of administration.

Hypoglycemia should be treated by the standard methods. In adults and older children, dextrose 50% is given at 1–2 mL/kg/dose. Bedside glucose testing is then performed and additional dextrose given if needed. In children, dextrose 25% is recommended at 2–4 mg/kg. Hypoglycemia in a child is occasionally the presentation of an inherited metabolic disorder,

and referral for further evaluation should be made when the history and physical are suggestive.

Hyponatremia has many causes, but diuretic use is commonly implicated in adults. In children common causes include administration of hypotonic fluids (most commonly in neonates) or GI disturbances (e.g., nausea/vomiting). Syndrome of inappropriate antidiuretic hormone secretion (SIADH) and other less common etiologies may be present. Generally speaking, water restriction and administration of normal saline (relatively hypertonic in this patient group) are sufficient for correction. Rapid correction of hyponatremia should be avoided as it may lead to central pontine myelinolysis.

> ☆ **TIPS AND TRICKS**
>
> In adult patients that have returned to normal neurological status, history and physical examination will predict the majority of the patients who will have laboratory abnormalities. Hypoglycemia and hyponatremia are the most commonly detected abnormalities in children and adults.

Acute severe head injury is a special circumstance. Even in patients who have not had a seizure, treatment for 1 week with an antiepileptic drug has been recommended with the intention of preventing early post-traumatic seizures. Phenytoin was previously the drug of choice for this indication, but recent studies have suggested levetiracetam is equally effective and may have a preferred side effect profile. If a seizure has occurred, longer antiepileptic therapy is generally employed.

Simple febrile seizures can recur in some children. Parents should be provided anticipatory guidance and first aid instruction for seizure management. Chronic antiepileptic medications are not recommended, as these seizures are considered provoked and are not associated with long-term adverse effects and/or an increased risk of epilepsy later in life.

In the presence of suspected CNS infection, antibiotics are often empirically administered. Depending on pretest probability of meningitis and age of the patient, if there is suspicion of acute bacterial meningitis medications might include dexamethasone, ceftriaxone, vancomycin, gentamicin, or ampicillin. Empiric acyclovir should be provided in cases of suspected viral encephalitis.

If a nontraumatic structural lesion is discovered on CT or on other imaging tests, this should be weighed in the decision to initiate anticonvulsant medications. Again, there are no studies to guide the clinician, but longer-acting antiepileptic drugs such as fosphenytoin or levetiracetam may be initiated.

## Outcomes

Acute symptomatic seizures are associated with increased mortality in the first 30 days, likely related to the precipitating condition. However, a first provoked seizure caused by an acute injury is unlikely to recur, with estimates of only 3–10%. For patients presenting in status epilepticus, the outcome is also linked to the precipitating cause. Generally, status epilepticus related to alcohol withdrawal or antiepileptic medication irregularity has a good prognosis, while status epilepticus following hypoxic insult, CNS infections, or electrolyte abnormalities has a poorer prognosis. Likely prognosis following a provoked seizure follows this same pattern.

## Conclusion

Acute symptomatic or provoked seizures occur at the time or within 7 days of an acute neurological, systemic, metabolic, or toxic insult. Determination of the suspected cause is guided mostly by the history or physical examination. If the patient has not returned to the baseline state, additional evaluations may be necessary, including laboratory work, neuroimaging, LP, or EEG, again with the indication for each suggested by the history and examination. Treatment of a provoked seizure should be directed at the underlying cause; benzodiazepine administration may be of use for seizure termination or in preventing short-term seizure recurrence.

## Bibliography

American Academy of Pediatrics. Committee on Quality Improvement, Subcommittee on Febrile Seizures. Practice parameter: Long-term treatment of the child with simple febrile seizures. *Pediatrics* 1999 June; **103**:1307–1309.

American College of Emergency Physicians Clinical Policies Committee. Clinical policy: Critical issues in the evaluation and management of adult patients presenting to the emergency department with seizures. *Ann Emerg Med* 2004; **43**:605–625.

D'Onofrio G, Rathlev NI, Ulrich AS, Fish SS, Freedland ES. Lorazepam for the prevention of recurrent seizures related to alcohol. *N Engl J Med* 1999; **340**:915–919.

Harden CL, Huff JS, Schwartz TH, et al. Reassessment: Neuroimaging in the emergency patient presenting with seizure (an evidence-based review): Report of the Therapeutics and Technology Assessment Subcommittee of the American Academy of Neurology. *Neurology* 2007; **69**:1772–1780.

Hirtz D, Ashwal S, Berg A, et al. Practice parameter: Evaluating a first nonfebrile seizure in children: Report of the Quality Standards Subcommittee of the American Academy of Neurology, the Child Neurology Society, and the American Epilepsy Society. *Neurology* 2000; **55**:616–623.

Krumholtz A, Wiebe S, Gronseth G, et al. Practice parameter: Evaluating an apparent unprovoked first seizure in adults (an evidence-based review): Report of the Quality Standards Subcommittee of the American Academy of Neurology and the American Epilepsy Society. *Neurology* 2007; **69**:1996–2007.

Pohlmann-Eden B, Beghi E, Camfield C, Camfield P. The first seizure and management in adults and children. *BMJ* 2006; **332**:339–342.

Schierhout G, Roberts I. Anti-epileptic drugs for preventing seizures following acute traumatic brain injury. *Cochrane Database Syst Rev* 2001; **4**:CD000173.

Subcommittee on Febrile Seizures AAP. Neurodiagnostic evaluation of the child with a simple febrile seizure. *Pediatrics* 2011; **127**:389–394.

Tunkel AR, Glaser CA, Bloch KC, et al. The management of encephalitis: Clinical practice guidelines by the infectious diseases society of America clinical infectious diseases. *Clin Infect Dis* 2008; **47**:303–327.

# Evaluating and Treating Status Epilepticus

Jeffrey Bolton[1] and Howard P. Goodkin[2]

[1]Department of Neurology, Boston Children's Hospital Division of Epilepsy, Harvard Medical School, Boston, MA, USA
[2]Division of Pediatric Neurology, Department of Neurology, University of Virginia, Charlottesville, VA, USA

Status epilepticus (SE) is the term applied to a prolonged, self-sustaining seizure or frequent, recurrent seizures that occur without a return to baseline. SE does not represent a single disease, nor does it represent a single seizure type. Although frequently the term "status" is used as a shorthand for an episode of generalized convulsive SE (e.g., tonic–clonic SE), the clinical manifestations of SE are broad, ranging from overt generalized or focal convulsive SE to nonconvulsive forms characterized by an alteration of consciousness (e.g., complex partial SE) to complete loss of consciousness (electrographic SE in the comatose patient in the ICU setting) in the absence of motor symptoms.

Given the multiple different clinical manifestations, it has proved hard to develop a universally accepted definition. Epidemiological definitions typically distinguish SE from self-limited seizures based on time durations of 30–60 min. Yet, it is neither practical nor appropriate to wait for 30 min or longer to initiate care in some SE types; therefore, a current operational definition for generalized convulsive SE has defined the duration as 5 min.

### ⚗ SCIENCE REVISITED

Studies investigating SE pathogenesis have demonstrated that SE is a dynamic, evolving process during which there are ongoing changes in the surface expression of several molecules including $GABA_A$ receptors, NMDA receptors, AMPA receptors, HCN channels, and potassium channels. These changes may account, in part, for the self-sustaining nature of SE and the inverse correlation between seizure duration and the effectiveness of current SE first-line therapies.

## Epidemiology and etiology

Status epilepticus is common, with an estimated annual incidence ranging from 15 to 50 episodes per 100,000 persons per year. Worldwide, these values translate to a minimum of 1 million episodes of SE per year.

Status epilepticus is most common at the extremes of life. In the classic prospective, population-based SE epidemiological study performed in Richmond, VA, the incidence was nearly 150 per 100,000 persons in children less than 1 year of age. The incidence dropped to less than 25 per 100,000 persons by 5 years of age until it increased again to greater than 50 per 100,000 persons after 40 years of age. This bimodal distribution has been observed across multiple prospective studies.

As noted earlier, SE is not a single disease but a symptom that can be the result of either a primary

*Epilepsy*, First Edition. Edited by John W. Miller and Howard P. Goodkin.
© 2014 John Wiley & Sons, Ltd. Published 2014 by John Wiley & Sons, Ltd.

central nervous system disorder or a secondary symptom from a systemic disorder. It occurs in both those with and those without a history of preexisting epilepsy. The range of precipitants is wide and varies by age. Common etiologies include cerebrovascular disease and anoxia, metabolic disturbances, trauma, tumor, fever, infection, and in those with epilepsy, noncompliance with antiepileptic medication or medication changes. In the Richmond study that included both children and adults, acute symptomatic causes accounted for 52% of the episodes, remote symptomatic causes accounted for 39%, and idiopathic/cryptogenic/unknown causes accounted for 5%. In the prospective North London study that included only children, acute symptomatic causes (including febrile seizures) accounted for 49%, remote symptomatic causes accounted for 16%, remote symptomatic causes with an acute precipitant accounted for 16%, and idiopathic/cryptogenic/unknown causes accounted for 19%.

## Convulsive status epilepticus

Attempts to develop a single classification system for the many seizure types of SE are ongoing. Currently, a simplified semiologically based system that divides SE broadly into convulsive and nonconvulsive forms is frequently informally employed.

Generalized convulsive SE is characterized by continuous or repeated tonic and/or clonic motor movements associated with loss of consciousness accompanied by an ictal electroencephalogram (EEG) pattern. Generalized convulsive SE may follow a dynamic progression of isolated recurrent seizures that wax and wane, ultimately evolving into a single continuous seizure. If seizures are refractory to treatment or left untreated, electromechanical dissociation may occur in which the motor component becomes more subtle, consisting of only minor jerking or twitching, while the EEG reveals persistence of a continuous or possibly periodic (i.e., periodic epileptiform discharges [PEDs]) ictal EEG pattern.

Focal motor SE without impairment of consciousness (i.e., epilepsia partialis continua [EPC]) can last for prolonged periods of time and is often refractory to medication. The motor manifestations of EPC are often clonic movements restricted to a single body region, commonly in the upper extremities. The differential diagnosis for this form of SE includes cerebral neoplasia (primary metastatic), cortical dysplasia, vascular lesion, focal infection, and inflammatory causes such as Rasmussen's syndrome.

## Nonconvulsive status epilepticus

The term nonconvulsive SE incorporates a number of different clinical situations. As described previously, nonconvulsive SE may represent the end stages of generalized convulsive SE. In addition, nonconvulsive SE also includes focal SE with impairment of consciousness (i.e., complex partial SE), absence SE, as well as the increasingly recognized state of unresponsiveness in the ICU associated with an ictal EEG pattern on bedside EEG monitoring. This condition is discussed in Chapter 32.

Complex partial SE should be considered in a patient with a persistent altered mental status ranging from slightly confused to nearly comatose. Motor symptoms are minor and typically manifest as automatisms. Patients in complex partial SE have been described as functioning in an "epileptic twilight state" or as the "wandering confused." They tend to cycle between periods of relative lucidness and episodes of motionless staring or complete unresponsiveness.

The term *spike–wave stupor* refers to a prolonged absence seizure causing the patient to present in a confusional state. Unlike complex partial SE, absence SE does not have cycling between responsive and unresponsive states, but instead tends to consist of mild persistently slowed mentation or lethargy. Although upon initial presentation absence SE may be difficult to differentiate from complex partial SE, an EEG will provide prompt clarification, demonstrating prolonged, often continuous, generalized 3-Hz spike-and-wave discharges. Subtle motor symptoms may be present, including myoclonic twitches of the eyelids or facial muscles. Absence SE occurs in children with primary generalized epilepsies. In adults, it may occur *de novo* (de novo absence in adults) as well as in the setting of benzodiazepine withdrawal or a prior history of absence seizures as a child.

There can also be focal forms of nonconvulsive SE without impairment of consciousness. These are characterized by a prolonged aura (aura continua) of sensory, special sensory, autonomic, or cognitive symptoms. The symptoms (e.g., dysesthesia, visual changes, fear) are dependent on cortical localization and can wax and wane over the duration of the prolonged seizure.

⚠ CAUTION!

It is important to consider psychogenic SE prior to commencement of second-line agents and intubation. If psychogenic SE is a possibility, an emergent EEG should be obtained.

## Management

In any medical emergency, adherence to a set of standard guidelines or protocol improves outcome; SE is no different. In all cases of SE, the goal should be prompt control of the seizure. There are four phases to SE management, independent of type: medical stabilization, antiepileptic drug (AED) administration until the episode is concluded, evaluation for an underlying etiology, and initiation or optimization of maintenance AED therapy (Figure 31.1).

Management starts with prompt recognition that the seizure is evolving into a prolonged seizure or repeated events without return to baseline. Once the diagnosis of SE has been made, the initial examination should be focused on respiratory and cardiovascular status (i.e., the ABCs of airway, breathing, and circulation). When possible, it is recommended that the patient be placed on cardiac monitoring and pulse oximetry, with frequent evaluation of vital signs and, if required, supplemental oxygen administration.

### First-line therapy

For the treatment of generalized convulsive SE and many cases of nonconvulsive SE, the benzodiazepines are the drugs of first choice as they have proved to be both safe and effective (Chapter 16). In the out-of-hospital setting, intramuscular (IM) midazolam, rectal diazepam, or a parenteral benzodiazepine should be used. In the emergency department or in-hospital setting, intravenous (IV) administration of the benzodiazepines is commonly used to ensure the rapid delivery of the maximal dose; however, some institutions have also turned to intranasal or IM administration of midazolam. For IV administration, lorazepam is often the drug of choice due to its relative rapid onset of action and long pharmacological effect.

EVIDENCE AT A GLANCE

The Rapid Anticonvulsant Medication Prior to Arrival Trial (RAMPART) was a randomized, double-blind, noninferiority clinical trial comparing IM midazolam to IV lorazepam in the prehospital treatment of SE by first responders. The results of the trial revealed equal efficacy and safety of IM midazolam in aborting seizures lasting over 5 min when compared to IV lorazepam. Advantages of IM midazolam include the ability to administer without IV access and better drug stability for storage in the field.

**Management**

- The ABCs (stabilization)
  - Airway: Stabilize and maintain the airway, remove obstruction
  - Breathing: Administer supplemental oxygen and provide mechanical ventilation as necessary
  - Circulation: Establish IV acess (consider thiamine and D50%)
  - Check fingerstick glucose
  - Commence continuous monitoring of vital signs (pulse, respiratory rate, blood pressure, pulse oximetry)
- Evaluation
  - Draw blood electrolytes including calcium, magnesium, phosphorus, serum transaminases, CBC, toxicology screen, and antiepileptic levels as indicated
  - Neurologic examination
  - Neuroimaging once stable (cranial CT or MRI, especially in the absence of a history of epilepsy)
  - Lumbar puncture if febrile
  - Emergent EEG if considering psychogenic seizures or nonconvulsive seizures or to monitor management

**Treatment***

| First-line (emergent) treatment | Second-line (urgent) treatment** | Refractory SE treatment | Alternative therapies |
|---|---|---|---|
| Lorazepam (IV) | Phenytoin (IV)/Fosphenytoin (IV,IM) | Pentobarbital | VNS |
| Diazepam (IV, PR) | Phenobarbital (IV) | Midazolam | Ketogenic diet |
| Midazolam (IM) | Valproate sodium (IV) | Propofol | Hypothermia |
| | Levetiracetam (IV) | Thiopental | ECT |
| | | Ketamine | Surgery |
| | | Inhalational anesthetics | Pyridoxine (infants) |
| | | Phenobarbital | |
| | | (Lacosamide; Topiramate) | |

*First-line (emergent) treatment should be initiated as soon as possible after recognition of SE. Second-line (urgent) and refractory SE treatment should proceed promptly, as required, after first-line therapies.
**Consider administration of second-line agent to prevent seizure recurrence even if seizure has terminated.
CBC, complete blood count.

**Figure 31.1.** Outline of treatment and evaluation of status epilepticus.

## Second-line therapy

To date, a randomized controlled trial evaluating the treatment of SE that is refractory to benzodiazepines has not been performed. Choices include first-generation agents such as phenytoin or phenobarbital as well as newer-generation AEDs such as valproate sodium and levetiracetam. Often, these agents are administered even if the benzodiazepines are successful, in an effort to reduce the probability of seizure recurrence immediately following benzodiazepine elimination.

> ### ☆ TIPS AND TRICKS
>
> For the patient >2 years old with a primary generalized epilepsy, the use of valproate sodium has been advocated as the initial secondary agent.

Many current protocols rely on phenytoin or its water-soluble prodrug, fosphenytoin, as the initial second-line agent. For IV loading in the absence of a central line, fosphenytoin offers several advantages over phenytoin including decreased cardiovascular side effects and the absence of associated purple glove syndrome. Although cardiovascular side effects are reduced with fosphenytoin, both medications may lead to hypotension, vasodilation, tachycardia, or bradycardia. Therefore, cardiovascular monitoring is recommended with IV loading of both medications. During the neonatal period, phenobarbital is preferred over phenytoin. For further discussion of these and other parenteral medications, the reader is referred to Chapter 18.

> ### ☆ TIPS AND TRICKS
>
> Even if overt convulsive activity terminates, electrographic seizures may persist in a patient with SE. For the patient who remains unresponsive following SE treatment, urgent bedside EEG recording will help differentiate between a postictal state and a continued nonconvulsive seizure.

## Third-line therapy and refractory status epilepticus

Refractory SE, defined as persistent SE despite treatment with appropriate doses of first- and second-line therapies, may occur in up to 30–40%

of cases. Common causes of refractory SE include infectious and antibody-mediated forms of encephalitis as well as a recently described syndrome, febrile infection-related epilepsy syndrome (FIRES). The medications used to treat refractory SE include continuous IV infusion of pentobarbital, midazolam, thiopental, lidocaine, propofol, or ketamine or inhalational anesthetics (e.g., isoflurane). The treatment and management of refractory SE is covered in Chapter 32.

> ### ☆ TIPS AND TRICKS
>
> In the child with refractory SE, a trial of pyridoxine should be considered because pyridoxine dependency can present with SE.

## Diagnostic evaluation

Within the emergency department or in the in-hospital setting, diagnostic studies are commenced in parallel with the treatment phase. Even in the field, it is important that emergency medical personnel perform a rapid assessment of blood glucose levels.

The diagnostic evaluation should be customized based on the details of the history and findings on physical examination. Laboratory studies that are often performed include electrolyte, calcium, magnesium, phosphorous, and blood glucose levels; a complete blood count; toxicology studies; and AED levels (if applicable). Any metabolic derangements should be corrected immediately. If the patient is febrile, blood culture and CSF studies should also be considered, followed by administration of meningitic antibiotic therapy.

Once the patient has been adequately stabilized, further diagnostic testing can be carried out. Patients with no prior history of seizure should undergo brain MRI and additional metabolic/infectious evaluation depending on clinical history.

## Prognosis

In recent studies, the mortality rate associated with SE has ranged from 4% to 37%. Even for those who survive an episode of SE, there is the potential to develop new neurological morbidity including intellectual dysfunction, motor abnormalities, and epilepsy. Like many situations in neurology, the prognosis depends on etiology and age, as the outcome is worse with acute precipitants and older age. Duration may also be a factor in determining SE outcome, with one prospective study finding a mortality of 32% for episodes of 60 min in duration or longer and only 2.7% for episodes of shorter duration. Therefore, prompt recognition and early termination of SE remains a cornerstone of improving the outcome.

## Bibliography

Brophy GM, Bell R, Classan J, et al. Guidelines for evaluation and management of status epilepticus. *Neurocrit Care* 2012; **17**:3–23.

Chin RF, Neville BG, Peckham, et al. Incidence, cause, and short-term outcome of convulsive status epilepticus in childhood: Prospective population-based study. *Lancet* 2006; **368**:222–229.

DeLorenzo RJ, Hauser WA, Towne AR, et al. A prospective, population-based epidemiologic study of status epilepticus in Richmond, Virginia. *Neurology* 1996; **46**:1029–1035.

Goodkin HP, Kapur J. The impact of diazepam's discovery on the treatment and understanding of status epilepticus. *Epilepsia* 2009; **40**:2011–2018.

Hocker SE, Britton JW, Mandrekar JN, Wijdicks EF, Rabinstein AA. Predictors of outcome in refractory status epilepticus. *Arch Neurol* 2012; **8**:1–6.

Kramer U, Chi C-S, Lin K-L, et al. Febrile infection-related epilepsy syndrome (FIRES): Pathogenesis, treatment, and outcome. A multicenter study on 77 children. *Epilepsia* 2011; **52**:1956–1965.

Loddenkemper T, Goodkin HP. Treatment of pediatric status epilepticus. *Curr Treat Options Neurol* 2011; **13**(6):560–573.

Lowenstein DH, Bleck T, Macdonald RL. It's time to revise the definition of status epilepticus. *Epilepsia* 1999; **40**:120–122.

Prasad K, Al-Roomi K, Krishnan PR, Sequeira R. Anticonvulsant therapy for status epilepticus. *Cochrane Database of Syst Rev* 2005; **19**:CD003723.

Raspall-Chaure M, Chin RF, Neville BG, Bedford H, Scott RC. The epidemiology of convulsive status epilepticus in children: A critical review. *Epilepsia* 2007; **48**:1652–1663.

Riviello JJ, Jr, Ashwal S, Hirtz D, et al. Practice parameter: Diagnostic assessment of the child with status epilepticus (an evidence-based review): Report of the Quality Standards Subcommittee of the American Academy of Neurology and Practice Committee of the Child Neurology Society. *Neurology* 2006; **67**:1542–1550.

Rosssetti AO, Milligan TA, Vulliémoz S, Michaelides C, Bertschi M, Lee JW. A randomized trial for the treatment of refractory status epilepticus. *Neurocrit Care* 2011; **14**:4–10.

Shorvon S, Relisi M. The outcome of therapies in refractory and super-refractory convulsive status epilepticus and recommendations for therapy. *Brain* 2012; **135**:2314–2328.

Silbergleit R, Durkalski V, Lowenstein D, et al. Intramuscular versus intravenous therapy for prehospital status epilepticus. *New Engl J Med* 2012; **366**:591–600.

Towne, AR, Pellock JM, Ko D, DeLorenzo RJ. Determinants of mortality in status epilepticus. *Epilepsia* 1994; **35**:27–34.

# Recognizing, Assessing, and Treating Seizures and Status Epilepticus in the ICU

**Nicolas Gaspard[1,2] and Lawrence J. Hirsch[2]**

[1]Computational Neurophysiology Laboratory, Yale University School of Medicine, New Haven, CT, USA
[2]Division of Epilepsy and EEG, Yale Comprehensive Epilepsy Center, Neurology Department, Yale University School of Medicine, New Haven, CT, USA

## Introduction

Seizures and status epilepticus (SE) are common in the ICU. This chapter presents a practical approach to the diagnosis and treatment of nonconvulsive seizures (NCSz) and refractory status epilepticus, the use of antiepileptic drugs (AEDs) in critically ill patients, and seizure prophylaxis.

## Epidemiology

Seizure is a common complication of critical illness. Clinical seizures, mostly generalized tonic–clonic seizures (GTCSs), occur in about 3% of patients admitted to an ICU. In those patients, the prevalence of NCSz – seizures with subtle clinical manifestations and purely electrographic seizures – is 15–20% overall. The risk is higher in certain populations such as those with acute brain injury, especially intracranial hemorrhage and CNS infection. NCSz or nonconvulsive status epilepticus (NCSE) occurs in almost half of patients treated for generalized convulsive status epilepticus (GCSE). There is a correlation between the degree of impairment of consciousness and the prevalence of seizures in the ICU,

with comatose patients having the highest rate. Children are also at higher risk.

## Etiology of seizures and status epilepticus in the ICU

Etiologies are diverse and are summarized in Table 32.1. The most common causes are drug withdrawal (AEDs, benzodiazepines, and barbiturates), acute stroke, anoxic brain injury, and metabolic/septic encephalopathy.

## Clinical manifestations and differential diagnosis

The manifestations of seizures and SE are protean. Of all the subtypes of seizures and SE described, the three semiologies most commonly encountered in the ICU are generalized tonic–clonic, myoclonic, and nonconvulsive.

The typical manifestations of GTCS are often altered in critically ill patients, and out-of-phase clonic movements, asymmetric seizures, or prolonged post-ictal states are frequent. If the seizure progresses to GCSE, the generalized clonic movements will become progressively less prominent as the patient transitions to NCSE, during which the motor activity may

*Epilepsy*, First Edition. Edited by John W. Miller and Howard P. Goodkin.

**Table 32.1.** Etiology of seizure and SE in the ICU.

*Acute brain injury*

    Ischemic stroke

    Intracerebral hemorrhage

    Subarachnoid hemorrhage

    Subdural hematoma

    Traumatic brain injury

    Anoxic brain injury

    Infections: meningitis, encephalitis, brain abscess

    Autoimmune/paraneoplastic diseases, including limbic encephalitis

    Head trauma: contusion, subdural hematoma

    Neoplasms: primary or secondary

    Hypertensive encephalopathy and posterior reversible encephalopathy syndrome (PRES)

    Demyelinating disorders

    Post-neurosurgical supratentorial procedure

*Metabolic abnormalities*

    Hyponatremia

    Hypocalcemia

    Hypophosphatemia

    Hypomagnesemia

    Hypoglycemia

    Nonketotic hyperosmolar hyperglycemia

    Renal failure

    Liver failure

    Vitamin deficiency (pyridoxine)

*Systemic infection/sepsis*

*Medications/drugs/toxins*

    Recreational drugs: cocaine, amphetamines, phencyclidine, heroin

    Antibiotics: beta-lactams (especially cefepime, ceftazidime, and imipenem), isoniazid (through pyridoxine deficiency)

    Antidepressants: bupropion

    Antipsychotics: clozapine, lithium

    Immunosuppressive drugs: cyclosporin A, tacrolimus

    Others: 4-aminopyridine, theophylline

*Alcohol withdrawal*

*Drug withdrawal*

    AEDs

    Benzodiazepines

    Barbiturates

*Chronic epilepsy*

ultimately be absent or limited to minor manifestations (see the following text).

> **⚠ CAUTION!**
>
> Almost half of patients that fail to regain consciousness after a treated episode of GCSE develop NCSE or NCSz.

Myoclonic seizures (MSz; epileptic myoclonus) and myoclonic status epilepticus (MSE) are characterized by bilateral myoclonic jerks affecting the face, the trunk, or the limbs. The jerks can be regular, symmetric, and synchronous, such as those that occur in anoxic brain injury, or multifocal, irregular, and sporadic, such as those that tend to occur in metabolic or toxic encephalopathy. The amplitude varies from very subtle to large. The differential diagnosis of epileptic myoclonus includes nonepileptic (subcortical and brainstem) myoclonus, which is also frequently encountered in acutely ill patients with multiple-drug regimens, anoxia, or metabolic imbalances. The differentiation can be difficult, especially in the absence of a clear EEG correlate to the jerks. As a rule, the presence of frequent myoclonic jerks with a nearly normal level of consciousness is incompatible with a diagnosis of MSE.

By definition, NCSz and NCSE have subtle or absent clinical manifestations. A thorough examination including careful observation of spontaneous eye and pupillary movements and of the face and limb extremities is needed. Seizures manifesting as pseudo-arousals, with eye opening and semi-purposeful movements, are not uncommon and are often overlooked (Figure 32.1). Autonomic dysfunction, including arrhythmias and blood pressure instability, is a possible manifestation.

The vast majority of seizures in critically ill patients are nonconvulsive. In fact, acute events with obvious clinical (mostly motor) manifestations are more likely to be nonepileptic and include clonus, tremor, shivering, nonepileptic myoclonus, and semi-purposeful movements.

## EEG in the management of seizures and status epilepticus in the ICU

EEG and continuous EEG (CEEG) monitoring are central to the diagnosis and treatment of seizure and SE, as recently stressed in the Neurocritical Care Society guidelines. Fifty percent of patients with NCSz will have their first seizure identified by a 1-h study, and 95% by a 24-h study. A longer duration of 48 or more hours is often needed in comatose patients and in patients with periodic discharges, as their first definite seizures are often delayed.

> **⚠ CAUTION!**
>
> Although GTCS and convulsive SE are easily recognized without EEG, most critically ill patients with seizures have only NCSz, which requires CEEG monitoring for detection.

The EEG during GTCS is usually difficult to interpret because of muscle artifact. When visible, the tonic phase is characterized by generalized, medium-high–voltage, approximately 10-Hz activity. This activity gradually slows as the clonic phase begins, becoming bursts of generalized polyspikes alternating with periods of attenuation. During the postictal period, the EEG shows generalized slowing and attenuation.

Several EEG patterns have been described in association with MSz and MSE. After anoxic brain injury, the EEG consists of generalized periodic discharges (GPDs) or a burst–suppression pattern, although sometimes there is no EEG correlate to post-anoxic myoclonus. The myoclonic jerks are usually synchronous with the GPDs or the bursts, and both increase with stimulation. In MSz and MSE of toxic and metabolic cause, jerks are often synchronous to multifocal spikes or spike-and-wave complexes.

The EEG patterns associated with NCSz and NCSE include a number of generalized and focal discharges. EEG criteria for definite NCSz have been published (see Table 32.2), but there are other patterns that can be seen in NCSz.

It is often difficult to distinguish ictal, interictal, and nonictal patterns in encephalopathic patients. Lateralized periodic discharges (LPDs; also known as periodic lateralized epileptiform discharges [PLEDs]) or GPDs are sometimes associated with clinical manifestations and in these cases have to be considered and treated as an ictal pattern. In most comatose patients, however, similar patterns lack any obvious clinical correlate, and it is impossible to infer their ictal nature. It is important to acknowledge this lack of certainty and avoid dogmatic and categorical views. We often refer to equivocal patterns as being on an interictal–ictal continuum, recognizing that they may

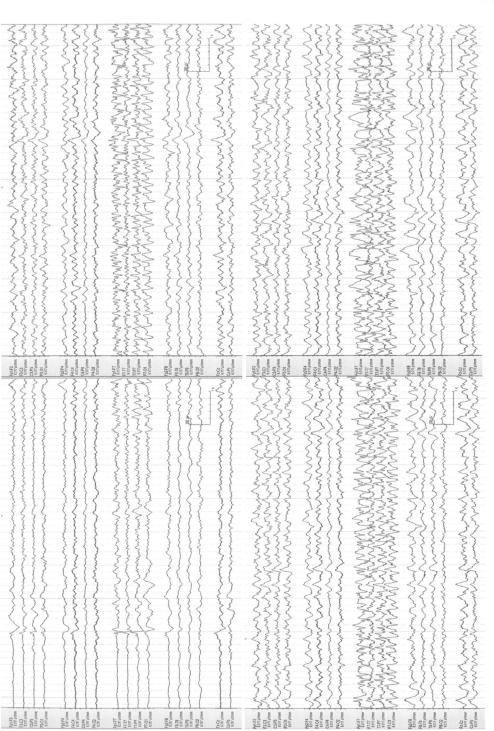

**Figure 32.1.** Left temporal seizure in a 22-year-old man with *Mycoplasma pneumoniae* infection-related refractory NCSE. Many seizures were purely electrographic. Some were accompanied by subtle manifestations, including pseudo-arousal, eye opening, and oral automatisms. NCSE was preceded by nonspecific prodromal symptoms (headache, low-grade fever, and photophobia) and a GTCS. He required sedation with anesthetic drugs (midazolam, propofol, ketamine, and finally pentobarbital) for about a month in addition to multiple AEDs. He had an excellent cognitive outcome (normal and high functioning) despite a prolonged course of SE. Consecutive pages of EEG are shown. High-pass filter is at 1 Hz, low-pass filter is at 70 Hz, and notch filter is off

**Table 32.2.** Criteria for the diagnosis of NCSz and NCSE.

Any pattern satisfying any of the primary criteria and lasting ≥10 s (for NCSz) or ≥30 min (for NCSE)

*Primary criteria*

1. Repetitive generalized or focal spikes, sharp waves, spike-and-wave complexes at ≥3/s
2. Repetitive generalized or focal spikes, sharp waves, spike-and-wave or sharp-and-slow wave complexes at <3/s and the secondary criterion
3. Sequential rhythmic, periodic, or quasiperiodic waves at ≥1/s and unequivocal evolution in frequency (gradually increasing or decreasing by at least 1/s, e.g., 2–3/s), morphology, or location (gradual spread into or out of a region involving at least two electrodes). Evolution in amplitude alone is not sufficient.

*Secondary criterion*

1. Significant improvement in clinical state or appearance of previously absent normal EEG patterns (such as posterior-dominant "alpha" rhythm) temporally coupled to acute administration of a rapidly acting AED. Resolution of the "epileptiform" discharges leaving diffuse slowing without clinical improvement and without appearance of previously absent normal EEG patterns would not satisfy the secondary criterion.

*Note*: These criteria are used for the diagnosis of definite NCSz, but there are many cases of NCSz that do not meet them; these criteria cannot be used to rule out NCSz/NCSE.
From Chong DJ, Hirsch LJ. Which EEG patterns warrant treatment in the critically ill? *J Clin Neurophysiol* 2005; **22**:79–91, with permission.

sometimes be ictal and sometimes not, even in the same individual at different times (Figure 32.2).

A useful approach in this situation is to perform a trial of a short-acting AED. An algorithm is proposed in Table 32.3. Concomitant electrographic and clinical improvement after administration of the drug strongly suggests the diagnosis of NCSE or NCSz. Absence of clinical improvement in the presence of electrographic improvement is inconclusive, as nonictal patterns, such as GPDs in the context of metabolic encephalopathy ("triphasic waves"), also respond to administration of benzodiazepines. The clinical improvement often lags behind EEG changes by hours (but usually <24 h). An important pitfall is that the administration of a sedative dose of benzodiazepine can blur the clinical improvement. Incremental administration of a small dose of a sedating drug (e.g., benzodiazepine) or use of a nonsedating drug is advised. The absence of EEG or clinical improvement does not exclude NCSz or NCSE, and the improvement in the EEG without clinical improvement does not help rule in or rule out NCSE.

## Other tests in the management of seizures and status epilepticus in the ICU

Given the previously mentioned limitations of the EEG in NCSE, we sometimes use imaging studies to help decide whether a pattern is likely ictal.

Prolonged seizures are associated with transient changes in MRI imaging, including increased signal in the cortex or hippocampus on T2-weighted, FLAIR, and diffusion-weighted sequences. Focal increase in brain perfusion or metabolism can also be demonstrated with perfusion CT, perfusion MRI, SPECT, or FDG-PET in the case of focal seizures or SE. Other changes can be identified with invasive brain monitoring such as cerebral microdialysis, although these techniques are not widely available and are not typically indicated.

## Treatment of seizures in the ICU

The treatment of seizures in critically ill patients is best initiated with an IV AED, which allows fast and reproducible loading. In the absence of published evidence or guidelines, the choice of treatment is mainly determined by the clinical situation, especially the presence of comorbidities and concerns about drug interactions and adverse effects (Chapters 18, 19, and 31). Fosphenytoin/phenytoin, valproate, levetiracetam, and lacosamide are all good choices. Several series have reported the safety and efficacy of all four medications, although no adequate comparative trial has been conducted. Plasma levels should be monitored, at least for valproate and phenytoin, including free phenytoin. It is probably better to

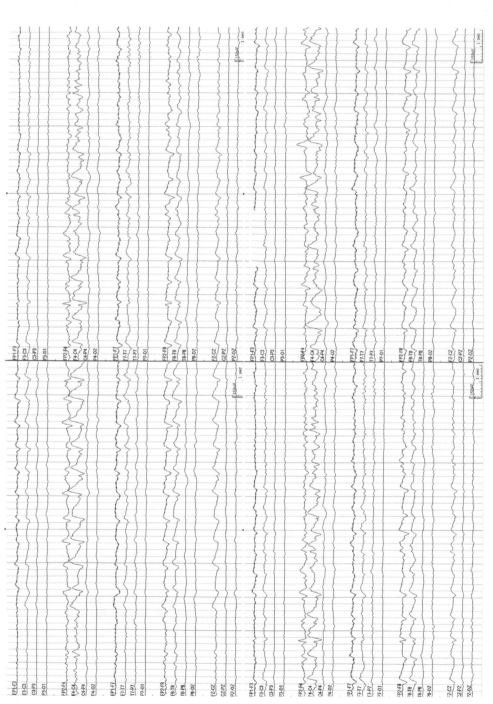

**Figure 32.2.** Right frontotemporal electrographic seizure in a 48-year-old man with traumatic brain injury and right hemispheric subdural hematoma. Despite drainage of the hematoma, the patient remained comatose. There were no clinical manifestations during the seizures, which consisted of rhythmic delta activity with superimposed fast frequencies, sometimes in a sharp-and-wave morphology. He was given AEDs, which led to immediate seizure control, and he progressively regained consciousness over the next 2 days. Electrographic *and* clinical improvement after treatment confirmed the condition's ictal nature. Four consecutive ~~pages~~ of EEG are shown. High-pass filter is at 1 Hz, low-pass filter is at 70 Hz, and notch filter is off.

**Table 32.3.** Antiepileptic drug trial for the diagnosis of NCSE.

*Indication*

- Rhythmic or periodic focal or generalized epileptiform discharges on EEG with neurological impairment

*Contraindication*

- Patients who are heavily sedated/paralyzed

*Monitoring*

- EEG, pulse oximetry, blood pressure, electrocardiography, respiratory rate with dedicated nurse

*AED trial*

- Sequential small doses of rapidly acting short-duration benzodiazepine such as midazolam at 1 mg or nonsedating IV AED such as levetiracetam, valproate, fosphenytoin, or lacosamide
- Between doses, repeated clinical and EEG assessment
- Trial is stopped after any of the following:
  - Persistent resolution of the EEG pattern (and examination repeated)
  - Definite clinical improvement
  - Respiratory depression, hypotension, or other adverse effect
  - A maximum dose is reached (such as 0.2 mg/kg midazolam, though higher may be needed if on chronic benzodiazepines)

The test is considered positive if there is resolution of the potentially ictal EEG pattern *and* either an improvement in the clinical state or the appearance of previously absent normal EEG patterns (e.g., posterior-dominant "alpha" rhythm). If EEG improves but patient does not, the result is equivocal.

*Note*: A negative or equivocal result does not rule out NCSE.
From Foreman B, Hirsch LJ. Epilepsy emergencies: Diagnosis and management. *Neurol Clin* 2011; **30**(1): 11–41, with permission.

divide the total daily dose into at least three administrations to favor stable plasma levels, especially for levetiracetam and lacosamide. Suggested doses, possible interactions, and adverse effects are summarized in Table 32.4. Adverse effects of IV valproate include hepatic toxicity, hyperammonemia (by functional impairment of the urea cycle), pancreatitis, thrombocytopenia, and platelet dysfunction. IV fosphenytoin/phenytoin should be administered under cardiovascular monitoring, given the risk of cardiac arrhythmia and hypotension. Potential hepatotoxicity is also a concern. Both levetiracetam and lacosamide have better safety and pharmacokinetic profiles and tend to be better choices in patients with significant comorbidities and multiple comedications. So far, they have not been proven to be superior to valproate or phenytoin, but small controlled trials indicate that levetiracetam used for the prophylaxis of seizures after traumatic brain injury (TBI) or subarachnoid hemorrhage (SAH) is associated with a similar efficacy and better tolerability than phenytoin.

**⚠ CAUTION!**

The use of valproate in children less than 2 years old is associated with a risk of hepatic toxicity and failure. Its use in this age group is not recommended.

It is important to recognize that the pharmacokinetics of many medications are significantly altered in critically ill patients. The stress response, increase in distribution volume, and compromised enteral absorption contribute to decreasing AED blood levels, while renal, hepatic, and cardiovascular failures contribute to their increase. Low plasma protein levels may also result in an increase in active, unbound ("free") levels of AED that are highly protein bound, such as phenytoin, valproic acid, most benzodiazepines (lorazepam having a lower bound fraction), propofol, and barbiturates. Hemodialysis and hemofiltration can remove AED from the circulating blood, especially hydrophilic

**Table 32.4.** Common agents used for the treatment of seizures and refractory SE in the ICU (see also Chapters 18 and 19).

| Drug | Loading dose | Maintenance dose | Level | Removed by dialysis | Interactions | Adverse reactions/ comments |
|---|---|---|---|---|---|---|
| *First-line treatment* | | | | | | |
| Lorazepam | 0.1 mg/kg up to 4 mg IV at 2 mg/min | N/A, repeat dose once if needed | N/A | No | — | |
| Midazolam | 0.2 mg/kg up to 10 mg IM, IN, or buccal | N/A, repeat dose once if needed | N/A | No | — | Sedation Respiratory depression |
| Diazepam | 0.2 mg/kg up to 20 mg PR (with PHT according to EFNS) | N/A, repeat dose once if needed | N/A | No | — | Hypotension |
| *Second-line treatment* | | | | | | |
| Phenytoin | 18–20 mg/kg IV up to 50 mg/min (25 mg/min in the elderly or patients with cardiovascular instability | 5–7 mg/kg/day PO/ IV, divided q 8h | Total: 15–20 µg/ mL Free: 1.5–2.5 µg/mL | <5% | Increases clearance of AEDs with hepatic elimination (CYP2B6, CYP2C9, and CYP3A4) | Cardiorespiratory depression Arrhythmia Hypotension Metabolic acidosis (PHT, diluted in propylene glycol) Infusion site injury (PHT) Nonallergic pruritus (FOS) |
| Fosphenytoin | 18–20 PE/kg IV up to 150 mg/min | 5–7 PE/kg/day PO/ IV divided q 8h | N/A | | | |
| Valproate | 20–40 mg/kg IV up to 3 mg/kg/min (probably safe up to 6 mg/kg/min) | 30–60 mg/kg/day, divided q 6h | 80–140 µg/mL | <20% | Displaces phenytoin from protein-binding sites | Hyperammonemia Thrombocytopenia Pancreatitis Hepatic toxicity in children <2 years |
| Levetiracetam | 2500–4000 mg IV up to 500 mg/min | 2–12 g/day PO/IV divided up to q 6h | 25–60 mg/L | 50% | — | No major adverse reaction |

| Drug | Loading dose | Maintenance dose | Level | Protein binding | Drug interactions | Adverse reactions |
|---|---|---|---|---|---|---|
| Lacosamide | 400 mg IV over 5 min | 400–600 mg/day IV divided q 12 h | Unknown | 50% | — | No major adverse reaction<br>May prolong PR interval |
| *Third-line treatment* | | | | | | |
| Phenobarbital | 20 mg/kg IV up to 60 mg/min | 1–4 mg/kg/day PO/IV divided q 6–8 h | 20–50 mg/mL | Yes | Increases clearance of AEDs with hepatic elimination (CYP2A6 and CYP3A4) | Sedation<br>Respiratory depression |
| Midazolam infusion | 0.2 mg/kg IV q 5 min until Sz control or maximum dose of 2 mg/kg | 0.1–2.9 mg/kg/h cIV | Titrate to desired level of EEG suppression | No | — | Sedation<br>Respiratory depression<br>Hypotension |
| Propofol infusion | 2 mg/kg IV q 5 min until Sz control or maximum dose of 10 mg/kg | 2–15 mg/kg/h cIV (limit to 5 mg/kg/h for treatment >48 h) | Titrate to desired level of EEG suppression | No | Potentiation of benzodiazepines | Sedation<br>Respiratory depression<br>Hypotension<br>Propofol infusion syndrome |
| Pentobarbital infusion | 5 mg/kg IV up to 50 mg/min q 5 min until Sz control | 1–10 mg/kg/h cIV | Titrate to desired level of EEG suppression | No | Increases clearance of AEDs with hepatic elimination (CYP2A6 and CYP3A4) | Sedation<br>Respiratory depression<br>Hypotension<br>Ileus, gastric stasis<br>Metabolic acidosis (diluted in propylene glycol)<br>Thrombocytopenia<br>Immunosuppression |
| *Alternative therapies* | | | | | | |
| Ketamine | 1.5 mg/kg IV q 5 min until Sz control or maximum dose of 4–5 mg/kg | 1.2–7.5 mg/kg/h cIV | Titrate to desired level of EEG suppression | Not known | Might potentiate GABA agonists | Hypertension<br>Possible rise in ICP |

(*Continued*)

**Table 32.4.** (*Continued*)

| Drug | Loading dose | Maintenance dose | Level | Removed by dialysis | Interactions | Adverse reactions/ comments |
|---|---|---|---|---|---|---|
| Topiramate | 100 mg q 12 h | 400–1600 mg/day PO divided q 6–8 h | Not known | Yes | Might potentiate GABA agonists<br><br>Weak CYP2C19 inhibitor and 3A4 inductor | Metabolic acidosis |
| Gabapentin | 300 mg q 8 h PO | 1800–3600 mg/day PO divided q 6–8 h | Not known | Yes | — | No major adverse reaction |
| Pregabalin | 75 mg q 12 h PO | 150–600 mg/day PO divided q 12 h | Not known | Yes | — | No major adverse reaction |
| Steroids | Methylprednisolone 1 g/ day during 3 days | 1 mg/kg/day and then taper | — | No | (−) Ketogenic diet | |
| IVIg | 0.4 g/kg/day for 5 days | No | — | No | — | |
| Plasmapheresis | 1 session qod for 5–7 days | Not known | — | — | Possible clearing of AEDs | |

FOS, fosphenytoin; PE, phenytoin equivalents; PHT, phenytoin; Sz, seizure.

drugs with a small protein-bound fraction, such as levetiracetam; in general, most AEDs (other than the highly protein-bound ones mentioned) will have about half of the drug cleared by these procedures, requiring supplemental doses afterwards. Finally, AED metabolism can be induced or inhibited by other medications, mainly but not only at the level of hepatic oxidation (the CYP proteins). Drug interactions are discussed further in Chapter 13.

There is no established strategy in case the first AED fails to control seizures. Switching to or adding a second AED are both acceptable options. In addition to starting an AED, the treatment of seizures should also include correction of metabolic factors that could contribute to lowering the seizure threshold, such as electrolytes or glucose imbalances, alkalosis, and renal and hepatic failure. Proconvulsive drugs and toxins (Table 32.1) should be avoided and even actively removed if possible.

---

### ☆ TIPS AND TRICKS

Although patients with early symptomatic seizures after acute brain injury carry a higher risk of developing epilepsy, most of them will not. There is thus no indication for long-term antiepileptic medication. No study has found that maintaining a patient on AEDs prevents development of epilepsy, but there are studies showing that the AEDs cause adverse effects and slow neurorehabilitation.

---

### Prevention of seizures in the ICU

Seizure prophylaxis with an AED should be reserved for selected populations of patients with acute brain injury (large or juxtacortical intracerebral hemorrhage, subarachnoid hemorrhage, and traumatic brain injury with parenchymal hematoma, cerebral contusion, or penetrating skull fracture). We do not usually recommend prophylaxis in other situations but strongly advise CEEG monitoring and initiation of treatment if seizures occur. There is no indication to pursue prophylactic AED for more than 1–2 weeks after the initial injury, except perhaps if high intracranial pressure persists and thus a seizure could be particularly harmful for the patient. Phenytoin, carbamazepine, and levetiracetam are all acceptable alternatives, although there is concern with side effects, allergies, and drug interactions with

phenytoin and carbamazepine, and carbamazepine is not available as an IV formulation. There is recent preliminary data that levetiracetam is not inferior to phenytoin for seizure prophylaxis and is better tolerated, although adverse behavioral effects are not unusual with levetiracetam.

### Management of refractory status epilepticus

Patients with GCSE that fail to respond to first- and second-line therapy should be admitted to an ICU with expertise in the treatment of refractory SE and access to CEEG. Chapter 31 provides an overview of treatment of SE. When SE is refractory, available guidelines for treatment advocate anesthetic agents. Three drugs are commonly used: pentobarbital (or thiopental, its prodrug, in Europe), propofol, and midazolam. All three have advantages and drawbacks, and it is still unclear if one of them is superior. Pentobarbital is usually very effective but is associated with a higher rate of adverse effects, especially prolonged cardiorespiratory depression. A concern with propofol is the risk of propofol-related infusion syndrome (PRIS).

---

### ✋ CAUTION!

The prolonged use (>48 h) of propofol at high dose (>5 mg/kg/h) increases the risk of developing PRIS, a rare but often lethal syndrome combining severe metabolic acidosis, arrhythmias, progressive cardiac failure and cardiovascular collapse, hyperlipemia, hepatomegaly, rhabdomyolysis, and acute renal failure. Concurrent use of catecholamines and steroids is a predisposing factor. Children are more susceptible to developing PRIS. Inadequate carbohydrate intake, such as that required by the ketogenic diet, also can precipitate the syndrome.

---

Treatment with anesthetic drugs should be performed under CEEG monitoring to adjust doses to the desired level of sedation and detect breakthrough and withdrawal seizures. Possible goals are seizure suppression or burst–suppression. Compared to seizure suppression, burst–suppression is associated with a lower (but not null) rate of breakthrough and withdrawal seizures and a higher rate of complications. There is no proven advantage for burst–suppression. With either goal, EEG should be monitored continuously for resurgence of ictal activity; seizures can arise out of burst-suppression and even from complete suppression. Current guidelines recommend maintaining sedation for at least 24 h without seizures detected and then slowly withdrawing the anesthetics over 24 h. Breakthrough seizures are managed by administering a new bolus and increasing the infusion rate (usually by 20%). In the case of withdrawal seizures, the sedative drug should be restarted at the maximal dose at which it was previously administered and continued for 24–48 h before attempting to taper it again. Switching to another sedative drug is a possible alternative. Pressors are often necessary during treatment of refractory SE.

If hypotension is a limiting factor, ketamine appears to be a good option. It acts mainly on the glutamate NMDA receptor and does not have significant cardiocirculatory depressant effects. On the contrary, it tends to elevate blood pressure. Although very little information about ketamine is available, it is fairly commonly used at some centers as an add-on sedative when further hypotension is not desirable. It should be used with caution in patients with known intracranial hypertension, as it has been associated with elevations in intracranial pressure.

---

### ⚗ SCIENCE REVISITED

In animal models, prolonged ictal activity is associated with acute and chronic molecular and cellular changes. In the acute phase or initiation phase, SE is sensitive to GABA agonists. However, internalization of GABA receptors starts to occur as early as 5 min after onset, while NMDA receptors are progressively overexpressed. This leads to a second, or maintenance, phase with distinct pharmacological sensitivity: GABA agonists are no longer effective, while NMDA antagonists, initially not efficient, become effective. The production, secretion, and response to various neuropeptides are also modified by prolonged ictal activity. Some of these changes may have potential therapeutic implications.

Finally, neuronal cell death, axonal and dendritic sprouting, and synaptogenesis have all been well documented after experimental SE. These cause a profound reorganization in neuronal networks that may play a major role in secondary epileptogenesis.

---

Refractory SE that fails to permanently respond to a course of anesthetic drugs has been termed malignant or super-refractory SE. Its treatment is extremely difficult and usually consists of a combination of AED and anesthetic drugs. In this setting, an immune etiology is often suspected, and treatment with AED is also often combined with immune modulators. There is no evidence or guidelines available, although many options have been proposed in small uncontrolled case series.

Recent years have seen the recognition of antibody-mediated forms of encephalitis manifesting as refractory seizures and SE, mainly the anti-NMDA and anti-voltage-gated potassium channel complex (anti-VGKCC, usually anti-LGI-1) syndromes. The anti-NMDA syndrome occurs more frequently in young women and adolescents. Behavioral and psychiatric symptoms often precede the seizures, which can be focal or generalized and evolve to SE. The encephalitis frequently evolves to coma and is associated with central respiratory failure, hemodynamic instability, and stereotypic orofacial dyskinesias. In half of cases, the EEG shows an unusual pattern of high-amplitude delta waves with superimposed beta activity, called "extreme delta brushes." About half of cases are paraneoplastic, typically associated with ovarian teratomas. The anti-VGKCC syndrome causes a more typical limbic encephalitis, which includes memory and other cognitive and behavioral changes in addition to seizures, and predominantly affects individuals over 50. The encephalitis is frequently preceded by potentially pathognomonic faciobrachial dystonic seizures, very brief spells that can mimic myoclonus or tics. Hyponatremia is another diagnostic clue. The syndrome is typically autoimmune and not associated with malignancy (especially when faciobrachial dystonic seizures are seen), but it can be associated with small-cell lung carcinoma, thymoma, or other neoplasms. In both syndromes, detecting antibodies in the serum or CSF confirms the diagnosis. Also, some may respond spectacularly to immune therapies. Steroids, immune globulins, plasma exchanges, rituximab, and cyclophosphamide have been used successfully.

The therapeutic approach to refractory NCSE significantly differs from the approach to refractory GCSE. NCSE carries a lower risk of severe systemic complications and a lower mortality rate. Aggressive treatment with sedative agents should be postponed, and sequential or additive trials of nonsedative AED should be attempted first. Older and newer AEDs are acceptable options, including AED with enteral administration (see Table 32.4). Their use, however, is supported only by small retrospective case series.

## Outcome

The outcome of seizures and SE in critically ill patients is determined primarily by their etiology. Age, longer duration of SE, subtle SE after GCSE, female sex, and a higher Acute Physiological and Chronic Health Evaluation (APACHE) score and comorbidity index are negative prognostic factors.

Between 25% and 50% of patients who survive an episode of SE will develop significant functional or cognitive disability. NCSz may also affect outcome after brain injury. They have been associated with increased cerebral blood flow and oxygen consumption, increased heart rate and blood pressure, hematoma expansion and midline shift after intracerebral hemorrhage, and increased intracranial pressure and metabolic demand after traumatic brain injury.

## Conclusions

The diagnosis and treatment of seizures and SE in the ICU remains a challenge. A high level of suspicion, careful examination, and the systematic use of CEEG in selected populations at risk are required to detect NCSz and NCSE, which represent the vast majority of seizures in this setting. Signs of NCSE and NCSz on the EEG are often difficult to distinguish from abnormal non-ictal patterns that characterize the acutely injured brain. The use of simple criteria or a trial of short-acting AED can sometimes clarify the situation. However, standardization and better characterization of EEG abnormalities seen in the critically ill are needed, as is a better understanding of their physiological implications. The use of invasive monitoring and of perfusion and metabolic imaging may advance our understanding.

Treatment options for refractory SE need to be studied in prospective controlled trials. In the meantime, guidelines recommend the use of anesthetic drugs and also advocate the need for CEEG to best manage those difficult cases. The treatment of NCSz and NCSE in critically ill patients also needs to be better studied.

## Bibliography

Alvarez V, Januel JM, Burnand B, Rossetti AO. Second-line status epilepticus treatment: Comparison of phenytoin, valproate, and levetiracetam. *Epilepsia* 2011; **52**(7):1292–1296.

Brophy GM, Bell R, Claassen J, et al. Guidelines for the evaluation and management of status epilepticus. *Neurocrit Care* 2012; **17**:3–23.

Chong DJ, Hirsch LJ. Which EEG patterns warrant treatment in the critically ill? Reviewing the evidence for treatment of periodic epileptiform discharges and related patterns. *J Clin Neurophysiol* 2005; **22**:79–91.

Claassen J, Mayer SA, Kowalski RG, Emerson RG, Hirsch LJ. Detection of electrographic seizures with continuous EEG monitoring in critically ill patients. *Neurology* 2004; **62**:1743–1748.

Claassen J, Perotte A, Albers D, et al. Nonconvulsive seizures after subarachnoid hemorrhage: Multimodal detection and outcomes. Annals of neurology. 2013; **74**(1):53–64.

Foreman B, Hirsch LJ. Epilepsy emergencies: Diagnosis and management. *Neurol Clin* 2011; **30**(1):11–41.

Foreman B, Claassen J, Abou Khaled K, et al. Generalized periodic discharges in the critically ill: A case–control study of 200 patients. *Neurology* 2012; **79**:1951–1960.

Mayer SA, Claassen J, Lokin J, Mendelsohn F, Dennis LJ, Fitzsimmons BF. Refractory status epilepticus: Frequency, risk factors, and impact on outcome. *Arch Neurol* 2002; **59**:205–210.

Meierkord H, Boon P, Engelsen B, et al. EFNS guideline on the management of status epilepticus in adults. *Eur J Neurol* 2010; **17**:348–355.

Vespa PM, O'Phelan K, Shah M, et al. Acute seizures after intracerebral hemorrhage: A factor in progressive midline shift and outcome. *Neurology* 2003; **60**(9):1441–1446.

Vespa PM, Miller C, McArthur D, et al. Nonconvulsive electrographic seizures after traumatic brain injury result in a delayed, prolonged increase in intracranial pressure and metabolic crisis. *Crit Care Med* 2007; **35**(12):2830–2836.

# Part VIII

# The Morbidity and Mortality of Epilepsy

# Mortality in Epilepsy

**Elizabeth J. Donner**

Division of Neurology, Department of Paediatrics, The Hospital for Sick Children
University of Toronto, Toronto, Ontario, Canada

## Introduction

Although most people with epilepsy live long lives, their risk of a premature death is increased compared to that of the general population. Both the Joint American Epilepsy Society/Epilepsy Foundation Task Force and the UK National Institute of Clinical Excellence Guidelines recommend that physicians discuss the risk of premature mortality with people with epilepsy as part of the delivery of comprehensive epilepsy education. A critical review of the relevant literature, including population-based studies and reports on epilepsy subgroups, is necessary to inform discussions of mortality with patients and their families.

> ⭐ **TIPS AND TRICKS**
>
> Despite the apprehension physicians feel about discussing mortality with their patients, people with epilepsy and their families report that they want to discuss mortality, especially the difficult issue of sudden unexpected death in epilepsy (SUDEP), with their physicians. There are several opportunities to discuss mortality and SUDEP in the course of epilepsy care. For example, upon witnessing a seizure, family members often wonder whether a seizure may be fatal, and they may initiate the conversation. A simple message can be used: Although people with epilepsy are at an increased risk of premature death, the best way to reduce that risk is to work with the healthcare team to reduce seizures.

## People with epilepsy have a two to three times increased risk of premature death

Population-based studies have demonstrated that people with epilepsy have a two to three times increased risk of premature death compared with that of the general population. A UK study that followed more than 1000 people for a median followup of greater than 20 years calculated an overall standardized mortality ratio (SMR) of 2.2. A similar study evaluated risk in people with chronic epilepsy of at least 4 years' duration and those with newly diagnosed epilepsy. In that study, the SMR was 3.1 for the chronic epilepsy group and 2.6 for the new-onset epilepsy group.

Standard mortality ratios are significantly higher for children than for adults with epilepsy, ranging from 5.3 to 9.0. The higher rate reflects the high mortality

*Epilepsy*, First Edition. Edited by John W. Miller and Howard P. Goodkin.

among children with significant neurological impairment as well as the overall lower mortality rate among children in the general population.

---

### 🔬 SCIENCE REVISITED

Study design determines how mortality is measured and reported. Population-based studies aim to include all people with epilepsy in a defined geographic area. These studies compare the rate of death among people with epilepsy to the rate of death in the general population as a *standardized mortality ratio* (SMR). The SMR is the ratio of observed deaths in the study population to expected deaths among people of the same age and sex in the general population. When there is no increased rate of death compared to the general population, the SMR equals one. It is only possible to calculate an SMR if there is available information about a reference population.

Cohort studies often report *case fatality rates* that describe the rate of death in a specific group. For example, a study may report a 12% case fatality among 120 adults who presented with status epilepticus, which means that 12% of the subjects died. Many studies report rates of death in *person-years*. One person-year is equal to one person living with epilepsy for 1 year. For example, the rate of SUDEP is estimated to be 1 in 1000 person-years. This means that if we follow 1000 people with epilepsy for 1 year, one will die of SUDEP.

---

Another way to describe premature mortality is to consider the life expectancy of people with epilepsy compared to that of people of the same age and sex in the general population. The life expectancy of people with idiopathic epilepsy is possibly reduced by up to 2 years, and the life expectancy of people with a symptomatic epilepsy can be reduced by as much as 10 years. Reduction in life expectancy declines over the duration of epilepsy. The longer a person survives with epilepsy, the higher the likelihood of survival.

In resource-poor areas of the world, the SMRs for people with epilepsy are even higher. For example, a study from rural China determined an SMR of 4.92, significantly higher than the SMR for epilepsy in European and North American studies. In the rural Chinese cohort, drowning was the leading cause of death.

## Risk factors for mortality in epilepsy

The strongest predictor of mortality in people with epilepsy is seizure etiology. Most of the increased risk of death in people with epilepsy is attributable to the inclusion of those with a secondary or symptomatic epilepsy (Table 33.1).

There is conflicting evidence on the risk of premature mortality in people with idiopathic epilepsy, as some studies have failed to demonstrate an increase in risk. Mortality risk in idiopathic epilepsy may occur later, as demonstrated by a large UK cohort in which followup at 14 years did not demonstrate an elevated SMR; however, when followup was extended up to 25 years, the SMR was elevated.

Beyond symptomatic etiology, the strongest risk factor for premature mortality is ongoing, persistent, poorly controlled seizures. Failure to obtain 5-year seizure remission was found to be the strongest risk factor for death by any cause in a long-term follow-up study of childhood-onset epilepsy. Younger age and recent diagnosis of epilepsy also increase risk. Nonadherence to antiepileptic drug (AED) therapy has been shown to be a significant risk factor, with an over three times increased risk of mortality.

Many other factors have been studied with conflicting results. Several reports suggest that males are at greater risk. In addition, generalized tonic–clonic seizures may increase risk; however, complex partial and myoclonic seizures have also been shown to increase risk, which is likely related to their underlying causes. Many factors that are associated with symptomatic epilepsy, such as cognitive impairment or developmental delay, and an abnormal neurological examination have also been found to increase mortality risk

---

### ★ TIPS AND TRICKS

For individuals with drug-resistant or surgically amenable epilepsy, surgical referral provides an opportunity to discuss mortality risk. Some studies have indicated that successful epilepsy surgery reduces mortality.

---

**Table 33.1.** Risk factors for mortality in epilepsy.

| Most important factors for mortality in epilepsy |
| --- |
| Symptomatic epilepsy |
| Persistent seizures |
| Poor adherence to AED therapy |

## Causes of death in epilepsy

The cause of death in a person having epilepsy may or may not be related to the epilepsy. Population-based studies have reported that people with epilepsy are at an increased risk of death due to cardiovascular disease, pneumonia, and cancer. Accidents and trauma also account for a significant proportion of deaths in this population. Suicide is an important concern given the high rates of psychiatric comorbidities, and people with epilepsy do have an increased risk of suicide. In children, most nonepilepsy-related deaths are due to respiratory complications associated with significant neurological impairment.

---

### ☝ CAUTION!

People with epilepsy have higher rates of anxiety and mood disorders, increasing the risk for suicide. Reports indicate that people with epilepsy have a two to three times increased risk of suicide. Certain anticonvulsant medications may also trigger or exacerbate mood and anxiety disorders in susceptible individuals. As such, it is imperative that healthcare practitioners assess people with epilepsy for suicidal ideation. Screening tools for suicidality are available for easy use in the ambulatory care setting.

---

Epilepsy-related deaths include those due to the underlying cause of the epilepsy and deaths directly due to a seizure. Deaths due directly to seizures and epilepsy include status epilepticus, accidents, and drowning due to a seizure, as well as SUDEP. The incidence of epilepsy-related deaths in a cohort of adults and children with newly diagnosed epilepsy followed for 40 years was found to be 6.8 per 1000 person-years within the first 2 years of diagnosis. The incidence of epilepsy-related deaths fell to 3.1 per 1000 person-years 2 years after diagnosis.

## Status epilepticus

A single, brief, self-limited seizure is rarely fatal; however, status epilepticus may be. Cohort studies of status epilepticus report case fatality rates between 10% and 30%, typically measured 30 days after onset. Most deaths occur in adults with acute symptomatic status epilepticus in the context of disorders such as anoxic encephalopathy and stroke. An age above 60 years is associated with significantly increased mortality from status epilepticus. In children, it is seldom fatal; studies report case fatality rates from 0% to 5%. In contrast to early mortality rates, long-term death rates are not increased with a past history of status epilepticus in adults or children with epilepsy.

## Sudden unexpected death in epilepsy

Although mortality in epilepsy may often be explained by an underlying condition, a proportion of deaths in people with epilepsy remain unexplained by circumstances and autopsy. Sudden death is nearly 24 times more likely in people with epilepsy than in the general population. The entity known as SUDEP is defined as a sudden, unexpected, witnessed or unwitnessed, nontraumatic, and non-drowning death in a patient with epilepsy, with or without evidence of a seizure and excluding documented status epilepticus. To meet criteria for SUDEP, postmortem examination should not reveal a toxicologic or anatomic cause of death (Table 33.2). The term *probable SUDEP* is used for cases that meet all criteria but for which no postmortem examination is available.

The overall risk of SUDEP is estimated to be 1 per 1000 person-years. Rates can be almost 10-fold higher, nearly 1 per 100 person-years, in populations with drug-resistant epilepsy. SUDEP occurs less frequently in childhood; reported rates of SUDEP in children range from 0.2 to 0.4 per 1000 person-years. There are several factors that may contribute to the lower rates of SUDEP in childhood, including a shorter duration of epilepsy and enhanced nocturnal supervision.

**Table 33.2.** Criteria for definite SUDEP.

| SUDEP |
|---|
| Deceased had epilepsy, defined as recurrent unprovoked seizures |
| Death was unexpected |
| Death occurred suddenly in benign circumstances |
| Death was not a consequences of trauma, drowning, or documented status epilepticus |
| Death may be witnessed or unwitnessed |
| Evidence of preceding seizure is not required |
| Postmortem examination does not reveal a cause of death |

In most cases of SUDEP, the deceased is found in the morning dead in bed, typically in the prone position. Although only a minority of deaths have been witnessed, in 50–90% of cases, there is evidence of a convulsive seizure, such as the presence of a tongue laceration, vomit, or disruption of the bed sheets. It should be noted that the presence of a seizure is not required to meet criteria for SUDEP, and there are documented witnessed cases in which a convulsive seizure was not seen. In a report of 10 witnessed cases of SUDEP in children, only five had a convulsive seizure at the time of death.

Several risk factors for SUDEP have been identified. A combined analysis of four case–control studies included 289 cases of definite or probable SUDEP and 958 living controls. Frequent generalized tonic–clonic seizures were found to be the strongest risk factors for SUDEP. Other identified risk factors included drug resistance, symptomatic epilepsy, younger age of epilepsy onset, longer duration of epilepsy, and male gender.

Early studies suggested a possible role of AEDs in SUDEP. However, the combined analysis demonstrated that when seizure frequency is considered, neither polytherapy nor any single AED is associated with an increased risk of SUDEP. Furthermore, a meta-analysis of 112 randomized AED placebo-controlled trials compared the rate of SUDEP among people receiving an add-on AED to that of those who received a placebo. The rate of SUDEP for adults receiving an add-on AED at the appropriate dose was 0.9 per 1000 people per year, while the rate of SUDEP for adults receiving an add-on placebo was 6.9 per 1000 people per year, suggesting that appropriate use of AED may decrease the risk of SUDEP.

Nocturnal seizures have also been identified as a significant risk factor for SUDEP. This risk is of particular interest, as there has been some evidence that increased nocturnal surveillance in the form of frequent nocturnal checks or the use of an auditory device may reduce SUDEP risk. More work is needed to evaluate the role of enhanced surveillance in SUDEP prevention before recommendations can be made to people with epilepsy and their families.

---

★ TIPS AND TRICKS

Given that young adults are at the highest risk of SUDEP, many practitioners choose to counsel young adults about the importance of AED

---

adherence and the avoidance of seizure triggers in reducing their risk at the time they leave the family home. People with epilepsy will learn about SUDEP and other risks of epilepsy as they seek out information about their disorder. The best way to ensure people with epilepsy have reliable, evidence-based information is to take the time to give them the facts.

## Conclusion

Physicians are often reluctant to consider the risk of mortality in people with epilepsy or discuss this risk with their patients because they perceive that little can be done to alter that risk. It is important to recognize that persistent ongoing seizures and poor adherence to AED therapy are strong risk factors for premature mortality. Comprehensive epilepsy care, including optimized medical management, early identification of drug-resistant epilepsy, and referral for surgical evaluation, is a critical step in lessening the extensive burden of seizures. The goal of seizure freedom should be regarded as an integral part of mortality risk reduction.

## Bibliography

Berg AT, Shinnar S, Testa FM, Levy SR, Smith SN, Beckerman B. Mortality in childhood-onset epilepsy. *Arch Pediatr Adolesc Med* 2004; **158**(12): 1147–1152.

Devinsky O. Sudden, unexpected death in epilepsy. *N Engl J Med* 2011; **365**(19):1801–1811.

Faught E, Duh MS, Weiner JR, Guérin A, Cunnington MC. Nonadherence to antiepileptic drugs and increased mortality. *Neurology* 2008; **71**:1572–1578.

Hesdorffer DC, Tomson T, Benn E, et al. Combined analysis of risk factors for SUDEP. *Epilepsia* 2010; **52**(6):1150–1159.

Hesdorffer DC, Tomson T, Benn E, et al. Do antiepileptic drugs or generalized tonic-clonic seizure frequency increase SUDEP risk? A combined analysis. *Epilepsia* 2012; **53**(2):249–252.

Lamberts RJ, Thijs RD, Laffan A, Langan Y, Sander JW. Sudden unexpected death in epilepsy: People with nocturnal seizures may be at highest risk. *Epilepsia* 2012; **53**(2):253–257.

Mu J, Liu L, Zhang Q, et al. Causes of death among people with convulsive epilepsy in rural West China: A prospective study. *Neurology* 2011; **77**(2):132–137.

Nashef L, So EL, Ryvlin P, Tomson T. Unifying the definitions of sudden unexpected death in epilepsy. *Epilepsia* **53**(2):227–233.

Neligan A, Shorvon SD. Prognostic factors, morbidity and mortality in tonic-clonic status epilepticus: A review. *Epilepsy Res* 2011; **93**(1): 1–10.

Neligan A, Bell GS, Johnson AL, Goodridge DM, Shorvon SD, Sander JW. The long-term risk of premature mortality in people with epilepsy. *Brain* 2011; **134**(Pt 2):388–395.

Nickels KC, Grossardt BR, Wirrell EC, Epilepsy-related mortality is low in children: A 30-year population-based study in Olmsted County, MN. *Epilepsia* 2012; **53**(12):2164–2171.

Rakitin A, Liik M, Oun A, Haldre S. Mortality risk in adults with newly diagnosed and chronic epilepsy: A population-based study. *Eur J Neurol*, 2010:**18**(3):465–470.

Sillanpää M, Shinnar S. Long-term mortality in childhood-onset epilepsy. *New Engl J Med* 2010; **363**(26):2522–2529.

Trinka E, Bauer G, Oberaigner W, Ndayisaba JP, Seppi K, Granbichler CA. Cause-specific mortality among patients with epilepsy: Results from a 30-year cohort study. *Epilepsia* 2013; **54**(3):495–501.

# Accidents in Epilepsy

**Allan Krumholz and Ana M. Sanchez**

Department of Neurology, Maryland Epilepsy Center, University of Maryland Medical Center, University of Maryland School of Medicine, Baltimore, MD, USA

## Introduction

Individual seizures usually are not very dangerous, but their unpredictability makes them increase the risk for accidents and injuries. This risk for accidents is the major reason for the many restrictions and limitations placed on people with seizures, the basis of much of the disability associated with epilepsy, and the cause of some of the adverse psychosocial consequences of epilepsy. Therefore, it is important for healthcare providers to carefully consider how best to manage epilepsy patients to ensure that they are optimally protected but their life activities are not unnecessarily limited. Indeed, people with epilepsy themselves note that many activities limited by accident risk, such as driving and employment, are among their major concerns (Figure 34.1).

## Epidemiology

Accidents are unexpected and unintended events leading to injury or death and are more common among individuals with epilepsy. Here we address nonfatal accidents and injuries, as Chapter 33 addresses mortality in epilepsy.

---

**EVIDENCE AT A GLANCE**

One large European prospective cohort study of children (over 5 years of age) and adults found that the risk for an accident at 12 months was 17% in individuals with epilepsy compared to 12% in controls, a significant difference. By 24 months, 27% had accidents compared to 17% of controls, again a significant difference. However, if one excluded accidents caused by seizures, the accident risk for people with epilepsy and controls was similar. Most accidents were minor, consisting of contusions and superficial wounds, but people with epilepsy had higher hospitalization rates.

---

Comorbid conditions may increase risk for accidents and injuries in adults and children with epilepsy. Individuals with epilepsy have a higher incidence of cognitive and motor impairment that may predispose them to accidents. For example, those with posttraumatic epilepsy may be prone to additional accident and injury. Other factors influencing accident risk are sedating and cognitive side effects of antiepileptic medications.

### Types of accidents and injuries

#### Burns

Individuals with epilepsy experience a higher rate of burn injuries. As many as 16% report suffering a seizure-related burn. Burns are more likely to occur

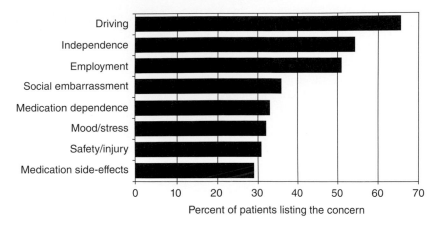

**Figure 34.1.** Concerns noted by patients with epilepsy. From Gilliam F, Kuzniecky R, Faught E, et al. Patient-validated content of epilepsy-specific quality-of-life measurement. *Epilepsia* 1997; **38**:233–236, with permission.

with complex partial seizures as opposed to generalized tonic–clonic seizures, with scald and contact burns (e.g., from a bath or iron) being the more common types. In cultures where open fires are used for cooking, burns associated with seizures are a common presentation of epilepsy.

### Falls and head injuries

It is reported that 45% of seizures are associated with a fall, which may then lead to head injury. The risk of head injury is higher with generalized tonic–clonic or myoclonic seizures. The most common seizure-related head injury is a concussion, accounting for 10% of injuries in people with epilepsy. Only a minority of head injuries are severe, causing intracranial bleeding or skull fracture.

### Drowning

Seizures pose a clear risk when individuals are in or near water, and people with epilepsy have a substantially higher risk of submersion injuries and drowning. In one retrospective study, 14% of adults with epilepsy reported a seizure while bathing or swimming. Submersion is more likely to be fatal than other accidents in children and adults with epilepsy. Most submersions occur in the bathtub or swimming pool, with most deaths occurring when a person with epilepsy is not properly monitored.

### Fractures

Fractures account for 11% of injuries in people with epilepsy. Although older antiepileptic medications

such as phenytoin, carbamazepine, phenobarbital, valproate, and primidone can decrease bone mineral density, there are not enough data to conclude that the increased risk of fracture is associated with specific drugs.

### Dental injury

Ten percent of people with epilepsy report a seizure-related dental injury. This is usually associated with falls and consists of losing teeth or fracturing the jaw.

### Soft tissue injury

Contusions, wounds, and abrasions are the most common injuries seen with seizures. These soft tissue injuries account for as much as 25% of seizure-related injuries. A retrospective study of children showed that scalp and facial bruises were the most common seizure-related injuries.

### Motor vehicle crashes

People with epilepsy have a nearly twofold increased risk for crashing, but that is for crashes of all causes, rather than just seizure-related ones. In fact, only 11% of all car crashes involving individuals with epilepsy are caused by seizures. Most result instead from the same cause of most crashes in the general population—namely, driver error. Studies of large populations confirm that the risk of crashing for individuals with epilepsy is not substantially higher than it is for other individuals who are not as strictly regulated, such as those with similar chronic medical conditions, including diabetes or hypertension, or certain higher-risk drivers, such as young males. Furthermore, the risk of motor vehicle crashes for individuals with epilepsy is far less than the risk of crashes related to alcohol. While a seizure during driving is dangerous, the risk of this happening is relatively limited and somewhat predictable, depending on how long an individual has been seizure-free.

## Work injuries

Employment is a major concern for people with epilepsy. Surveys indicate that epilepsy is the medical disability viewed least favorably by prospective employers. Accident risk is a major consideration. Unemployment rates for people with epilepsy in the USA vary from 12% to 50%, depending on epilepsy type and associated medical, psychological, and social issues. Misconceptions about epilepsy contribute to these employment problems. Most people with epilepsy are actually capable of functioning at a high level, and accident and absence rates of workers with epilepsy are not higher than those of other employees. Current social and legal trends are combating discrimination against people with medical disabilities such as epilepsy to bring down barriers to employment.

## Safety and prevention

### Driving

Every US state permits those with controlled seizures to drive. The person with epilepsy is legally obligated to report his or her condition to the Department of Motor Vehicles. Physicians are required to report that a person has epilepsy only in a minority of states. Specific standards are available online (www.epilepsyfoundation.org). In general, states limit driving for those at greatest risk for seizures while driving. The standard for determining that risk is the duration of time a person with epilepsy has had no seizures, with the accepted period varying from 3 to 12 months, depending on individual US state rules. Emphasis on the seizure-free interval is widely supported, with a 3-month seizure-free interval recommended in a consensus statement from the American Academy of Neurology, the American Epilepsy Society, and the Epilepsy Foundation. Several favorable and unfavorable modifiers were proposed to modify the duration of the required seizure-free interval for driving with epilepsy (Table 34.1).

**Table 34.1.** AAN, AES, EF consensus on driving and epilepsy.

| General principles: |
|---|
| • A seizure-free interval should be stated: 3 months is preferred |
| • Both favorable and unfavorable modifiers could alter this interval (individualized determinations) |
| • Physicians should not be required to report patients to the DMV (physician immunity) |
| • Patients should be responsible for self-reporting |

| *Favorable modifiers:* |
|---|
| • Seizures during medically directed medication change |
| • Seizures related to a reversible acute illness |
| • Simple partial seizures that do not interfere with consciousness or motor function |
| • Seizures with persistent prolonged auras |
| • Purely nocturnal seizures |
| • Sleep-deprived seizures |

| *Unfavorable modifiers:* |
|---|
| • Noncompliance with medication, medical visits, and/or lack of credibility |
| • Recent alcohol or drug abuse |
| • Prior bad driving record |
| • Prior crashes due to seizures |
| • Frequent seizures after seizure-free interval |

Source: Anonymous. Consensus statements, sample statutory provisions, and model regulations regarding driver licensing and epilepsy. American Academy of Neurology. American Epilepsy Society, Epilepsy Foundation of America. *Epilepsia* 1994; **35**:696–705.

### Work

Most jobs are suitable for people with epilepsy. Most categorical prohibitions should be avoided and are usually not legal in the USA, although a small number of jobs require them (Table 34.2). When medical advice is sought regarding the suitability of particular jobs for people with epilepsy, the response should take into account the job requirements and that individual's seizure history. For jobs with a high physical risk to the worker or others, the details of the work should be examined to reduce this danger to an acceptable level. Only when such risk reduction cannot be achieved are restrictions on the employment justified and potentially legal.

**Table 34.2.** Jobs and careers for which epilepsy-specific standards and rules or restrictions exist.

| |
|---|
| Commercial driving (especially for interstate commerce) |
| Airplane pilots |
| Bus drivers |
| Military service |
| Law enforcement officers (varies by state) |

The Americans with Disabilities Act (ADA) specifically prohibits exclusion of qualified people with epilepsy from employment opportunities unless they are actually unable to perform the job. Consequently, categorical prohibitions on employment of people with epilepsy in any capacity, previously widespread, are now illegal for most employers.

After someone with active seizures begins work, it may be advisable for that person to inform selected coworkers of the problem so that panic and other inappropriate responses to seizures are avoided. When seizures are likely in the workplace, education of coworkers and supervisors may help avoid or deal with misunderstandings. The Epilepsy Foundation has specific resources to help with employment and legal support.

### Sports and recreation

Individuals with epilepsy should be able to participate in most types of sports. Yet some sports may require additional safety precautions. Organized sports are to be encouraged, and there is no evidence that contact sports worsen seizure frequency. Reasonable supervision is required for swimming, and additional safety measures may be considered for sports such as rock climbing, gymnastics, or horseback riding. Relatively few sports are discouraged in people with epilepsy. The list of discouraged sports includes such activities as sky diving, rock climbing without a harness, and scuba diving, because a seizure in those situations would be particularly dangerous.

### Home

A person with epilepsy may modify the home to improve safety without sacrificing independence or privacy. To avoid burns, the microwave oven may be used preferentially over the stove. If the stove must be used, then the back burner is preferable. In the bathroom, while showers are safer than baths, one should ensure that drains work. In regard to burns and scalding, there are safety devices to control water temperature. Ladders and some power tools should be avoided by individuals at risk for seizures.

**⚠ CAUTION!**

Because of the risk of drowning in the event of a seizure, a person with epilepsy should be counseled to take showers instead of baths and leave the door unlocked.

### Child care (new parents)

New parents with epilepsy may have increased seizure frequency due to sleep deprivation. Mothers or fathers with epilepsy may be understandably anxious about having a seizure when alone and caring for the young child. Steps to improve safety include using an infant seat or chair for feedings, not allowing babies to sleep in the bed with the parent, changing diapers on the floor as opposed to a table, giving the baby sponge baths on the floor with a separate bowl of water, using an umbrella stroller to limit the time spent carrying the baby around the house, and creating a fenced play area where the child will stay safe if the parent has a seizure. Importantly, new parents with epilepsy should enlist the help of others in caring for an infant or toddler.

**★ TIPS AND TRICKS**

*Medication compliance*: Improving medication compliance can improve seizure control and thereby decrease risk of seizure-related injury. Ensuring medication compliance is particularly challenging for individuals with mental handicaps and may require assistance of family and friends as well as written or electronic reminders.
*Alarms*: Seizure alarms, medical alert systems, and medical bracelets may improve safety. "Seizure dogs" are specifically trained to respond to a seizure by barking or otherwise alerting that a person is having a seizure. However, there is no scientific evidence that such dogs can actually predict seizures.

> *Protective headgear:* Helmets are more commonly prescribed in people with cognitive impairment and atonic seizures to safeguard against head injury, but there is little evidence in the literature that supports the use of protective headgear.

## Future perspectives

Many existing guidelines, standards, and rules for safety and prevention of accidents in people with epilepsy and seizures are based on expert opinion and are not evidence based. This is because few of the needed prospective population-based studies have been performed. Also, safety recommendations and rules should be subject to ongoing prospective research to monitor and test these standards and ensure that they achieve the goal of maintaining balance between protecting people with epilepsy from the risk of accidents caused by seizures and allowing them to participate optimally in society.

## Bibliography

Ahmad BS, Hill KD, Gorelik A, Habib N, Wark JD. Falls and fractures in patients chronically treated with antiepileptic drugs. *Neurology* 2012; **79**: 154–151.

Anonymous. Consensus statements, sample statutory provisions, and model regulations regarding driver licensing and epilepsy. American Academy of Neurology. American Epilepsy Society, Epilepsy Foundation of America. *Epilepsia* 1994; **35**: 696–705.

Asadi-Pooya AA, Nikeresht A, Yaghoui E, Nei M. Physical injuries in patients with epilepsy and their associated risk factors. *Seizure* 2012; **21**:165–168.

Beghi E, Cornaggia C. Morbidity and accidents in patients with epilepsy: Results of a European cohort study. *Epilepsia* 2002; **43**:1076–1083.

Dasgutpa AK, Saunders M, Dick DJ. Epilepsy in the British Steel Corporation: An evaluation of sickness, accident and work records. *Br J Ind Med* 1982; **39**:145–148.

Gilliam F, Kuzniecky R, Faught E, Black L, Carpenter G, Schrodt R. Patient-validated content of epilepsy-specific quality-of-life measurement. *Epilepsia* 1997; **38**:233–236.

IOM (Institute of Medicine). *Epilepsy Across the Spectrum: Promoting Health and Understanding.* Washington, DC: The National Academies Press, 2012.

Kirsch R, Wirrell E. Do cognitively normal children with epilepsy have a higher rate of injury than their nonepileptic peers? *J Child Neurol* 2001; **16**:100–104.

Krumholz A. Driving issues in epilepsy: Past, present, and future. Current review in clinical science. *Epilepsy Curr* 2009; **9**:31–35.

Krumholz A, Hopp J. Legal and regulatory issues for people with epilepsy. In: Noseworthy J. ed. *Neurological Therapeutics: Principals and Practice,* 3rd ed. London: Martin Dunitz Ltd, 2009.

Sneed RC, Stencel C. Protective helmets for children with special health care needs. *South Med J* 2001; **94**(5):519–521.

Spitz MC. Injuries and death as a consequence of seizures in people with epilepsy. *Epilepsia* 1998; **39**(8):904–907.

Tomson T, Beghi E, Sundqvist A, Johannessen SI. Medical risks in epilepsy: A review with focus on physical injuries, mortality, traffic accidents and their prevention. *Epilepsy Res* 2004; **60**:1–16.

Wirrell E. Epilepsy-related injuries. *Epilepsia* 2006; **47**(Suppl. 1):79–86.

# Medical Comorbidity in Epilepsy

**Kimberly L. Pargeon and Sheryl R. Haut**

Epilepsy Management Center, Einstein-Montefiore, Bronx, NY, USA
Department of Neurology, Montefiore Medical Center, Albert Einstein College
of Medicine, Bronx, NY, USA

Many patients with epilepsy have comorbid medical conditions, which often complicate the treatment of seizures and affect quality of life. Disorders are comorbid if they occur in the same person more frequently than chance alone would suggest. Comorbid conditions in epilepsy occur in a number of forms: medical disorders that coexist with or increase the risk for epilepsy and are related to a common pathophysiology; conditions that arise as a direct result of epilepsy treatment; and conditions otherwise unrelated to epilepsy that complicate epilepsy treatment. These relationships can have important diagnostic and treatment considerations, and a broad familiarity is essential for anyone who cares for patients with epilepsy.

## Conditions that coexist with epilepsy or increase epilepsy risk

### Migraine headaches

The comorbidity of migraine and epilepsy presents both diagnostic dilemmas and treatment opportunities. Persons with either migraine or epilepsy appear to be more than twice as likely to also have the other disorder, and epilepsy and migraine share many similarities. Both are chronic disorders with episodic attacks, with a return to baseline between episodes. Both disorders are thought to be related, at least in part, to neuronal hyperexcitability, with some shared genetic influences. Similar triggers for migraine headaches and seizures include changes in stress levels and hormonal conditions, such as those that occur with menstruation. Considerable treatment overlap exists, possibly related to the shared pathophysiology, and antiepileptic drugs (AEDs) are often used for migraine prophylaxis, both with FDA approval (valproate sodium and topiramate) and off-label.

The sensory, motor, and cognitive characteristics of epilepsy and migraine may overlap and present diagnostic challenges, particularly if visual symptoms are present (Table 35.1). Furthermore, postictal headaches are frequently migrainous, and headache can occasionally be the sole or most predominant clinical manifestation of epileptic seizures. Seizures may also occur during or within an hour of migraine aura, in a condition that some have referred to as migralepsy. When a diagnostic dilemma arises, the EEG may be helpful in distinguishing migraine from seizure.

### ☆ TIPS AND TRICKS

When using a single medication to treat comorbid disorders, be sure to dose appropriately for both disorders. For example, target dosing for topiramate in migraine is 50–100 mg daily, but the epilepsy dosing is sometimes higher, in the 50–400 mg range.

*Epilepsy*, First Edition. Edited by John W. Miller and Howard P. Goodkin.
© 2014 John Wiley & Sons, Ltd. Published 2014 by John Wiley & Sons, Ltd.

## ⚜ SCIENCE REVISITED

Familial hemiplegic migraine (FHM) is an autosomal dominant form of migraine characterized by hemiparesis during the migraine aura. Three major genetic loci involved in FHM are also associated with epilepsy: *CACN1A*, which codes for a neuronal P-/Q-type calcium channel and is associated with some focal epilepsies; *ATP1A2*, which codes for a Na/K ATPase and has been identified in families with benign familial infantile convulsions; and *SCN1A*, which codes for a sodium channel and is implicated in a wide spectrum of epileptic disorders from generalized epilepsy with febrile seizures + type 2 (GEFS + 2), a mild form of epilepsy, to the more severe myoclonic epilepsy of infancy (SMEI).

### Stroke

Stroke has been well established as a risk factor for epilepsy, and it is one of the most common etiologies for new-onset seizures in the elderly. Seizures can occur in 6–15% of patients in the first 1–2 weeks immediately following a stroke. Factors that are associated with a higher risk of acute seizures include hemorrhagic stroke, subarachnoid hemorrhage, cortical localization, stroke recurrence, and larger infarcts with greater disability. Studies have been contradictory as to whether early or late initial seizures better predict development of chronic epilepsy.

Patients with epilepsy who are taking warfarin can be at risk for either embolic or hemorrhagic stroke due to drug interactions with certain AEDs, particularly agents interacting with hepatic cytochrome P450 enzymes. Drug interactions between warfarin and AEDs are described in detail in Chapter 13.

## ⚠ CAUTION!

Although acute seizures are not seen in the majority of stroke patients, clinicians should be mindful of this complication in a select group of patients, particularly those with large, cortically based infarcts and especially in patients with hemorrhagic infarcts.

### Polycystic ovarian syndrome

There is an increased incidence of polycystic ovarian syndrome (PCOS) in epilepsy, affecting as many as 10–25% of women with epilepsy, with or without treatment with AEDs. PCOS has several key characteristics, including polycystic ovaries; disruption of normal menstruation, ranging from irregular cycle intervals to amenorrhea; and hyperandrogenism, which can clinically manifest as hirsutism, acne, and alopecia. The link between epilepsy, AED use, and PCOS remains controversial, particularly in relation to valproate sodium. The question often raised is whether valproate sodium directly causes PCOS or instead increases certain risk factors, such as excess weight or insulin resistance. Further, long-term treatment with valproate sodium may increase risk of developing aspects of PCOS such as hyperandrogenism but not overt disease. PCOS may contribute to the increased rate of infertility in women with epilepsy and is an important consideration when treating young women who have epilepsy.

**Table 35.1.** Distinguishing visual symptoms in seizure and migraine.

| | Visual symptoms | |
|---|---|---|
| | **Migraine with aura, acephalgic migraine** | **Seizure** |
| Color | Black and white (may be colored) | Colored |
| Positive symptoms | Linear or flash, zigzag | Circular, spherical |
| Localization | Begin at center, expand to hemianoptic field | Hemifield |
| | | Same spatial localization each episode, may cross |
| Scotoma | Common, often follows positive visual symptoms | Uncommon |
| | | "Postictal Todd's" scotoma may occur |

## Conditions related to epilepsy treatment

### Fractures and reduced bone density

Patients with epilepsy are at higher risk for fractures for multiple reasons, including seizure-related falls, imbalance of gait from medication side effects, and neurological deficits leading to decreased mobility. However, an important culprit appears to be bone loss that may be related to osteopenia or osteoporosis due to certain AEDs, particularly the enzyme-inducing agents (Chapters 12 and 19). Decreased bone mineral density may be caused by AEDs either by accelerated bone loss in adults or by poor bone accrual in children. It has been reported that the odds of a broken bone increase by 4–6% for every year of AED use; the risk for any fracture increases by 40% per decade, and the risk for seizure-related fractures increases by 60% per decade.

Currently, there are no official recommendations for timing and type of screening measures for bone health. For those at higher risk of fracture, routine and regular screening should include bone mineral density measurements with dual-energy X-ray absorptiometry (DEXA) as well as serum 25-OH-vitamin D. There are also limited data on appropriate calcium and vitamin D supplementation. The Institute of Medicine recently recommended a daily adult vitamin D intake of 600 international units (IU) with a maximum of 4000 IU (Table 35.2).

### ☆ TIPS AND TRICKS

Most patients with epilepsy are unaware of the risk of bone loss with use of certain seizure medications. Clinicians should remember to discuss these risks and to screen for bone density, especially with those who have been taking AEDs associated with bone loss for many years.

### ⚙ SCIENCE REVISITED

Cytochrome P450-inducing agents such as phenytoin and phenobarbital tend to be associated with the most significant effects on bone health, thought to be due to increased vitamin D metabolism. However, these effects have also been reported with valproate, an enzyme inhibitor, so the full pathophysiological mechanism remains unknown.

### Vascular/metabolic risk

Patients with epilepsy appear to be at increased risk for diseases such as hypertension, dyslipidemia, cardiac conduction abnormalities, and diabetes. Epilepsy monotherapy with strong enzyme-inducing agents, including carbamazepine or phenytoin, or with valproate sodium for more than 2 years has been shown to alter biomarkers correlating with accelerated development of atherosclerosis, including increased common carotid artery intima thickening; increased high-sensitivity C-reactive protein; and alterations in levels of cholesterol, folate, and total homocysteine. Carbamazepine specifically can be associated with occasional cardiac conduction abnormalities, as can phenytoin, but it also has been occasionally associated with accelerated atherosclerosis in children, and infrequently it can induce hypertension during initiation.

### ☆ TIPS AND TRICKS

Carbamazepine and other enzyme-inducing AEDs have been linked to elevated total cholesterol and LDL in children and adults and should be periodically screened in at-risk populations.

## Conditions that affect epilepsy treatment

### Hepatic disease

Hepatic disorders can significantly affect epilepsy treatment. The liver metabolizes most AEDs and is the primary producer of albumin. The active forms of highly protein-bound drugs such as phenytoin and carbamazepine are the unbound, freely circulating forms. The increased proportion of unbound AED with low albumin levels in liver disease will lead to increased free levels and possible adverse effects. Hepatic diseases can variably affect blood flow to the liver via the hepatic artery and portal veins, differentially affecting how AEDs reach the liver and thus their metabolism. Furthermore, parenchymal disease of the liver can alter enzymes in the cytochrome P450 system, which can affect the metabolism of common AEDs including phenytoin, carbamazepine, oxcarbazepine, and benzodiazepines.

Ideal AED therapy for patients with liver dysfunction would be, if possible, a single agent with little protein binding that is primarily renally excreted with

Table 35.2. Recommended daily intake of calcium and vitamin D by age.

| Life stage group | Calcium | | | Vitamin D | | |
|---|---|---|---|---|---|---|
| | Estimated average requirement (mg/day) | Recommended dietary allowance (mg/day) | Upper level intake (mg/day) | Estimated average requirement (IU/day) | Recommended dietary allowance (IU/day) | Upper level intake (IU/day) |
| Infants 0–6 months | a | a | 1000 | b | b | 1000 |
| Infants 6–12 months | a | a | 1500 | b | b | 1500 |
| 1–3 years old | 500 | 700 | 2500 | 400 | 600 | 2500 |
| 4–8 years old | 800 | 1000 | 2500 | 400 | 600 | 3000 |
| 9–13 years old | 1100 | 1300 | 3000 | 400 | 600 | 4000 |
| 14–18 years old | 1100 | 1300 | 3000 | 400 | 600 | 4000 |
| 19–30 years old | 800 | 1000 | 2500 | 400 | 600 | 4000 |
| 31–50 years old | 800 | 1000 | 2500 | 400 | 600 | 4000 |
| 51–70-year-old males | 800 | 1000 | 2000 | 400 | 600 | 4000 |
| 51–70-year-old females | 1000 | 1200 | 2000 | 400 | 600 | 4000 |
| >70 years old | 1000 | 1200 | 2000 | 400 | 800 | 4000 |
| 14–18 years old, pregnant/lactating | 1100 | 1300 | 3000 | 400 | 600 | 4000 |
| 19–50 years old, pregnant/lactating | 800 | 1000 | 2500 | 400 | 600 | 4000 |

a For Infants, adeqate Intake is 200 mg/day for 0–6 months of age and 260 mg/day for 6–12 months of age.
b For Infants, adeqate Intake is 400 IU/day for 0–6 months of age and 400 IU/day for 6–12 months of age.

Source: © The Institute of Medicine (2011), reproduced with permission.

**Table 35.3.** Dosage adjustments of AEDs in renal impairment and dialysis.

| Antiepileptic agent | Dose adjustment in renal failure |
|---|---|
| Carbamazepine | Almost entirely cleared by hepatic metabolism and not susceptible to dialysis |
| Felbamate | Forty to 50% excreted unchanged in the urine; unlikely to be readily dialyzed; specific dosage recommendations not available |
| Gabapentin | Almost 100% excreted unchanged in the urine and readily dialyzed; maintenance dose reduced in proportion to reductions in creatinine clearance; supplementary dose after dialysis recommended |
| Lacosamide | Low plasma protein binding (<15%) with some metabolism through CYP2C19 but about 95% elimination through the urine; maintenance dosage likely reduced with reductions in creatinine clearance but no specific recommendations available |
| Lamotrigine | Half-life prolonged 50% in renal insufficiency; 20% in bodily stores removed by 4h of hemodialysis; specific dosage recommendations not available |
| Levetiracetam | Almost 100% excreted unchanged in the urine and readily dialyzed; maintenance dose reduced in proportion to reductions in creatinine clearance; supplementary dose after dialysis recommended |
| Oxcarbazepine | Active metabolite 25% excreted in urine; extent to which active metabolite cleared by dialysis unknown; maintenance dose reduced in moderate renal insufficiency |
| Phenobarbital | Twenty-five percent excreted unchanged in urine and dialyzable; dosage adjustment is based upon plasma levels; supplementary dose after dialysis is often required |
| Phenytoin | Primarily cleared by hepatic metabolism and not susceptible to dialysis; unbound fraction can increase in renal failure |
| Pregabalin | About 90% excreted unchanged in the urine and readily dialyzed; likely similar to gabapentin, with reduction of maintenance dose in proportion to reductions in creatinine clearance and supplementary dose after dialysis recommended |
| Tiagabine | Almost entirely cleared by hepatic metabolism and not susceptible to metabolism |
| Topiramate | Seventy percent excreted unchanged in urine and dialyzable; maintenance dose requires reduction in mild-to-moderate renal insufficiency; cleared during dialysis at a rate that is four to six times that of a control patient; supplementary dose recommended |
| Valproate | Almost entirely cleared by hepatic metabolism and not susceptible to dialysis; unbound fraction can increase in renal failure |
| Zonisamide | Cleared by both renal and hepatic routes; creatinine clearance of less than 20mL/min is associated with an increase in the mean plasma concentration of 35%; extent to which drug is cleared by dialysis is unknown |

Adapted from Boro A, Haut S. Medical comorbidities in the treatment of epilepsy. *Epilepsy Behav* 2003; 4:S1–S12. Other updated information from http://www.pdr.net.

less hepatic metabolism. Levetiracetam and pregabalin are examples (Chapter 19). Potent cytochrome P450-inducing agents such as phenytoin should be avoided if possible, but if used, free levels should be followed, although AEDs should always be titrated towards a goal of effective and tolerated dosages, not to a specific "therapeutic" serum level. In addition, tests such as aspartate aminotransferase (AST), alanine aminotransferase (ALT), and coagulation panels may be helpful for gauging hepatic function.

**☝ CAUTION!**

Phenytoin metabolism is more likely to be altered in *acute hepatitis* than in *chronic cirrhosis*; it is 95% metabolized by the liver, mostly by CYP2C9 and CYP2C19. Fosphenytoin is converted to phenytoin via phosphorylases, and its conversion is slightly faster in the context of liver disease due to decreased binding of fosphenytoin to plasma proteins.

**★ TIPS AND TRICKS**

Patients with low albumin levels can have alterations of the free or active levels of phenytoin. The Sheiner–Tozer equation can be used to correct for low albumin observed in hepatic or renal disease:

$$C_{corrected} = \frac{C_{observed}}{\left[0.9 \cdot (Alb. / 4.4)\right] + 0.1}$$

### Renal disease

Seizures in the context of renal disease, particularly in patients undergoing dialysis, may be related to severe uremia or electrolyte disturbances. These states can lead to uremic encephalopathy or dialysis disequilibrium syndrome, with symptoms ranging from irritability, mild confusion, and headaches to the extreme of seizures, coma, or even death. Dialysis disequilibrium syndrome is more common in patients recently started on dialysis and is thought to be due to cerebral edema.

The comorbidity of epilepsy and renal disease can pose treatment complications, particularly for patients taking AEDs with high protein binding. Changes in protein binding are associated with renal insufficiency, resulting in increased free fractions of highly protein-bound drugs such as phenytoin. Dosing adjustments for AEDs in renal failure are presented in Table 35.3. Dialysis complicates epilepsy treatment further, as patients taking AEDs may have seizures following dialysis due to rapid clearance of the drugs. A significant determiner of a drug's degree of renal excretion is its water solubility. As the glomerular filtration rate decreases, dosage requirements for water-soluble drugs such as gabapentin will decrease, but this will have little effect on more lipid-soluble drugs, such as carbamazepine. AEDs are generally cleared by dialysis via diffusion down their concentration gradient. As such, drugs that are highly water soluble with low protein binding and smaller volumes of distribution are more easily dialyzed. Clinicians should be aware of the need to adjust dosing of certain AEDs, especially levetiracetam, gabapentin, and topiramate, in the setting of dialysis (Table 35.3).

## Conclusion

The treatment of epilepsy is often complicated by comorbid medical conditions. The clinician who is familiar with these comorbidities will be well equipped to choose optimal antiepileptic therapies, adjust dosing schedules appropriately, and monitor outcomes effectively.

## Bibliography

Ahmad BS, Hill KD, O'Brien TJ, Gorelik A, Habib N, Wark JD. Falls and fractures in patients chronically treated with antiepileptic drugs. *Neurology* 2012; **79**:145–151.

Barri YM, Golper TA. Seizures in patients undergoing hemodialysis. Literature review current through August 2012 and topic last updated on October 14, 2011. Available at www.uptodate.com (accessed on September 18, 2012).

Bladin CF, Alexandrov AV, Bellavance A, et al. Seizures after stroke: A prospective multicenter study. *Arch Neurol* 2000; **57**:1617–1622.

Boggs JG. Seizure management in the setting of hepatic disease. *Curr Treat Options Neurol* 2011; **13**:333–345.

Boro A, Haut S. Medical comorbidities in the treatment of epilepsy. *Epilepsy Behav* 2003; **4**:S1–S12.

Chuang YC, Chuang HY, Lin TK, et al. Effects of long-term antiepileptic drug monotherapy on vascular risk factors and atherosclerosis. *Epilepsia* 2012; **53**(1):120–128.

Haut S, Bigal M, Lipton RBL. Chronic disorders with episodic manifestations: Focus on epilepsy and migraine. *Lancet Neurol* 2006; **5**(2):148–157.

Institute of Medicine (IOM). 2011. *Dietary Reference Intakes for Calcium and Vitamin D*. Washington, DC: The National Academies Press. Available at http://www.iom.edu/vitamind (accessed on September 18, 2012).

Pack AM. Implications of hormonal and neuroendocrine changes associated with seizures and antiepileptic drugs: A clinical perspective. *Epilepsia* 2010; **51**(Suppl. 3):150–153.

Pack AM. Treatment of epilepsy to optimize bone health. *Curr Treat Options Neurol* 2011; **13**:346–354.

So EL, Annegers JF, Hauser WA, O'Brien PC, Whisnant JP. Population-based study of seizure disorders after cerebral infarction. *Neurology* 1996; **46**(2):350–355.

Verrotti A, D'Egidio C, Mohn A, Coppola G, Parisi P, Chiarelli F. Antiepileptic drugs, sex hormones, and PCOS. *Epilepsia* 2011; **52**(2):199–211.

# Cognitive Effects of Chronic Epilepsy

**Daniel L. Drane**

Departments of Neurology and Pediatrics, Emory University School of Medicine, Atlanta, GA, USA
Department of Neurology, University of Washington School of Medicine, Seattle, WA, USA

## Introduction

Seizures can transiently disrupt neural networks, leading to brief cognitive and sensorimotor dysfunction. Epilepsy can have chronic effects upon functioning associated with permanent structural changes in the brain. For most with epilepsy, particularly those with well-controlled seizures on antiepileptic drugs (AEDs), the chronic cognitive effect of seizures will be mild. At the other end of the spectrum, however, there are individuals with profound impairment of cognitive functions, ranging from isolated deficits related to the region of the seizure focus to global disability from widespread changes in brain structure and function.

## Measuring cognitive function

Neuropsychological assessment is useful for establishing baseline cognitive function against which change can be measured. This is helpful for evaluating cognitive complaints when they arise, for assessing disease progression, and for determining the effect of treatment. Neuropsychological assessment is mandatory for patients undergoing epilepsy surgery and is particularly important for those with poorly controlled seizures. Such assessment can be important for academic and vocational planning, for the provision of rehabilitative services, and to confirm localization of seizure onset zone for surgical planning.

Table 36.1 and 36.2 contain lists of cognitive and emotional domains that are typically assessed in the context of epilepsy and some of the more common measures employed. There are no standard test batteries used routinely to assess epilepsy, although some core tests are recommended by the NIH's Common Data Elements project to facilitate comparisons between clinical centers. For evaluating change over time, some groups use reliable change indices (RCIs) or other statistical procedures (e.g., standard regression-based scores) to control for practice effects, although these methods can also obscure meaningful change if not used appropriately. The optimal neuropsychological report assesses whether or not there are factors causing a variable performance (e.g., interictal epileptiform discharges, motivational issues), considers the effects of AEDs, and highlights any localizing or lateralizing features of the results. Recommendations should include appraising the risk of decline in cognitive performance as it relates to treatments such as surgery and the possible benefit of rehabilitation strategies or social services for patients with deficits.

**Table 36.1.** Core neurocognitive functions to be assessed in epilepsy patients and suggested tests.

| Neurocognitive domains | Within-domain areas to emphasize during assessment | Possible tests to consider |
|---|---|---|
| Language | • Naming (e.g., visual, auditory/naming to description, category-related)<br>• Verbal fluency (semantic, letter, and action)<br>• Screen reading and other core language tasks | • Boston Naming Test, Columbia Auditory Naming Test, Category-Related Naming Tests<br>• Category Fluency Tasks (e.g., animals, supermarket items), D-KEFS Verbal Fluency, Controlled Oral Word Association Test, Action Fluency<br>• Recognition Reading Subtest of the Wide Range Achievement Test (WRAT), American Version of the National Adult Reading Test (AMNART), Wechsler Test of Adult Reading, Token Test, Sentence Repetition |
| Attention | • Primary attention (auditory and visual)<br>• Complex attention (auditory and visual)<br>• Sustained attention (auditory and visual) | • Digit Span Forward (WAIS), Picture Completion (WAIS)<br>• Digit Span Backward and Letter-Number Sequencing (WAIS), Trail Making Tests, Spatial Span<br>• Continuous Performance Test (not used as commonly by most epilepsy centers) |
| Visual processing | • Visuoperception<br>• Visual-spatial<br>• Object recognition | • Visual Object and Space Perception Battery (VOSP), Facial Recognition Test<br>• Judgment of Line Orientation, VOSP<br>• Famous Faces Test, Category-Related Object Recognition Tests |
| Constructional praxis | • Graphomotor copying tasks<br>• Assembly tasks | • Copying Simple Shapes (e.g, Greek Cross, Necker Cube), Rey Complex Figure Test (Copy)<br>• Block Design (WAIS) |
| Memory and learning | • Auditory/verbal learning, memory retention, and recognition<br>  ■ List learning tasks<br>  ■ Contextual memory<br>  ■ Associative learning<br>• Visual learning, memory retention, and recognition<br>  ■ Simple geometric designs<br>  ■ Face recall<br>  ■ Complex visual designs<br>  ■ Spatial recall<br>  ■ Remote recall | • Rey Auditory Verbal Learning Test, California Verbal Learning Test, Verbal Selective Reminding Test<br>• Logical Memory Subtest (Wechsler Scales), Reitan Story Memory<br>• Verbal Paired Associates (VPA) Subtest (Wechsler Scales; WMS-III VPA appears less helpful than other versions, as it eliminated the easier word pairs)<br>• Visual Reproduction (Wechsler Memory Scales; older versions appear to be more useful for lateralization than the 3rd edition)<br>• Face Recall/Hospital Facial Recognition Task; Twins Test<br>• Rey Complex Figure Test, Taylor Complex Figure<br>• Route Learning Paradigms<br>• Information Subtest (WAIS), Autobiographical Memory Measures |

*(Continued)*

**Table 36.1** (*Continued*)

| Neurocognitive domains | Within-domain areas to emphasize during assessment | Possible tests to consider |
|---|---|---|
| Executive control processes | • Complex problem solving | • Wisconsin card sorting test, Brixton Spatial Anticipation Test, Iowa Gambling Task |
| | • Response inhibition | • Color–Word Interference (Stroop) Test, Hayling Test, Go/No-Go Tasks |
| | • Complex attention/mental flexibility | • Trail Making Test, Mental Control (WMS) |
| | • Abstract reasoning | • Similarities Subtest/Matrix Reasoning Subtest (WAIS) |
| | • Generative fluency tasks (verbal and visual) | • D-KEFS Verbal Fluency, D-KEFS Design Fluency, 5-Point Design Fluency |
| | • Metacognition | • Cognitive Estimation Tasks |
| General intellectual functioning | • Verbal and performance IQ | • WAIS (various editions) |
| | | • Wechsler Abbreviated Scale of Intelligence |
| Academic achievement | • Reading recognition | • WRAT—Reading Recognition |
| | • Reading comprehension | • Gray Oral Reading Test (GORT) |
| | • Mathematical skills | • WRAT—Arithmetic |
| | • Spelling ability | • WRAT—Spelling |
| Symptom validity testing | • Determine task engagement. This can be disrupted due to issues including poor motivation as well as the impact of acute seizures and epileptiform activity | • Word Memory Test |
| | | • Medical Symptom Validity Test |
| | | • Victoria Symptom Validity Test |
| | | • "Embedded" Measures of Task Engagement[a] |

*Note:* WAIS, Wechsler Adult Intelligence Scale; WMS-III, Wechsler Memory Scale 3rd edition; MCG, Medical College of Georgia.

[a]Embedded measures of task engagement refer to attempts to use improbable performances on standard clinical tests in order to recognize possible test invalidity.

**Table 36.2.** Sensory, motor, mood and personality, and quality of life variables to be assessed in epilepsy patients and suggested tests.

| Neurocognitive domains | Within-domain areas to emphasize during assessment | Possible tests to consider |
|---|---|---|
| Sensory | • Visual, auditory, and tactile acuities | • Snellen Eye Chart<br>• Extinction to Double Simultaneous Stimulation<br>• Tactile Form Recognition<br>• Reitan–Klove Sensory Examination |
| Motor | • Handedness<br>• Gross motor speed<br>• Fine motor speed and dexterity<br>• Grip strength<br>• Psychomotor speed | • Edinburgh Handedness Scale<br>• Finger-Tapping Test<br>• Grooved Pegboard Test<br><br>• Hand Dynamometer<br>• WAIS Subtests (e.g., Symbol Search, Digit Symbol) |
| Mood and personality | • Mood and emotional status<br>• Psychopathology<br>• Personality features<br>• Somatizational/ conversion profile | • Minnesota Multiphasic Personality Inventory (2nd edition or Restructured Form)<br>• Personality Assessment Inventory (PAI)<br>• Brief Self-Report Inventories (e.g., Beck Depression and Anxiety Scales)<br>• Mini Psychiatric Inventory (MINI) |
| Quality of life | • Adjustment to seizures and treatment (e.g., AEDs, surgical intervention)<br>• Satisfaction with social support and vocational and interpersonal functioning | • Quality of Life in Epilepsy (QOLIE)<br><br>• Washington Psychosocial Seizure Inventory (WPSI) |

*Note*: WAIS, Wechsler Adult Intelligence Scale; AEDs, antiepileptic drugs.

## Causes and mechanisms of cognitive dysfunction associated with epilepsy

Structural lesions can disrupt both local and global neural networks, generally resulting in predictable cognitive deficits. Structural lesions are common, often representing the etiology of the epilepsy (e.g., tumors, dysplasia). Sometimes lesions such as hippocampal atrophy in temporal lobe epilepsy (TLE) reflect the chronic effect of epileptiform activity upon the brain. Some patients also have structural lesions from prior surgical intervention.

Functional impairment of brain networks can also occur from transient chemical and electrical disruptions of brain circuitry from interictal and ictal abnormalities, synaptic and ion channel abnormalities, and medication side effects. When the functional disruption of brain circuitry is potentially reversible and not from a structural lesion, effective management of the underlying process can improve cognition (e.g., changing an AED causing adverse effects, decreasing epileptiform discharges, or altering synaptic neurotransmitter availability).

Mounting evidence indicates that cognitive functions are supported by large-scale distributed neural networks of varying complexity. The less complex systems mediate basic sensory and motor processing, while higher-order cognitive functions such as semantic memory and language are supported by interactions between widespread distributed neural systems. Cortical and subcortical gray matter structures function as processing nodes in these networks, which are then connected by white matter tracts. As already discussed, epilepsy and its treatments produce structural and functional disruption of these networks, as do the underlying neurological processes that cause the epilepsy and other associated comorbidities. Uncontrolled seizures themselves alter brain structure and function, as reflected by gray and white matter volumetric changes and altered functional connectivity demonstrated by resting state fMRI and diffusion tensor imaging (DTI). Disease-related variables such as seizure duration and frequency determine the severity of these brain changes.

---

### ♜ SCIENCE REVISITED

Diffusion tensor imaging studies demonstrate white matter changes in both cerebral hemispheres of TLE patients, with the greatest disruption on the side ipsilateral to seizure onset and in regions closest to the seizure onset zone. The severity of these abnormalities correlates with seizure duration and frequency and is believed to reflect reduced axonal density or myelin abnormalities. These abnormalities persist even if seizures become controlled. Altered white matter connectivity may occur in both cerebral hemispheres following surgical resection to treat epilepsy. These white matter alterations result in decreased brain connectivity and increased cognitive dysfunction.

---

Understanding the mechanistic structure of cognitive dysfunction and its causes can help to predict the nature and potential magnitude of cognitive impairment of a given patient, to estimate future cognitive trajectory, and to anticipate the effect of different treatments. The epilepsy neuropsychologist uses this framework to predict and optimize cognitive and psychiatric outcome and determine the patient's needs for rehabilitative, mental health, or social services. This process involves thinking through the multitude of neural processes that can go awry in epilepsy and the various disease and treatment-related factors that can disrupt them.

## Patterns of cognitive dysfunction associated with epilepsy

Understanding and predicting cognitive function and its trajectory of change requires a general knowledge of the various seizure classification schemas and some key disease-related variables such as age of seizure onset. Such schemas typically group patients by seizure etiology, seizure type, and epilepsy syndrome. We will consider each schema and its relationship to cognition in turn.

1. *Seizure etiology* The symptomatic epilepsies generally exhibit the worst baseline cognitive functioning, although there is increasing recognition that the idiopathic "benign" epilepsies of childhood often also exhibit at least mild dysfunction.

   *Symptomatic* epilepsies (structural/metabolic/immune epilepsies, Chapter 2) have a pattern of cognitive impairment typically driven by the primary injury or neurological disease, although seizures may also contribute progressively. Knowledge of the location and extent of the underlying lesion causing these epilepsies provides information about which cognitive functions might be compromised. For example, left TLE patients with typical left hemisphere language lateralization often experience problems with auditory/verbal memory and learning, naming, and semantic fluency. Of course, such potential deficit patterns are also modified by information from other schemas. For example, those with early age of seizure onset may have reorganized function and are thus less likely to have these deficits than those with later seizure onset.

   *Idiopathic* epilepsy (genetic epilepsy, Chapter 2) is associated with cognitive dysfunction that may arise from more subtle abnormalities in cellular physiology and also directly from seizures. Because they lack obvious structural lesions, these patients tend to have less severe cognitive dysfunction than those with symptomatic epilepsy or cryptogenic epilepsy (epilepsy of unknown etiology, Chapter 2). Patients with genetic epilepsy can have focal or generalized seizures, with different patterns of cognitive deficits.

2. *Seizure type* Seizures are typically classified as either focal or generalized. Please see Chapter 2 for a detailed description of seizure classification. Cognitive deficits tend to be greatest for those

experiencing the largest, most disruptive generalized seizures; for example, someone with generalized tonic–clonic seizures is likely to experience more cognitive dysfunction than someone with only absence or simple partial seizures. Knowledge of seizure type is relevant for judging cognitive impairment, which will reflect underlying brain regions involved in a given seizure. Most individuals experience stereotyped patterns of seizures, meaning that the same brain regions are repeatedly disrupted. Focal seizures tend to produce more circumscribed patterns of cognitive dysfunction than seizures with generalized onset. However, more recent studies demonstrate that even focal seizures often disrupt large-scale brain networks far beyond the seizure onset zone, even without secondary generalization. For example, volumetric MRI demonstrates that patients with TLE have significant reduction in parietal, frontal, and temporal neocortical thickness and white matter volumes, as well as decreased thalamic volumes as compared to normal. Through PET and magnetic resonance spectroscopy, prefrontal metabolic abnormalities have also been shown in TLE, although many of the metabolic abnormalities will normalize if seizures improve. For example, frontal hypometabolism in patients with TLE will frequently reverse if seizure freedom is achieved after anterior temporal lobectomy. Much of the cognitive improvement seen after seizure control likely results from the reduction of such widespread effects, allowing these broader brain regions to return to normal patterns of function.

With focal seizures, the brain region affected by structural and electrophysiological disruption will dictate the nature of cognitive deficits that occur. For example, occipital lobe seizures are more likely to be associated with visual dysfunction, while frontal lobe seizures may be characterized by impairment in executive control processes (e.g., organization, planning, response inhibition, problem solving, and complex attention), aspects of comportment and personality, and motor performance. In patients with focal seizures that secondarily generalize, broader dysfunction and impairment of primary attention and processing speed are more likely.

Patients with generalized seizures often have cognitive deficits involving executive functions, in keeping with the fact that MRI volumetric studies in this group demonstrate frontal lobe atrophic changes. Otherwise, there is a tendency for these patients to have broader, global dysfunction, worse in those experiencing status epilepticus or larger convulsive seizures. There are also generalized epilepsy syndromes occurring with baseline global brain dysfunction (including mental retardation), sometimes associated with progressive decline.

3. *Epilepsy syndromes*: The same basic rules apply regarding the effect of seizure type, etiology, and other disease-related and psychosocial variables on cognitive function. Familiarity with each epilepsy syndrome is useful, as patterns of cognitive functioning are among the defining criteria for several of them. For example, acquired aphasia involving both receptive and expressive speech during the first decade of life is a key component of *Landau–Kleffner syndrome* (Chapter 21), an epileptic syndrome with epileptiform discharges in the temporoparietal regions. *Lennox–Gastaut* and *West syndromes* (Chapter 21) typically present with mental retardation and autistic-like behavior. Even seemingly more benign focal epilepsy syndromes, such as benign epilepsy of childhood with centrotemporal spikes(Chapter 21), may be associated with cognitive fluctuations and academic problems.

## Epilepsy treatments and cognition

Many treatments such as AEDs and neurosurgery can also worsen cognitive function, regardless of epilepsy type. It has been long known that AEDs can have a negative effect on cognitive function, although this effect is generally considered to be small when recommended dosages and therapeutic blood levels are not exceeded and when polypharmacy is avoided. However, certain AEDs can affect cognition more severely in a subset of patients. In addition, some AEDs such as valproate sodium can adversely impact neurodevelopment. Questions remain as to whether AED treatment can result in chronic changes in brain structure and function. Epilepsy surgery can also lead to deficits when resected regions were relatively healthy and functional or when destruction of fiber pathways decreases network connectivity.

## ✋ CAUTION!

Topiramate and zonisamide can lead to significant reversible cognitive dysfunction, including problems with verbal fluency, executive functions, and attention in a subset of individuals. These drugs also have the potential to reduce the effect of amobarbital, interfering with the results of the intracarotid amobarbital (Wada) procedure.

## Cognition over the life span in epilepsy

Emerging research has recently demonstrated that cognitive, behavioral, and psychiatric compromise often precedes seizure onset in both children and adults. Deficits at onset may include attention, executive function, memory, processing speed, and visual–spatial and constructional ability. In addition, nearly half of children with new-onset, idiopathic, or generalized epilepsy experience more psychiatric problems prior to their first recognized seizures than do age-matched controls. These problems include depression, anxiety, and attention deficit hyperactivity disorders. Although MRI structural abnormalities, outside of those causing symptomatic epilepsy, have been less consistently observed in new-onset patients, there is evidence of restricted white matter development compared to controls 2 years after seizure onset.

Neurodevelopmental factors can affect cognition. For example, early-life seizures originating in the language-dominant cerebral hemisphere can lead to reorganization of function within the same hemisphere or to the contralateral one, leading to compensated cognitive performance.

Some patients with poorly controlled epilepsy experience progressive decline in function. Patients with an earlier age of seizure onset and a longer duration of seizures tend to show worse cognitive functioning than those with briefer seizure durations. While early studies were usually cross-sectional and lacked adequate control groups, more recent studies demonstrate that patients with uncontrolled epilepsy often show declines in memory. In addition, aging also affects patients with epilepsy, with some indication that refractory epilepsy is associated with higher risk for developing dementia. As noted earlier, some epilepsy syndromes show progressive changes in neuroimaging in addition to cognitive decline over time.

## EVIDENCE AT A GLANCE

One longitudinal study demonstrated that at least 20–25% of patients with poorly controlled TLE experienced significant cognitive decline over 3–7 years. This group with the worst outcome was older, had the longest duration of epilepsy, took more medications, and had more abnormal brain volumes. Of note, a lack of practice effects upon repeat testing was also observed for nearly the entire sample of TLE patients (i.e., the vast majority failed to show the expected gains typically observed in healthy controls undergoing repeat testing).

## Effect of interictal and subclinical epileptiform activity on cognitive function

In addition to the effects of actual seizures, emerging research over the past decade offers strong support for the claim that interictal epileptiform discharges can have a pronounced, albeit transient, influence on cognitive function. Once again, focal discharges tend to produce restricted cognitive impairment, while more widespread discharges can affect wider regions of brain function, potentially leading to significant deficits that are not present to the same degree in the absence of these discharges. Assessment of function during these events can help characterize the patient's seizure focus, and failure to recognize the influence of such activity can lead to erroneous conclusions about cognitive functioning.

## Conclusions

The severity, pattern, and progression of cognitive dysfunction in patients with epilepsy are determined by many factors, including underlying disease pathology, duration and type of seizures, chronic AED exposure and other treatment effects, psychosocial variables, and neurodevelopmental and aging effects. Measuring cognitive functions and understanding these modulating factors allow appropriate interventions and provide understanding of the potential for change in cognitive function with treatment and its likely trajectory over time. Reducing seizures, particularly achieving a seizure-free state, may reduce cognitive impairment and decline.

## Bibliography

Aldenkamp AP. Effect of seizures and epileptiform discharges on cognitive function. *Epilepsia* 2007; **38**:S52–S55.

Bernhardt BC, Worsley HK, Evans AC, Bernasconi A, Bernasconi N. Longitudinal and cross-sectional analysis of atrophy in pharmacoresistant temporal lobe epilepsy. *Neurology* 2009; **72**:1747–1754.

Bonilha L, Rorden C, Appenzeller S, Carolina Coan A, Cendes F, Min Li L. Gray matter atrophy associated with duration of temporal lobe epilepsy. *Neuroimage* 2006; **32**:1070–1079.

Cortez MA, Perez Velazquez JL, Snead OC, 3rd. Animal models of epilepsy and progressive effects of seizures. *Adv Neurol* 2006; **97**:293–304.

Ebus S, Arends J, Hendriksen J, et al. Cognitive effects of interictal epileptiform discharges in children. *Eur J Paediatr Neurol* 2012; **16**:697–706.

Elger CE, Helmstaedter C, Kurthen M. Chronic epilepsy and cognition. *Lancet Neurol* 2004; **3**:663–672.

Helmstaedter C, Kurthen M, Lux S, Reuber M, Elger CE. Chronic epilepsy and cognition: A longitudinal study in temporal lobe epilepsy. *Ann Neurol* 2003; **54**:425–432.

Hermann BP, Seidenberg M, Bell B. The neurodevelopmental impact of childhood onset temporal lobe epilepsy on brain structure and function and the risk of progressive cognitive effects. *Prog Brain Res* 2002; **135**:429–438.

Hermann B, Jones J, Sheth R, Dow C, Koehn M, Seidenberg M. Children with new-onset epilepsy: Neuropsychological status and brain structure. *Brain* 2006; **129**(Pt 10):2609–2619.

Hermann B, Seidenberg M, Lee E-J, Chan F. Cognitive phenotypes in temporal lobe epilepsy. *J Int Neuropsychol Soc* 2007; **13**:12–20.

Hermann B, Meador KJ, Gaillard WD, Cramer JA. Cognition across the lifespan: Antiepileptic drugs, epilepsy, or both? *Epilepsy Behav* 2010; **17**(1):1–5.

Kemmotsu N, Girard HM, Bernhardt BC, et al. MRI analysis in temporal lobe epilepsy: Cortical thinning and white matter disruptions are related to side of seizure onset. *Epilepsia* 2011; **52**:2257–2266.

Marco M, Trimble MR. Antiepileptic drug-induced cognitive adverse effects: Potential mechanisms and contributing factors. *CNS Drugs* 2009; **23**:121–137.

Vlooswijk MCG, Vaessen MJ, Jansen JFA, et al. Loss of network efficiency associated with cognitive decline in epilepsy. *Neurology* 2011; **77**:938–944.

# Recognizing and Treating Psychiatric Comorbidity in Epilepsy

**Jay Salpekar**

Center for Neuroscience and Behavioral Medicine, Children's National Medical Center, George Washington University School of Medicine, Washington, DC, USA

## Introduction

Since the days of Hippocrates, scholars have understood that psychiatric comorbidity is significantly overrepresented in patients with epilepsy. Epidemiology studies consistently report that psychiatric illness is more common with epilepsy than with other common diseases such as asthma or diabetes – each of which involves noteworthy lifestyle changes and, in the case of asthma, sudden symptom exacerbation. Today, the common intersection of neurological and psychiatric symptoms is well accepted, and comprehensive care for persons with epilepsy includes thorough psychiatric assessment and treatment.

Although the awareness of treatment needs is well established, it has been challenging to resolve whether psychiatric illness is coincidental or associated with the underlying epilepsy. Psychosocial stress and stigma have a large impact upon patients' lives and may independently lead to dysfunction. Adding to the complexity is the effect of treatment. Historically, antiepileptic drugs (AEDs) have been viewed as causing cognitive and affective symptoms, even while these same drugs have appeared to be effective treatments for psychiatric conditions.

Although the evidence is limited, the paradigm for understanding the etiology of psychiatric comorbidities has shifted in the last decade. Now it is more widely recognized that psychiatric symptoms reflect an intrinsic process resulting from chemical or physiological changes in key brain regions. In many cases, the same pathophysiological mechanisms may lead to both psychiatric symptoms and seizures. Most importantly, interdisciplinary neuropsychiatric approaches to treatment have greatly informed the management strategies available to clinicians.

## Identification of psychiatric illness

Although it is a cliché, the most important step in managing psychiatric comorbidity is to look for it in the first place. Many clinicians are hesitant to ask questions about psychiatric symptoms out of fear of being obliged to solve problems they may feel ill equipped to manage. However, the evidence is compelling that the presence of psychiatric comorbidity has a negative impact upon treatment outcomes for epilepsy itself. In many cases, the psychiatric comorbidity may be more damaging to quality of life than the seizures themselves. Thus, it is in everyone's interest to ask the questions and proactively address psychiatric comorbidity. Psychiatric conditions will persist and adversely affect treatment outcome, whether a clinician strives to identify them or not.

*Epilepsy*, First Edition. Edited by John W. Miller and Howard P. Goodkin.
© 2014 John Wiley & Sons, Ltd. Published 2014 by John Wiley & Sons, Ltd.

**Table 37.1.** Screening questions for depression.

| | |
|---|---|
| 1. | Do you often feel unhappy? |
| 2. | Do you feel hopeless about the future? |
| 3. | Have you ever thought that life was not worth living? |
| 4. | Do you think that you would be better off dead? |
| 5. | Have you thought about doing something to kill yourself? |

A starting point for history taking is the simple acknowledgment that psychiatric symptoms often co-occur with epilepsy. Direct history taking during an office visit often yields higher-quality information than the use of rating scales. Addressing the subject in a straightforward, matter-of-fact way puts patients at ease and avoids any untoward insinuation regarding "flawed" character traits. An approach of universal screening is usually the most successful.

---

### ☆ TIPS AND TRICKS

Successful conversation starters for screening for psychiatric comorbidity:
 "We now understand that with epilepsy, parts of the brain dealing with emotions or thinking may also be affected. So we are asking all of our patients about problems with nervousness or mood. Have you noticed any feelings of depression or mood swings?"
 "Epilepsy can sometimes cause stress in people's lives. How are you managing?"
 "Parts of the brain that cause seizures can sometimes cause sad feelings too. Has that ever happened to you?"

---

A positive response justifies further inquiry, most effectively accomplished in a progressive, stepwise manner. In the case of depression screening, any "yes" answers to the questions in Table 37.1 warrant asking the next question on the list.

### Treatment approaches

The most prudent treatment approach for psychiatric illness comorbid with epilepsy is to use principles established for patients without epilepsy. Comprehensive care for psychiatric illness often includes a combination of psychiatric medications, psychotherapy, and vocational or educational support.

However, the initial step in managing psychiatric comorbidity may be to optimally manage epilepsy and adeptly select AEDs with beneficial psychotropic effects. Judicious selection of AEDs may represent the most intuitive initial step for treatment of psychiatric comorbidity.

In addition to medications, psychotherapy and social support may be extremely effective in improving the course of psychiatric illness. Social isolation is a common phenomenon for children and adults with epilepsy. Psychotherapeutic efforts to provide social and family support are related to medication compliance for children and adults with epilepsy and may improve outcome for patients following surgical treatment. Engaging children and adolescents in cognitive behavioral therapy appears to improve social competence.

### Antiepileptic drugs

Antiepileptic drugs are broad-spectrum, versatile medications that effectively treat many behavioral target symptoms, including impulsivity, rage outbursts, and mood lability. AEDs are commonly used as first-line or adjunctive agents for major depression and bipolar disorder. Carbamazepine, valproic acid, and lamotrigine have long been key medication treatments for mood disorders without epilepsy, and these medicines have class I level evidence for efficacy in bipolar disorder. Ultimately, seizure and behavior control may go hand in hand; optimizing AED treatment may offer the best chance at symptom control for epilepsy and psychiatric symptoms. As in the treatment of epilepsy, low doses of adjunctive AEDs may be synergistic and lead to improved behavior.

Impulsivity lies at the core of many psychiatric illnesses, including bipolar disorder, attention deficit hyperactivity disorder (ADHD), and substance abuse. AEDs serve to reduce neuronal hyperexcitability, making them ideal treatments for psychiatric illness in which impulsivity is a significant concern. In several small studies, anticonvulsant drugs were effective treatments for agitation, dysphoria, anxiety, and irritability in the context of epilepsy. The initial strategy for clinicians facing behavior problems in the context of epilepsy may be to optimize AED treatment, selecting agents that have proven to be robust "mood stabilizers."

Psychiatric side effects from AED treatment are common. Although psychiatric and behavioral problems may potentially be associated with any medicine, the risk with some medicines has been more commonly reported. Phenobarbital increases the possibility of depression, irritability, and disinhibition. Irritability has also been associated with levetiracetam. Impairments in short-term memory, verbal fluency, and cognitive processing speed have been reported with topiramate. However, it should be noted that behavioral symptoms may be misattributed as side effects instead of signs of a comorbid psychiatric illness that would be an appropriate target of anticonvulsant medicine.

## Seizure risk and psychiatric medications

Although psychiatric medications have commonly been viewed as increasing the risk for seizures, the reality is that the risk is low for most medicines commonly used today. Few psychiatric medicines appear to pose a significant risk for decreasing seizure threshold, especially for epilepsy that is well controlled. For seizures that occur less often than once a month, risperidone and methylphenidate have been shown in controlled studies to have no appreciable effect upon seizure threshold. Selective serotonin reuptake inhibitors (SSRIs) also appear to pose a low risk for decreasing the seizure threshold.

**CAUTION!**

Psychiatric medications that significantly increase seizure risk are clozapine, chlorpromazine, clomipramine, high doses of bupropion, and toxic doses of tricyclic antidepressants.

## Depression and anxiety

Depression is the most common psychiatric illness associated with epilepsy and is proving to be the strongest predictor of quality of life in patients with epilepsy, even more than seizure frequency or severity. It is worrisome that depression is often unrecognized and undertreated. Suicide has been reported as responsible for 10% of deaths in adults with epilepsy as compared to 1% in the general population. Recent FDA precautions have raised concern about AEDs as a class of drugs leading to increased risk of suicidal thoughts and behaviors. However, this risk has not been isolated independent of comorbid depression.

Anxiety is a broad-symptom category and may be expressed in specific situations, as in social phobia or panic disorder, or more globally, as in generalized anxiety disorder. Anticipatory anxiety regarding possible seizures is often present to some extent, though it may not rise to the level of a formal psychiatric illness. Social anxiety symptoms such as isolation and fear of being in public places are often noted. Anxiety is also notable as an experiential phenomenon in patients whose seizures involve the amygdala. Sensations of fear or anxiety may occur in the context of a seizure aura or throughout the ictal period. Anxiety and depression are often associated with one another, especially in younger patients, and treatment approaches are very similar.

Some people have anxiety and depressive symptoms restricted to a peri-ictal state. For others, symptoms are present all the time. Although the time course may differ, the high level of comorbidity strongly implies that a complex interaction between epilepsy and depression may be occurring, with symptom expression occurring bidirectionally in many cases. The presence of depression appears to predict a greater risk of developing epilepsy, as much as a sixfold increase in older adults. Persistence of depressive symptoms predicts suboptimal response to AEDs.

**SCIENCE REVISITED**

Temporal lobe structures such as the hippocampus and amygdala are common locations for seizure foci and also crucial structures involved in the neural circuitry of depression. Temporal lobe epilepsy is particularly associated with depression.

When assessing depression, it is most important to establish whether symptoms represent a significant departure from a patient's usual state of health.

**Table 37.2.** Typical depressive symptoms across the life span.

| Symptom | Children | Adolescents | Adults |
|---|---|---|---|
| Sleep | Equivocal | Increased – may be phase shifted | Decreased – often middle or terminal |
| Appetite | Equivocal | Decreased – may be increased for anxious patients | Decreased |
| Energy | May be increased, tantrums or restlessness | Decreased | Decreased, even for family activities |
| Social interaction | Disruptive behavior in social settings | Withdrawal from family and friends | Isolation |
| Substance abuse | Uncommon | Common, alcohol less common than other substances | Common, alcohol primarily |
| Work and school function | Disinterest | Drop in grades, apathy | Absenteeism, lack of motivation |
| Somatic complaints | Common, especially GI | Common, especially headaches | Less common |
| Suicidality | Uncommon | Ideation common; gestures may be impulsive | Planning or preparatory behavior common |

GI, gastrointestinal.

Specific neurovegetative symptoms may vary depending upon age and social circumstances, but the underlying theme is usually markedly diminished interest in usual activities and feelings of hopelessness and a negative outlook for the future. Common symptoms throughout the life span are described in Table 37.2.

## Use of antidepressant medication

For moderate-to-severe depressive symptoms or for any signs of suicidality, antidepressant medication may be indicated. SSRIs are the mainstay for treatment of depression and are well tolerated by persons with epilepsy. Several important principles for management are described as follows:

1. To minimize potential side effects, start with a low dosage regardless of age or weight.
2. Side effects of increased energy, sleep disruption, and gastrointestinal (GI) effects emerge in the first 1–2 weeks. Antidepressant "improved mood" effects typically do not begin until 2–4 weeks. Allow several weeks to elapse before increasing the dosage.
3. The risk for suicide is higher in the first weeks of treatment, as the energy level increases but the therapeutic effects on mood have not yet begun.
4. Follow up frequently, especially in the first 2 months of treatment. Weekly visits are appropriate, especially for younger patients.
5. Make safety agreements with patients and contingency plans with caregivers.
6. If patients become activated, agitated, or restless, consider discontinuing the medication.
7. Monitor suicidality at every contact.

> ★ **TIPS AND TRICKS**
>
> **Picking an SSRI**
> Assess whether the patient has activated/anxious symptoms as opposed to psychomotor slowed/fatigued symptoms
>
> - Need more activation
>   - Fluoxetine
>   - Sertraline
>   - Duloxetine
> - Need less activation
>   - Citalopram
>   - Mirtazapine
>   - Escitalopram

## Attention deficit hyperactivity disorder (ADHD)

Attention deficit hyperactivity disorder is the most common psychiatric condition in pediatrics and also the most common comorbidity accompanying epilepsy in school-aged children. Prevalence ranges from 20% to 38% depending upon assessment methods and sampling. The ADHD subtypes are predominantly inattentive, predominantly hyperactive or impulsive, and combined type. Symptoms of absence epilepsy may appear similar to ADHD-primarily inattentive subtype and are a common differential diagnosis. Attention difficulties may also accompany absence epilepsy and partial epilepsy localized to the frontal lobe. As is the case for depression, a bidirectional relationship has been considered such that ADHD increases risk for seizures and that more patients with epilepsy have ADHD.

Despite the frequency of this comorbidity, in-depth treatment studies are scarce. One obstacle has been the view that stimulant drugs may decrease seizure threshold. However, as reviewed earlier, this belief has not been supported in published studies.

Methylphenidate is available in short-acting and in time-release preparations and has been the most frequently studied treatment for children with ADHD comorbid with epilepsy. Although the safety and efficacy of methylphenidate in children with uncontrolled seizures remain uncertain, current evidence suggests that using the extended release formulation in children with well-controlled epilepsy is safe and effective.

## Intellectual and developmental disability (IDD)

The presence of epilepsy in children and adults with intellectual and development disability (IDD) ranges from 30% to 50% depending on classification. Some groups report that complex partial seizures and temporal lobe EEG abnormalities may be particularly common with autism. Improved behavior and cognition have been reported in children treated with AEDs even without the presence of distinct seizure episodes.

Aggressive behavior is a common reason for urgent referrals. In this situation, clinicians may feel pressure to treat with medications, usually antipsychotics or sedative medications. However, urgent treatment with a medication is often not required, as the incident may reflect environmental factors or emotional reactivity. Therefore, it is imperative to obtain as much detail as possible regarding the disruptive behavior, with a goal of determining how much of the behavior reflects underlying neurological impulsivity versus situational reactivity. For example, a young adult with epilepsy and IDD who has reactive aggression only at mealtime or other transition times may not require medications to manage the behavior. Instead, an astute caregiver may be able to redirect the disruptive behavior with distraction or verbal prompting. On the other hand, if a patient is unpredictably impulsive and disruptive regardless of context, then the behavior may reflect deficits in brain function, thus justifying the use of medication to target underlying neurological impulsivity. A model for determining treatment necessity for disruptive behavior is outlined in Figure 37.1.

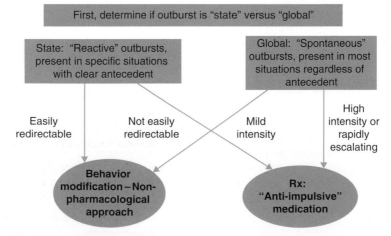

**Figure 37.1.** Approach to management of behavior problems resulting from impulsive reaction.

## Conclusion

Psychiatric comorbidity with epilepsy is common and can be more debilitating than the epilepsy. The etiology of psychiatric comorbidity is still difficult to resolve, but interdisciplinary management from both neurologists and psychiatrists is well indicated for many. The treatment of common psychiatric comorbidities associated with epilepsy such as ADHD, depression, anxiety, and IDD is similar to that utilized for patients without epilepsy. Most psychiatric medications may be used safely in persons with epilepsy; exacerbation of seizures is uncommon. Clinicians who proactively identify and treat psychiatric comorbidity will find that treatment outcome for epilepsy is improved and overall quality of life is greatly enhanced. Future studies will inform treatment strategies associated with specific epilepsy factors.

## References

Barry JJ, Ettinger AB, Friel P, et al. Consensus statement: The evaluation and treatment of people with epilepsy and affective disorders. *Epilepsy Behav* 2008; **13**(Suppl. 1):S1–S29.

Goncalves EB, Cendes F. Depression in patients with refractory temporal lobe epilepsy. *Arq Neuropsiquiatr* 2011; **69**:775–777.

Hamiwka L, Jones JE, Salpekar J, Caplan R. Child psychiatry. *Epilepsy Behav* 2011; **22**:38–46.

Hesdorffer DC, Hauser WA, Annegers JF, Cascino G. Major depression is a risk factor for seizures in older adults. *Ann Neurol* 2000; **47**:246–249.

Hesdorffer DC, Kanner AM. The FDA alert on suicidality and antiepileptic drugs: Fire or false alarm? *Epilepsia* 2009; **50**:978–986.

Jones JE, Hermann BP, Barry JJ, Gilliam FG, Kanner AM, Meador KJ. Rates and risk factors for suicide, suicidal ideation, and suicide attempts in chronic epilepsy. *Epilepsy Behav* 2003; **4**(Suppl. 3):S31–S38.

Kanner AM. Depression in epilepsy: A complex relation with unexpected consequences. *Curr Opin Neurol* 2008; **21**:190–194.

Loring DW, Marino S, Meador KJ. Neuropsychological and behavioral effects of antiepilepsy drugs. *Neuropsychol Rev* 2007; **17**:413–425.

Post RM, Denicoff KD, Frye MA, et al. A history of the use of anticonvulsants as mood stabilizers in the last two decades of the 20th century. *Neuropsychobiology* 1998; **38**:152–166.

Rogawski MA, Loscher W. The neurobiology of antiepileptic drugs for the treatment of nonepileptic conditions. *Nat Med* 2004; **10**:685–692.

Salpekar JA, Conry JA, Doss W, et al. Clinical experience with anticonvulsant medication in pediatric epilepsy and comorbid bipolar spectrum disorder. *Epilepsy Behav* 2006; **9**:327–334.

Torres AR, Whitney J, Gonzalez-Heydrich J. Attention-deficit/hyperactivity disorder in pediatric patients with epilepsy: Review of pharmacological treatment. *Epilepsy Behav* 2008; **12**:217–233.

# Index

Note: Page numbers in *italics* refer to Figures; those in **bold** to Tables.

*Epilepsy*, First Edition. Edited by John W. Miller and Howard P. Goodkin.
© 2014 John Wiley & Sons, Ltd. Published 2014 by John Wiley & Sons, Ltd.